Animals, Diseases, and Human Health

Animals, Diseases, and Human Health

Shaping Our Lives Now and in the Future

**Radford G. Davis,
DVM, MPH, DACVPM, Editor**

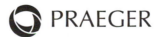

PRAEGER

AN IMPRINT OF ABC-CLIO, LLC
Santa Barbara, California • Denver, Colorado • Oxford, England

Copyright 2011 by ABC-CLIO, LLC

Library of Congress Cataloging-in-Publication Data

Animals, diseases, and human health : shaping our lives now and in the future / Radford G. Davis, editor.
     p. ; cm.
  Includes bibliographical references and index.
  ISBN 978-0-313-38529-2 (hardcopy : alk. paper) —
ISBN 978-0-313-38530-8 (eISBN)
    1. Zoonoses.   2. Human-animal relationships.   3. Human ecology.
I. Davis, Radford G.
    [DNLM: 1. Zoonoses—transmission.   2. Animal Assisted Therapy.
3. Animal Welfare.   4. Bonding, Human-Pet.   5. Communicable
Diseases, Emerging—transmission.   6. Communicable Diseases,
Emerging—veterinary. WC 950]
  RA639.A55   2011
  614.5'6—dc23   2011026322

ISBN: 978-0-313-38529-2
EISBN: 978-0-313-38530-8

15 14 13 12 11   1 2 3 4 5

This book is also available on the World Wide Web as an eBook.
Visit www.abc-clio.com for details.

Praeger
An Imprint of ABC-CLIO, LLC

ABC-CLIO, LLC
130 Cremona Drive, P.O. Box 1911
Santa Barbara, California 93116-1911

This book is printed on acid-free paper ∞

Manufactured in the United States of America

Contents

Introduction   vii
Radford G. Davis, DVM, MPH, DACVPM

1. Allergies to Pets   1
   A. McKenzie André, MD, MPH, and
   Zandra Hollaway André, DVM, MPH, DACVPM

2. Pets in Health-Care Settings   13
   Louisa J. Castrodale, DVM, MPH, DACVPM

3. Dog Bites and Dangerous Pets   33
   Kira A. Christian, DVM, MPH, DACVPM

4. Animal Abuse, Cruelty, Neglect (and the
   Connection to Human Violence)   51
   Miranda Spindel, DVM, MS, and
   Lila Miller, BS, DVM

5. Emerging Diseases   71
   Tegwin K. Taylor, DVM, MPH, DACVPM

6. Wildlife Trade, Demand, and Health   99
   Kristine M. Smith, DVM, DACZM

7. Immunocompromised, High-Risk Populations and Animals   119
   Radford G. Davis, DVM, MPH, DACVPM

8. Zoonoses of Concern from Dogs   139
Carina Blackmore, MS Vet. Med., PhD, DACVPM

9. Zoonoses of Concern from Cats   161
Ken Thorley, BVSc, MVS, MACVSc

10. Zoonoses of Concern from Small Mammals   181
Jeffrey L. Rhody, DVM

11. Zoonoses of Concern from Pet Birds   201
Niklos Weber, DVM, DABVP (Avian, Canine, Feline)

12. One Health   219
Radford G. Davis, DVM, MPH, DACVPM

13. The Future: Modern Animal Biotechnology   239
Larisa Rudenko, PhD, DABT,
Jeffery Jones, DVM, PhD, and
Evgenij Evdokimov, PhD

Index   263

About the Editor and Contributors   283

Introduction

Radford G. Davis, DVM, MPH, DACVPM

Why read this book? Because we live in a world where, seen or unseen, animals impact our lives in countless ways, some for the betterment of our physical and mental health, and some that can cause us harm. With 7 billion people on the planet, we humans have a great effect on all living things, our environment, and ultimately on disease. We share our living space with livestock, with dogs and cats and other pets, but also with a great variety of wildlife; therefore, we share diseases too. Today, it is recognized that the health of animals and the health of people are wedded, that we cannot have full understanding of a disease, its impact, or its prevention without understanding its epidemiology in animals, in humans, and what, if any, role the environment has. Of course, what we do to our environment does impact health, of that there is no doubt. Climate change is real, and the results will continue to impact each of us, our domestic animals, and wildlife, directly or indirectly, for much of the foreseeable future.

Understanding the diseases of animals that can be transmitted to people is an important first step in selecting the best pet and also in reducing the burden of disease in people. But, as you may guess, understanding is not enough—we must work to address the causes of disease, disease emergence, and disease spread. To do this means that we must address the drivers of disease—that is, the things that lead to diseases emerging and becoming a problem. This may mean improving education, reducing poverty, modifying agricultural practices, changing government policy, rethinking drug use in the human and veterinary medical fields—the list is indeed long, but worthy of our best efforts. The One Health concept recognizes the overlap of animal health, human health, and the environment and takes a broad look at health and disease and the drivers of each.

In some countries, animals become family members, sleep in our beds, and receive advanced veterinary care. In other countries, animals are more a source of food, draft power, currency, and livelihood. We need to concern ourselves with the diseases we can get from animals, but we needn't overreact. This book can help you with those concerns. Whether we are bringing animals into nursing homes for visits, choosing the best pet for a child, or helping a person with AIDS to understand the real risks of pet ownership, we shouldn't lose sight of the tremendous benefits animals have for us, both the physical benefits as well as the psychological ones.

From this book you will learn about the diseases you might acquire from animals and how to prevent them. You will learn why you have allergies to a cat; you will come to understand the link between animal abuse and human violence; and you will see why some animals are simply too dangerous to keep as pets. With each chapter you read, you will come to comprehend how animals and human health are connected.

What of the future? The future holds promise, some mystery, and some answers into how animals affect human health, and vice versa. It is certain that, no matter what, animals will always have some influence on our health and well-being, and even our economy, no matter where we live, what our occupations are, how many animals we own, or what we eat. With over 9 billion people expected to be living on Earth by 2050, there is no better time than now to broaden our vision and understanding and redouble our efforts into the relationship between the health of animals and humans and the environment and find solutions that will protect the health of all species.

Chapter 1

Allergies to Pets

A. McKenzie André, MD, MPH, and
Zandra Hollaway André, DVM, MPH, DACVPM

INTRODUCTION

Millions of us own pets—dogs, cats, horses, rabbits, ferrets, iguanas, and the list goes on. People and their pets form unique bonds, so much so that these animals are often considered family members. The human-animal bond has many different forms of relationships, including companionship, protection, and service. The benefits of these relationships have been well documented in the literature. Unfortunately, so have the disadvantages, namely allergies. Allergies to animals have been recorded for typical pets, such as dogs and cats and more exotic nontraditional pets such as chameleons.[1]

There are many types of allergies, including indoor, outdoor, skin, and eye allergies. Many people with allergies usually have more than one type. Approximately 40 million Americans have indoor and outdoor allergies as their primary allergy, and of these nearly 10 million sufferers are allergic to dander (material shed from the bodies of animals such as dried skin or hair), the most common of pet allergies.[2]

WHAT ARE ALLERGIES?

Allergies are an acquired, abnormal immune response to a substance, usually a protein, which normally does not cause a reaction but instead is recognized as foreign and subsequently elicits an immune response. Allergy symptoms develop when these proteins are carried through the air and come in contact with the lining of the respiratory tract. Allergies can have mild to severe manifestations, from sneezing and itchy eyes to difficulty breathing, asthma attacks, and even death. These manifestations are not always proportionate to the amount of exposed allergen. A person with a severe animal allergy can experience a reaction in a public place from exposure to pet dander that is carried on a pet owner's clothing. Although allergies cannot be cured, they can be controlled with prevention and proper treatment.

Allergy and Hypersensitivity

An allergy can also be referred to as hypersensitivity or atopy. Hypersensitivity reactions refer to exaggerated responses to foreign proteins by the body's normal immune system. According to the Coombs and Gell classification system, which describes immune responses by the mechanism of tissue injury, there are four types of hypersensitivity reactions depending on the key mediator for the reaction. These four categories are named Type I, Type II, Type III, and Type IV. Almost all pet allergies are Type I hypersensitivity reactions mediated by a class of antibodies referred to as IgE. Antibodies, a type of protein also known as immunoglobulins, are produced by white blood cells and help identify foreign materials within the body for elimination. There are five main classes of antibodies. Besides IgE, there are also IgG, IgA, IgM, and IgD antibodies. All antibodies have the same general structure made up of two heavy chains and two light chains. At the end of the light chains there is a section that is highly variable. This region helps each antibody target a specific protein. Immune reactions occur when antigens (foreign proteins) combine with antibodies to trigger a response. The type of response depends on the type of antibody and where in the body it occurs. Sometimes you will hear the word atopy used interchangeably with allergy or hypersensitivity. Atopy actually refers to a predisposition to have exaggerated IgE-mediated immune responses. Thus, atopic individuals are prone to suffer Type I hypersensitivity reactions.

For people prone to allergies, the first time they are exposed to an unrecognized protein (allergen) they produce antibodies. These antibodies, once formed, will be distributed throughout the body and will stick to special cells in the body. The body is now sensitized. The next time that the body is exposed to the allergen these sensitized cells will release their contents into the bloodstream. These contents include several proinflammatory compounds such as histamine, which cause such localized symptoms we normally associate with allergies as eye redness, itching, runny nose, and nasal congestion. These same compounds, when released in the respiratory tract, can cause edema (swelling) and bronchial constriction, which can lead to wheezing and difficulty breathing.

CAUSES OF ALLERGIES TO PETS

Allergies to pets are similar to other allergies in that they represent an excessive or abnormal reaction to a usually innocuous naturally occurring substance or allergen. These allergens are really very small pieces of protein. Although it is not entirely understood why some people develop allergies and others do not, there is some evidence to suggest that the tendency to develop allergies is hereditary. If a person's parents suffer from allergies, there is a good chance that their children will also suffer from allergies.

It is unclear what role sensitization and the age of first pet exposure plays in the development of allergies. There was a thought that the earlier you exposed a child to pets, the less likely they would be to develop pet allergies; however, studies have looked at people who grew up with pets starting at a young age and the data is mixed. "For cat ownership, the results are inconsistent between studies of similar design, with some studies suggesting an increase in risk and others a decrease among cat owners. For dogs, results are more consistent, generally suggesting that owning a dog has no effect or indeed may be protective against the development of specific sensitization to dog and allergic sensitization in general."[3] Given the lack of conclusive findings, there are no recommendations regarding the proper time to expose children to pet and/or pet allergens.

It is a common misconception that people with allergies are reacting to the animal hair or fur. This is not correct. Pet allergies can be caused by exposure to animal dander, urine, dried saliva, or hair. Allergies to pets are actually hypersensitivity reactions to proteins present in these substances. All living creatures (even humans) produce dander. For people allergic to birds, the feathers and droppings are triggers. The scales from reptiles can also be the causative agent for those allergic to reptiles.[1] A multitude of proteins can be found in dander, urine, dried saliva, hair, feathers, bird droppings, and scales, and specific proteins in each of these cause allergic symptoms, whereas hair and feathers can be more of a skin irritant rather than a trigger of a true allergic response. These proteins are quite small and cannot be seen by the naked eye. In fact, they are so small and light they can float in the air for long periods of time. These particles, while suspended, come to rest on furniture, walls, curtains, and clothes and eventually find their way into a person's nasal passages or are inhaled into the bronchial passages.

All cats and dogs naturally produce dander despite the common myth that dogs with shorter hair do not cause allergies. Different species shed more skin cells than others. If there is an association with longer-haired pets and allergies, it most likely lies in the fact that pets with more hair or fur have the capacity to accumulate or hold onto more dander. There are also allergenic proteins found in cat and dog saliva. Cats are generally more allergenic than other pets because they are constantly grooming themselves and are literally covered in dried saliva. They then proceed to rub against furniture and people, depositing allergens on the upholstery and clothes. Cat allergies are often caused by a potent allergenic protein found in the saliva of cats called Fel d 1. This particular protein is the predominant culprit for allergic reactions to cats. People's reaction to protein can be variable. Some people may develop allergies to feline protein other than Fel d 1, which could explain why one person may have different reactions to different breeds or sexes of cats.

Unlike cats, all dogs do not produce the same universal allergens. There are some differences between breeds. In addition, there is variation in the amount of dander produced by different dogs. Dogs with nonshedding coats generally produce less dander than dogs that have coats that shed a lot. According to the American Kennel Club, examples of breeds with nonshedding coats are Bedlington terrier, bichon frise, Chinese crested, Irish water spaniel, Kerry blue terrier, Maltese, poodles, Portuguese water dog, schnauzer, soft-coated wheaten terrier, and xoloitzcuintli.

There are some species of dogs that produce a lot of drool, which can accumulate on carpeting. Once the saliva dries the proteins can then aerosolize and become suspended in the air, especially during cleaning and vacuuming. Urine is another potential source of allergens. The urine accumulates on the pet's fur and once it dries becomes aerosolized. In addition, the location of the cat litter boxes can be a potential source of the allergens in the household if they are placed in the main living areas of the house or near air vents.

In addition to dogs and cats, many other types of pets may be triggers for allergies, including horses, rabbits, guinea pigs, hamsters, gerbils, rats, and mice. Just as with dogs and cats, the pet's hair is not the culprit; it is the proteins found in the dander, urine, and dried saliva. If hay or wood shavings are used for an animal's bedding, as is the case with horses, rabbits, hamsters, or other pocket pets, the bedding could be the trigger for the allergies due to all of the accumulated urine. Because these animals do not typically roam free in the household, there tends to be less environmental contamination in the home, leading to fewer allergens to respond to. In this case, the allergens would be confined to the cage or stall.

SYMPTOMS OF PET ALLERGIES

Allergy symptoms, which usually occur within a few minutes of exposure, typically occur when the allergen comes in contact with mucous membranes of the eyes and nose. However, if the person has only mild sensitivity, then the allergy symptoms can be delayed for several days. Table 1.1 lists some of the common symptoms associated with pet allergies.

These symptoms, if more severe, can be associated with facial pressure and pain, difficulty sleeping, and swollen and blue-colored skin under the eyes. In young children, your only clue may be the observation of frequent upward rubbing of the nose. Of course, not everyone will have all these symptoms. Some people with pet allergies may also experience such skin symptoms as redness or a rash after a pet scratch or lick. Direct contact with an allergy-causing pet may trigger allergic dermatitis symptoms, which may include itchy skin or raised red patches (hives). It is important to remember that different people can have varying sensitivities to the same allergen. The time it takes to develop a reaction, the amount of exposure required, and severity of the symptoms are really individualized. If the allergen levels are low, symptoms may not appear until after several days of contact with the pet.

Respiratory symptoms associated with pet allergies include difficulty breathing with associated shortness of breath and coughing, which can lead to difficulty sleeping. In severe cases, there can be a whistling or wheezing sound heard when a person breathes out due to narrowing of the airway. There may even be chest tightness or pain. It is important to remember that the breathing difficulties can come on quite quickly and that this should be considered a medical emergency. The respiratory concern is heightened for people with asthma, who are at an increased risk for respiratory problems due to allergies. In fact, for about 20–30 percent of people with asthma, cat contact can trigger a severe asthma attack.[2] Cat allergies can also lead to chronic asthma. A member of a household who suffers from asthma should consult with their physician to review their medication regimen and evaluate the risks associated with living with pets, especially cats.

Table 1.1

Common Pet Allergy Symptoms

Sneezing
Runny nose
Nasal congestion
Itchy, red, or watery eyes
Postnasal drip
Itchy nose, roof of mouth, or throat
Cough

Allergic bird owners can also suffer from allergic alveolitis, also known as hypersensitivity pneumonitis or bird fancier's lung. This is not a communicable disease passed between animals and humans because no infectious agent is transmitted, but it is an allergic process that is recognized as one of the major threats to human respiratory health from avian species.[4] Exposure to bird dander, for example when cleaning the cage, can trigger this allergic response.

WHEN TO SEE A PHYSICIAN

Depending on the symptoms manifested, it may be difficult to recognize a pet allergy. Most people will recognize severe allergic reactions that come on fast and involve sneezing or trouble breathing. For people who have such milder reactions as nasal congestion, a slight cough, or scratchy throat, a pet allergy may be harder to identify. For parents of young children, diagnosis of pet allergies may be even more difficult, given that pet allergies can present with symptoms that are similar to many other childhood illnesses. For example, in infants, the runny nose or cough that is assumed to be from an illness may really be because of allergies. If there is any chance that an allergy may be the cause, then you should schedule an appointment with your physician. Some of the clues the physician will be looking for include:

- Nasal symptoms, such as a runny nose or congestion that occur only after certain exposures (e.g., playing with a dog or having a cat sit on a lap).
- Persistent nasal or respiratory symptoms that last longer that a typical virus or cold.
- When symptom occurrence is associated with certain locations. For example, if symptoms resolve when you go to work or if a child's symptoms are worse at school, then an evaluation may be necessary.
- If you have a pet at home and the symptoms never really go away.
- If you experience pain or tenderness in the nasal cavity or have any difficulty breathing, chest tightness, wheezing, swelling of lips or throat, hives, or a generalized rash, then you should see a physician immediately.

If you already know you have allergies, see your physician if:

- You do not know what is causing the allergy. Remember that people can have allergies to multiple substances, and a household pet may not be responsible for all of a person's symptoms.

- If you are on medication for another illness.
- If the symptoms continue to persist even after taking over-the-counter medications.
- If you start to experience side effects from medications.

Finally, it is important to remember there are a lot of different over-the-counter medications. These medicines treat symptoms associated with allergies, but do not provide a cure. Parents should be careful when administering such medications to their children and should look for medications specifically made for children. Children should not receive adult medications in smaller doses.

WHAT TO EXPECT AT A PHYSICIAN'S VISIT

In many cases, a diagnosis of pet allergy can be made from a careful description of the symptoms and living environment. Your physician will spend a lot of time asking you to describe your symptoms. He will want to know if there are any aggravating factors or situations when your symptoms are better or worse. Your physician will then perform a standard medical history, and ask about other medical conditions. This will be done for two reasons: first, to rule out any other potential causes for the symptoms, and, second, to see if there are other medical conditions that predispose you to having allergic reactions (e.g., asthma). There will also be a discussion about your family history, since hypersensitivities can be inherited. The physician will usually perform a physical exam targeting areas where you may be experiencing symptoms, including the eyes, nose, throat, and any areas on the skin where there may be a rash. He will also listen to the lungs to determine the quality of breath sounds and any signs of wheezing.

1.1. DID YOU KNOW?

- Common cockroaches are known to be a cause of allergies, and it is not because they are dirty. They harbor various kinds of mold that people can be allergic to.
- The large and docile Madagascar hissing cockroach, a favorite exotic pet, harbors 14 types of mold in its feces or on its body.
- People who are allergic to mold should always wash their hands carefully after handling these creatures.

After getting a full patient history and performing a physical exam, a diagnosis of a specific pet allergy may be identified. If the cause of the allergy symptoms is still unclear, then your physician will schedule another appointment for allergy testing. There are several different tests that can be used to determine if your symptoms are due to an allergy. The goals of testing are twofold. First, the physician will want to make sure that the symptoms are truly related to allergies. Second, he would like to identify the specific allergen so that it can be avoided in the future. The testing is based on the fact that people who suffer from allergies produce antibodies to specific allergens. The presence of these antibodies can help identify the particular allergen that causes the symptoms.

Diagnostic Tests

Your physician may recommend having a skin or blood test in order to diagnose the allergy. These tests are useful because, in addition to identifying a particular allergen, the test can help quantify the severity of your sensitivity to that allergen. The skin test is usually more sensitive and less expensive than the blood tests. The skin test can be performed in one of two ways. Neither method is particular painful, but they may be slightly uncomfortable. In both methods the patient is basically being exposed to small amounts of allergens in a defined area on the skin. In most cases, these tests will be done by an allergy specialist.

The physician will review your history and determine a list of potential allergens. There can be many potential allergens found in the household, so your physician will likely test for allergies to dust mites, pollens, and molds. To conduct the test, your physician will identify a fairly large area of skin where he or she will introduce the different allergens they will be evaluating. This area is usually located on the forearm or on the back (especially with children). On a skin test they may test up to 25 antigens at one time. In the skin prick method a small needle containing a small amount of the allergen in pricked into the skin. If you are allergic to that allergen then you may develop redness, itchiness, or hives at the site of the prick that corresponds to that allergen. The result is usually apparent within a few minutes. The skin patch method is similar but involves taping metal discs (each containing a different allergen) to your skin for two to three days. Again, if the test is positive, when they remove the skin patch there will be areas of redness or itching corresponding to the allergen that caused the reaction.

There are times when the skin tests are not ideal for testing for allergies. If a person is on antiallergy medication, has a history of severe reaction to a particular allergen, or is prone to eczema, the results of the skin tests may be hard to interpret. In those cases a blood test will be performed.

The blood test for allergies is called the radioimmunoassay test, or RAST. This blood test can identify the presence as well as quantify the amount of an allergen-specific antibody. The RAST test is scored on a scale from zero to six. This scale ranges from undetectable to extremely high levels of IgE antibody. The scale will also approximate severity of symptoms during an allergic reaction. RAST testing is more expensive than either of the skin test methods, but many allergens can be evaluated from one blood sample.

If your main allergic symptoms cause difficulty breathing, such as an asthma exacerbation, your physician may recommend challenge (also known as provocation) testing. In this test, you will be placed in a controlled environment and exposed to the allergen by breathing. If you begin to develop symptoms, the medical staff is in place to quickly reverse the symptoms. This test should only be performed in the presence of experienced health-care professionals.

Finally, if it is still unclear whether you have allergies, your physician may recommend a trial separation from your pet to see if symptoms improve. Because animal dander can stay in the environment for a long time, the separation could be at least several months long with a thorough cleaning of the household expected in the interim. Often, this is the only way to prove to owners that their pets are causing the problem.

Treatment

The treatment of pet allergies is the same as for other allergies. Thus, the mainstay of treatment is identification and avoidance of the cause of the allergies. This may prove difficult, however. Protecting yourself against pollen, for example, is a lot different than saying good-bye to a trusted pet and family member. There are ways to treat the symptoms of pet allergies, and, depending on the severity of symptoms, this may be all that is needed.

Minor allergy symptoms can often be treated by such over-the-counter remedies as antihistamines, which will help reduce the redness and itching of eyes as well as the runny nose associated with stuffed nasal passages. Eye drops that contain sodium cromoglicate and/or antihistamines can target eye symptoms. Nasal sprays that contain sodium cromolyn, antihistamines, or steroids (prescription only) can also reduce the inflammation and stuffy feeling in the nasal passages during an attack. These products usually work best before being exposed to an allergen. Decongestants can be used to reduce symptoms after they have already started, but are usually quite short acting. If allergy symptoms are severe, then a physician may prescribe steroids either nasally, orally, or, in the case of severe allergic reactions, via injection. These will help cut the body's response to the allergen. Long-term treatment with steroids is not a solution because patients can develop severe side effects to the medication.

Another treatment option involves a series of repeated injections of small amounts of the allergy-inducing agent to create tolerance (hyposensitization) against known allergy-inducing substances. This prevents the immune system from producing too much histamine. Such treatment can be very intensive, requiring a period of weekly injections for several months followed by a yearly regimen for up to five years. It requires strict adherence and coordination by a physician.

HOUSEHOLD REMEDIES AND PREVENTION

We are constantly being exposed to pet allergies in our day-to-day contacts with other people or from just being outside. These allergens enter into our workplaces and homes, usually on our clothes. Once allergens are in the home environment they can stay around for months. These particles are not only microscopic and light but also extremely sticky, which means they can be very hard to remove. Fortunately, for most people with allergies this exposure is usually not of sufficient quantity to cause symptoms.

For pet owners, discovering that you or someone in your family has a pet allergy can be traumatic. How a person copes with this news is not dissimilar to the loss of a loved one. The only surefire way to control allergies is to limit a person's exposure to the pet or, sadly, remove the pet from the home. For people who have severe allergies, this may be the only reasonable solution. However, if allergies are mild, we can choose to keep our valued pets with some extra steps and simple rules, ensuring they remain a part of the family for years to come. We can categorize these steps into three groups: things we can do in our home, things we can do for our pets, and things we can do for ourselves.

Things We Can Do in Our Homes

- Remove carpets or install carpets with low pile that are less prone to accumulating pet dander.
- If you have carpets, vacuum the rugs frequently using a HEPA (high efficiency particulate air) filtered vacuum cleaner that removes and traps airborne allergens. HEPA filters capture much smaller particles that standard vacuums tend to recirculate back into the air.
- Use of chemicals such as tannic acid or benzyl benzoate, numerous commercial carpet cleaners, or steam vapor cleaners that can be used on floors and carpets have been shown to reduce the presence of allergens.

- Remember to clean drapes and curtains as well as carpets because allergens can deposit on these as well and stay for months.
- Consider allergen-free material for bedding.
- If you do not want to change your couch to one with hypoallergenic material, you can consider using plastic covers.
- Use hot water (140 degrees Fahrenheit) to wash pillows, bed covers, linens, and mattress pads every 7 to 14 days.
- Keep the home well ventilated.
- Invest in a good HEPA air filter cleaner or purifier for your home.
- Remember to clean out air filters regularly.
- Keep litter boxes and cages away from main living areas and/or air vents in homes with central air.

Things We Can Do for Our Pets

- Keep your pets outdoors as much as possible, especially if someone has severe pet allergies.
- Keep pets off upholstered furniture and bedding.
- Keep pets out of rooms with carpets or at least designate a room in the home as pet-free (usually this is the bedroom).
- Bathe your pet regularly (weekly is best) with dander-control pet shampoo to reduce dander.
- Brush your pets outdoors to remove excess hair and to keep from spreading allergens in the air. If you are allergic, have a nonallergic friend or family member do the brushing.
- Provide a well-balanced diet for your pets, which will help prevent or reduce hair loss and will subsequently lead to less accumulation of allergens in the home.

Things We Can Do for Ourselves

- After playing with pets, people with allergies should wash their hands and be careful not to rub their eyes before washing.
- Do not mix clothes worn when playing with pets with clean clothes before washing them.
- When dusting, use a damp cloth to keep from aerosolizing particles.

CONCLUSION

Allergies to pets can have a profound effect on the lifestyles of owners and family members. Anything that keeps us from enjoying their company and companionship can be very hard to accept. Pet allergies are common. However, with some understanding, planning, and simple precautions, people who suffer from pet allergies can still enjoy the company of pets in their homes.

FURTHER READING

Apfelbacher CJ. Contact to cat or dog, allergies and parental education. *Pediatric Allergy and Immunology* 2010;21:284–91.

Everyday Health Website. Pet Allergies: Worst Animal Offender. Available at: http://www.everydayhealth.com/allergies-pictures/pet-allergies.aspx

Kalstone S. *Allergic to Pets? The Breakthrough Guide to Living with the Animals You Love*. New York: Bantam Dell; 2006.

Mayo Clinic Website. Pet Allergy. Available at: http://www.mayoclinic.com/health/pet-allergy/ds00859

REFERENCES

1. Phillips J, Lockey R. Exotic pet allergy. *Journal of Allergy and Clinical Immunology* 2009;123:513–15.
2. Asthma and Allergy Foundation of America Website. Pet Allergies. Available at: http://www.aafa.org/display.cfm?id=9&sub=18&cont=236.
3. Simpson A, Custovic A. Pets and the development of sensitization. *Current Allergy and Asthma Reports* 2005;5:212–20.
4. Gorman J, Cook A, Ferguson C, et al. Pet birds and risks of respiratory disease in Australia: A review. *Australian and New Zealand Journal of Public Health* 2009;33:167–72.

Chapter 2

Pets in Health-Care Settings

Louisa J. Castrodale, DVM, MPH, DACVPM

INTRODUCTION

Ask any pet owner if they think pets can make you happier or healthier and they will undoubtedly say yes. The emotional connection of pets to their owners is that powerful—just think about those people who refused to move out of harm's way during natural disasters because they refused to abandon their pets. This chapter reviews the history of pets exerting a healing influence on humans in more formal health-care settings, describes some of the specific effects that have been seen, reviews guidelines that were developed to minimize transmission of diseases or occurrence of other adverse health effects, including some examples of those potential diseases, and concludes with some thoughts on what we may see in the future with pets in health-care settings.

HISTORY OF PETS AS THERAPY

Long before the development of formal programs that brought pets into health-care settings, there were anecdotal reports of animals providing some form of comfort to people who were physically or mentally ill. Two recent papers, written by Hooker et al.[1] and Jorgenson,[2] chronicle reports of the history and evolution of animals in the human health-care arena. These reports include stories of animals the Quakers used to promote healing in the late 1700s and the famous nurse Florence Nightingale's recognition of the value of pet animals in providing companionship to chronically ill people in the late 1800s. Dogs were used to benefit the health and welfare of mentally ill patients and recovering veterans in the early 20th century, but formal research that quantified or more precisely described the benefits of pet therapy did not begin until the 1960s.[1,2]

In the early 1960s, Dr. Boris Levinson, a child psychiatrist, began to observe improved outcomes among patients who had controlled interactions with animals as part of their therapy. Although initially discounted, his work using dogs to put his pediatric patients at ease and the associated documentation of the positive results were noticed and eventually expanded to other venues where psychiatrists incorporated aspects of pet therapy into their own treatment regimens. In the 1970s, pets began to be brought to nursing homes or residential long-term care settings with other researchers documenting improvements to the physical and emotional well-being of elderly patients.

In the 1980s and 1990s, increasingly more research was published to demonstrate more specific clinical physical and emotional effects of pet interactions with patients. Accordingly, there was a corresponding increase in the development of formal programs involving animal visits in health-care settings, like acute care hospitals or pediatric cancer centers, where the animals were brought into contact with more medically fragile patients. Not surprisingly, as research increased on benefits, there was the accompanying slow and steady development of guidelines from various organizations, such as the Centers for Disease Control and Prevention (CDC), the American Veterinary Medical Association (AVMA), and the Association for Professionals in Infection Control and Epidemiology (APIC), to address the potential of pets to share infections with, or otherwise adversely impact the health of, patients they were visiting. Infection control guidelines for such programs were created in a somewhat patchwork manner by agencies with different areas of expertise until a consensus document addressing health and safety concerns for pets visiting health-care settings was published in 2008.[3] This collaborative effort brought together the viewpoints of these various professional organizations and disciplines plus those people involved in pet therapy organizations to consolidate knowledge and guidelines into a single comprehensive document.

DEFINITIONS

Animal-Assisted Intervention

Animal-assisted intervention (AAI) is an umbrella term that can be used to generally describe the use of animals that are intended to provide an interaction with a human for a proposed health benefit. Within AAI, there are two main categories. One category is animal-assisted activities (AAA), which refers to situations where volunteers take their pets to visit hospitals, nursing homes, or other types of facilities for the purpose of being petted and interacting generally with the residents or patients. The second category is animal-assisted therapy (AAT), which refers to more specific and structured interactions, where health-care professionals or certified therapists use an animal as a treatment modality with written, individualized treatment programs that contain specific, documented goals tailored to the patient's ability and wellness plan.

Hand Hygiene

Hand hygiene is a critical component of any infection control program, whether the aim is to minimize the transmission of infectious agents between people, or from animals to people (or vice versa). There are two main options for hand hygiene in a health-care setting: good old-fashioned hand washing with running water and soap, or hand-sanitizing sprays, gels, foams, or rubs. Waterless hand washing is a practical and acceptable option given available resources, but hands that are visibly soiled or contaminated with proteinaceous material should preferably be washed with soap and water. Although the term hand hygiene is often used to formally refer to particular circumstances, the practice really applies to any setting (even at home) where people have opportunities to touch animals, and, more importantly, where people have opportunities to touch other people, because the vast majority of infectious conditions that people will experience in their lifetimes are going to originate from other human beings.

Health-Care Settings

For the purposes of this chapter, a health-care setting means any hospital, nursing home, or supervised living or long-term care facility that is formally recognized by local authorities. There are different kinds of animals that may become involved in therapy situations. In some settings, like a nursing home or a long-term care facility, animals may also reside at the facility and deliver more ongoing and informal benefits of therapy. Or there may be a more formal program at a children's hospital, for example, in which animals come for periodic and organized visits to deliver individualized attention to a specific patient.

Infection Control

Infection control refers to a general discipline designed to minimize the development and spread of infections within a health-care setting. Larger health-care facilities usually have an infection control department and dedicated staff that monitor and carry out the practices and procedures that keep patients, residents, and staff safe. Policies are based on national and international guidelines and relate to such situations as how to prevent a patient hospitalized with a contagious airborne disease from infecting other people, or how devices and materials should be appropriately disinfected. The main responsibility for applying these procedures or overseeing them falls to the infection preventionist who has formal training in infection control. The infection preventionist should be centrally involved with any facility's AAI program. This person or this department should be consulted to develop a written policy for animal visits that is tailored to the demographics of that health-care setting and consistent with its other infection control policies.

Service Animals

Animals involved in AAI are separate from service animals specially trained to belong to a specific owner and perform a specific function tailored to the owner's need. For example, service dogs might open doors, turn on lights, assist the hearing or visually impaired, or provide an early warning for an owner's seizure. These animals (but not AAI animals) are granted privileges, such as free access to airplanes or buildings by federal law.

Zoonoses

Zoonoses are infectious diseases that are naturally transmitted between animals and humans. Sometimes the animal is overtly diseased, like with a virus such as rabies, and passes that to a human through a bite. Other times, the zoonotic pathogen might be something that is normally present in an animal, like *Salmonella* in a reptile, and is not necessarily causing any signs or symptoms in that animal.

BENEFITS TO HUMAN HEALTH AND WELL-BEING

While the informal benefits of companionship, happiness, and sometimes exercise from owning pets are common knowledge, and for many people the reason to own a pet, there has been formal research on more specific physiological and psychological effects of involving animals in the healing and/or palliative care process. Much of the research that has been published and is ongoing relates to programs that involve nursing practice. This is probably not coincidental because the framework for integrating AAI into a more standard treatment program rests on the idea of a holistic approach to complicated medical conditions that may have both a physical and emotional component without a single easy treatment. The increase in recognition of the benefits of AAI on health in general and the recognition of the impact that mental status can have on physical symptoms and healing will likely also increase the application and scope of AAI in the future.

A 2009 publication gives a comprehensive list of studies through 2008.[4] Presented below are some highlights of that list as well as some more recent studies divided into a few distinct categories of effects and patient populations.

Physiological Effects

Since the 1980s, there have been some general studies demonstrating that contact with, or being in the presence of, animals can reduce people's blood pressure and relieve stress, which can then indirectly promote the healing process. More recent studies among people with cardiac disease or hypertension have shown measurable effects of interactions with animals on indicators that are used to measure, monitor, or prognosticate diseases or conditions. One example is a 2007 study that compared hospitalized patients with advanced heart failure who received a visit from a therapy dog to patients who received a visit from a human volunteer and to patients who did not receive any special visit. Results suggested that patients with the dog visits had significantly lower cardiopulmonary measures compared with the other two groups. The benefits to improved measures are twofold, in that patients have improved function, which may in turn allow for a reduction in medications that are intended to produce a similar effect.

Psychological Effects

In addition to effects on physiology, interactions with pets have also been demonstrated to impact levels of anxiety and depression. These are, of course, important factors that then indirectly play into the physical status of a person who is ill and can complement efforts to treat physical aspects of disease or dysfunction. For example, one study evaluating the use of therapy animals in effecting a change in cancer patients' self-perception of health found qualitative results suggesting that those people who received animal visits were more likely over time to report benefits to self-perception of health and increases in sense of coherence, which refers to one's ability to endure stressful life events.[5]

Mental Illness

Studies related to mental illness and the benefits of pet ownership have been published, and it is not surprising that, given the benefits mentioned above, AAI could have positive impacts on people who are hospitalized with serious mental illness. A 2009 study among inpatients with schizophrenia that evaluated self-esteem, psychiatric symptoms, self-determination, and emotional symptoms found that patients who received controlled interactions with animals over time showed significant improvements in many clinical aspects of schizophrenia.[6] As with most of the studies, the results are preliminary given the small number of patients involved, and effects may depend on a patient's previous interactions with animals; however, even small results can be encouraging findings for chronic conditions that may be more successfully managed by a combination of therapeutic modalities.

Impacts on Long-Term Care Facility Residents

Although residents in long-term care nursing facilities may experience some of the benefits described above, they are also a more special population than those hospitalized for possibly a more transient period or health condition. There is a growing body of research looking at ways to improve the quality of life for this population, which may spend many years in these settings. Many elderly persons in nursing homes suffer from dementia, and activities may be designed to improve mentality acuity or even just mental comprehension and engagement. For example, a study was designed to demonstrate the effect on dementia from various kinds of dog-related stimuli. Although results were modest and subject to the previously mentioned limitations, residents with moderate dementia experiencing contact with live dogs (as opposed to pictures or videos) demonstrated increased vocalization and more meaningful conversation.[7] Similarly, residents of long-term care facilities who may not have frequent visitors have issues with loneliness. Another study sought to demonstrate whether visits from animals over time could impact the quantitative measure of loneliness. Although the impacts were shown to be greatest among those people who had previously owned pets, residents showed a decrease in loneliness scores after a program of animal visitation.[8] Interestingly, not all findings have been positive. There have been some studies in long-term care settings that have anecdotally reported unexpected anxiety when an animal is taken away or when an animal has movement restrictions in the facility.

Interaction with Medications

Because animals can have impacts on cardiovascular function or other physiologic parameters, this may alter the body's demand for regulatory medications. Some studies have shown that pets can help reduce or complement the amount of medications or dosing schedules. A study looking at the effect of pain perception on children undergoing surgical procedures found that the calming, distractive effect of animal visits was noticeable, such that these interactions could function as adjuncts to opiates prescribed for pain relief or medications needed to relieve anxiety.

AAI PROGRAMS AND ASSOCIATED ENTITIES

There are numerous programs within the United States and other nations that provide training, registration, and standards for dogs involved with AAI (see Table 2.1 at the end of the chapter). Each has individualized protocols and guidelines for the animals involved with their particular programs. They can help with locating, training, and coordinating volunteers for the animals.

In many cases, health-care facilities use external agencies to provide visiting or therapy animals and rely on them to ensure that the animals are appropriate and that the handlers have been trained sufficiently. AAI organizations should have explicit, written policies to protect the health of patients and animal handlers, and records should be kept for each AAI animal, including results of temperament testing, veterinary exams, vaccination records, and a log of all visits.

Most animal handlers will have a limited understanding about zoonoses and routine infection control practices. AAI organizations should provide formal, basic training of handlers in infection control, how to read an animal's body language, and how to protect patient confidentiality. When setting up a visiting program, the AAI organizations, and later possibly the specific AAI team that will be involved, should schedule meetings with the infection preventionist (or designee) of the health-care setting to discuss expectations and protocols.

The best-known and established AAI organization in the United States is the Delta Society Pet Partner Program. They can help groups that are interested in starting an AAI program with guidelines and templates for developing different kinds of programs (see Table 2.1).

Not necessarily specific to AAI or therapy dogs, there are other organizations that can provide training of animals in the fundamentals of good behavior that would be prerequisites for entry into any AAI program, for example, the Canine Good Citizen test created by the American Kennel Club (AKC). Started in 1989, AKC's Canine Good Citizen (CGC) Program is a certification program that is designed to reward dogs who have good manners at home and in the community. The CGC Program is a two-part program that stresses responsible pet ownership and basic good manners for dogs. Some therapy dog groups use the completion of the CGC Program as a partial screening tool or as a basis for the dog's evaluation.

Although not a specific AAI agency, the concept of integrating animals into long-term care facilities is enshrined in the ideals of the Eden Alternative homes, which strives to create a more homelike situation for elders who would otherwise be in long-term care facilities with an institutional feel. These Eden group settings are intended to create an elder-centered community that supports close and continuing contact with plants, animals, and children (see Table 2.1).

CURRENT LAWS

Each state or locality might have different regulations that dictate rules and standards for AAI activities and whether they are permissible in various settings. Health-care institutions need to check and make sure they follow those regulations. Animal associations or organizations wishing to begin a program also need to make sure they are acting within these legal bounds. Usually, local animal control authorities or environmental health staff from the appropriate public health authority would be able to direct interested agencies to the relevant rules. Many local laws dictate requirements for licensing and vaccinations that would be prerequisites for any animals in that jurisdiction.

Beyond the state and local laws, most health-care settings will have internal policies related to infection control, many of which are extensions of guidelines of the Joint Commission on Accreditation of Healthcare Organizations (JCAHO), a national accrediting body for hospitals to ensure that they comply with federal standards, including those related to infection control. Beyond those, any facility engaging in AAI should have individualized written and approved policies that govern approved AAI agencies, policies about visits, coordination with volunteers, approval of visits by medical staff, and so on.

GUIDELINES FOR AAI VISITS TO HEALTH-CARE SETTINGS TO MINIMIZE HEALTH AND SAFETY RISKS

The intent of AAI activities is to effect positive benefits, but animals can present disease risks to humans, especially medically fragile ones, but careful planning can ensure acceptable outcomes. The popularity of animal-assisted interventions in human health-care settings has been steadily increasing in the past few decades, with many hospitals and long-term care facilities allowing some form of animal visitation with their patients and residents. Most animals that visit are part of a formal AAI program, interacting with many patients over time. Less frequently, pets that belong to residents, patients, and their families or friends may visit with specific familiar individuals on a temporary basis.

In order to protect the health of patients, animals, and their handlers, the potential risks of infection and injury associated with animals visiting hospitalized or residential-living people need to be acknowledged and managed appropriately. Some potential adverse health efforts to consider are injury from bites, trips, or falls, or scratches; allergies from planned or incidental contact with animals; and concerns for transfer of infectious pathogens, including conditions such as methicillin-resistant *Staphylococcus aureus* (MRSA) or *Clostridium difficile*. A summary of the 2008 guidelines developed to minimize health and safety risks for AAI visits to health-care settings is described below.[3]

Characteristics of Therapy Animals

Good therapy animals do not need to be a specific breed or even a purebred animal. They need to be friendly and like people and be well-trained and responsive to commands. The animal's ability to calmly accept unusual or new circumstances is essential to being a good therapy animal. Animal handlers must be able to communicate with their animals in a gentle, positive manner and recognize their animal's particular signs of stress. AAI animals receive significant training and desensitization to learn how not to respond to a wide variety of unusual sights, sounds, smells, touches, and situations. Given the time needed for training and the increased predictability of behavior as animals mature, most successful AAI animals are at least one year old.

Sources and Species of Animals

Animal handlers must ensure that their animals are of suitable temperament and health for visiting people who may be at high risk of injury or of acquiring infections from the animals. Patients' pets are potentially suitable for visiting that patient provided that care is taken to restrict encounters to only that patient, that the animal is under a handler's control at all times, and the pet is of a suitable species (i.e., a small domesticated animal). Given that the patient already has a history of exposure to the animal, the pet is presumed to be of lesser risk of producing adverse health effects to that person than an unknown animal.

For animals or pets involved in formal AAI programs, suitable animal species are those small companion animals that can be trained and domesticated. Animals that are not suitable include those species identified as being of higher risk of causing human infection or injury, such as reptiles, amphibians, monkeys, rodents, hedgehogs, prairie dogs, or other recently domesticated wild animals. Animals obtained directly from the wild or obtained directly from an animal shelter or similar facility are not suitable because of their unknown or predictable behavior or health history. AAI animals should be adults, litter-trained, and part of an organized AAI program.

Temperament and Behavior of AAI Animals

All animals involved in AAI activities should successfully complete a standard temperament evaluation that has been specifically designed to evaluate the behavior of AAI animals under conditions that they might encounter in health-care settings. The evaluation process should assess an animal's reactions toward strangers, to loud and/or novel stimuli, to angry voices and potentially threatening gestures, to being crowded, to being patted and hugged, to having a tail pulled and being handled roughly, and to other animals. Animals should also be evaluated for their ability to readily obey handler's commands.

Behavior evaluators should have experience in assessing animal behavior and degree of training and have successfully completed a course or certification process in evaluating temperament. Evaluators should have experience with AAI programs and appreciate the types of challenges that animals may encounter in health-care settings. If possible, animal-handler teams should be evaluated in a health-care setting to make sure that classroom obedience translates to the real world. The handler must also be able to feel comfortable and calm in settings where people may be seriously ill or dying and may have a dramatically altered appearance. Animals should be regularly reevaluated, especially as they get older or if they start behaving erratically or showing such health problems as loss of hearing or sight, which might impact how they respond in a health-care setting.

AAI animals should enjoy interacting with people and appear relaxed in their presence, as demonstrated by relaxed body postures, tail position, and respiration. A useful tool for determining a dog's suitability for participating in AAI before a formal temperament evaluation is the validated self-report survey, C-BARQ (Canine Behavioral and Research Questionnaire), developed by researchers at the University of Pennsylvania (see Table 2.1). Inappropriate animal behavior includes aggressive acts (biting, snapping, swatting, or scratching), which may be provoked out of fear or other motivations, other potentially injurious actions such as mouthing or jumping up on people, and poor responses to handlers' commands. If someone wanted to consider enrolling his or her animal in AAI, completing the C-BARQ could be a helpful first hurdle to clear.

Health Screening of AAI Animals

Dogs and cats involved in AAI should be vaccinated against rabies as required by local law. For the protection of both animals and people, animals should not be brought to health-care facilities if they are displaying certain symptoms or signs, such as vomiting or diarrhea, sneezing or coughing of unknown or suspected infectious origin, open wounds, skin infections or hot spots, or showing signs of heat.

AAI animals should be regularly evaluated by a licensed veterinarian who can provide informed counsel about recommended vaccinations and other routine medications appropriate for the local risk of diseases, such as ectoparasite control for fleas and ticks and endoparasite control for intestinal or systemic worms. Animal owners should let veterinarians know if their animals are involved in AAI programs so that veterinarians can be aware of potential exposures to and risk from patients in health-care settings. There are educational materials for veterinarians to give owners about consideration for pets for immunocompromised people, the principles of which are relevant to AAI animals (see the CDC's Healthy Pets website in Table 2.1). Veterinarians also need to be aware that AAI animals are at risk of acquiring infectious organisms from the people and environments that they visit and should consider the possibility of hospital-associated pathogens such as MRSA and other multidrug-resistant bacteria when treating infections in these animals. A more detailed and comprehensive list of specific recommendations for veterinarians seeing patients involved in AAI is available.[9]

Routine laboratory screening for asymptomatic carriage of specific, potentially zoonotic microorganisms, including bacteria such as MRSA, is not recommended. Some screening may be required by an individual institution based on guidance from their risk managers or suggested by checklists provided by accreditation evaluators. By only allowing AAI animals to visit if they are well and without symptoms, with the knowledge that carriage of certain bacteria can be transient, and with all involved parties adhering to fastidious hand hygiene, there is no blanket public health recommendation to obtain routine screening cultures. In situations where epidemiological evidence suggests that an AAI animal might be involved in transmission of an infectious disease, special studies could be developed in conjunction with public health authorities, infection control departments, and veterinarians that might involve laboratory testing to determine what might have happened.

Reports have shown that raw meat-based diets and treats can be contaminated with enteric pathogens, such as *Salmonella*, that can subsequently be shed by animals in their stool. Therefore, animals involved in AAI should not be fed any raw foods or treats of animal origin within the past 90 days to avoid possibly shedding pathogenic bacteria while in the presence of medically fragile patients. Actually, every animal owner should avoid feeding raw food diets, particularly if there is a medically fragile person in the home.

Animal Handlers

Animal handlers are vital to ensuring that established protocols are followed, such as encouraging patients to engage in hand hygiene before and after handling animals and advising health-care setting staff if unusual incidents occur. AAI animal handlers frequently visit with more than one patient sequentially in a day. Consequently, animal handlers should be considered a volunteer in the health-care setting and should be held to the same standards for infection control practices as other volunteers. In addition, the animal handler may be asked to complete a confidentiality contract.

For animals that belong to a patient, the animal handler, who is usually a friend or relative, needs to make sure that the animal has minimal contact with anyone else in the facility regardless of the attention that will naturally be paid to the novelty of an animal in health-care settings. Visits from these owned animals must be prearranged and approved by the staff at a health-care setting, including the patient's medical provider. The animals must be under strict control at all times and in compliance with the facilities' policies. Unlike formal AAI animals, individually owned patient animals may not be oriented to a health-care setting and their behavior and disposition unknown or unpredictable, especially if they perceive their owner to be in distress. The infection control staff or the governing policies for AAI in general at the facility would likely require those vaccinations (e.g., rabies) that are also legally required by the local jurisdiction's animal control authority.

Most handlers of AAI animals will be part of a formal AAI program that has training policies and procedures, including lessons about zoonoses acquisition and transmission; basic infection control practices (including proper clean-up and disposal of animal wastes); reading an animal's body language to identify signs of physical discomfort, stress, fear, or aggression; patient confidentiality; and a basic orientation to the facility, including key players such as the infection preventionists, as well as instructions for how and which facility staff to contact before and during a visit to ensure that the visit goes smoothly.

Prior to visiting, animal handlers must comply with the health-care setting's policies for human health screening requirements in place for their volunteers and employees. During the visits, handlers must practice personal hand hygiene in accordance with the health-care setting's policies for volunteers and employees. Handlers need to be on alert for higher risk exposure contacts, such as patients allowing themselves to be licked, patients failing to practice hand hygiene, or patients otherwise handling the animal in a manner that might increase the likelihood of frightening or harming the animal or the animal harming a patient accidentally.

Preparation for Visiting

Animals' coats should be combed prior to visiting to remove as much loose hair, dander, and other debris as possible, and nails should be trimmed and without sharp edges. Animals should be recently washed and clean before a visit and free of excessive odors (i.e., not heavily groomed with potentially allergenic sprays). Related accessories, such as carriers or animal leashes, harnesses, and collars should be visibly clean and odor-free. Simple short leashes should be used instead of leashes with spikes or retractions, which could cause injuries to patients petting the animals. AAI animals should be identified with a clean noticeable scarf, collar, harness or leash, tag, or other special identifier that is readily recognizable by staff and other visitors. Dogs should be given an opportunity to urinate and defecate prior to entering the health-care setting. Wastes should be disposed of according to the policy of the particular facility.

Visits should be preauthorized, preferably with written consent from the patient or his agent for the visit, so that all involved are not surprised by the activity. Patients need to be carefully assessed to determine whether visiting with animals will provide some benefit to them, and that the risk of adverse effects for either the patients or the animals with which they will interact is minimal. Patients may not know anything about potential health hazards associated with interacting with animals. Animals should only visit with patients who have clearly expressed an interest. It is also important when presenting the opportunity to patients that the involved parties understand the boundaries of the visit, such as the estimated visit duration and limitations to contact—that is, refraining from licking. All immunocompromised patients should be assessed by their primary health-care providers to determine whether visiting with an animal would be appropriate.

Animal handlers should obtain oral permission from other individuals in the room prior to entering for visitation. Similarly, before entering an elevator with an animal, the handler should ask the other passengers for permission. Animals should not be allowed to visit in rooms shared by people with known or suspected fears of animals or animal allergies. Animals should not be allowed into certain parts of the facility including food or medication preparation or storage areas, intensive care units, operating rooms, isolation quarters, and neonatal nurseries.

2.1. DID YOU KNOW?

Animals might have the most beneficial impact on patients' health by what they don't do. When a young patient who was hospitalized for depression and risk of suicide was asked what he liked best about animal visits, he replied that the dog never asked him, "How are you feeling?"

Source: Personal communication to the author by Mary Troll, coordinator of Providence Alaska Medical Center Pet Therapy Program. Used with permission.

During the Visit

Visits from an AAI animal should be relatively short (less than an hour) to minimize the likelihood of adverse events associated with animal fatigue. Visits should be shorter if the animals show any signs of fatigue, stress, thirst, overheating, or urges to urinate or defecate, or if the patient (or patients if sharing a room) appear agitated or upset by the interaction. On the day of the visit, animal handlers should make sure that they are feeling well, and refrain from visiting if they have newly developed symptoms of a possible communicable disease, such as a worsening cough or sneezing, runny nose, fever, diarrhea and/or vomiting, or undiagnosed rash. This also applies to AAI animals. Even if a visit has been long planned and eagerly anticipated, if either the handler or the animal wakes up with new symptoms, it is best to reschedule the visit for a time when the team is feeling well.

Animals must be controlled at all times while visiting, which includes using leashes or pet carriers when transporting and making sure that patients' room doors are closed and containment is achieved so no inadvertent visiting can occur. Handlers should be mindful to avoid other activities that divert their attention away from the animal.

Animal handlers should discourage patients, health-care workers, and facility staff from shaking the animal's paw. Animals should also be prevented from licking patients and anyone else, and anyone who is licked should wash their hands afterward. Patients should not be visited while they are eating or drinking, and should not snack during their interactions with the animal. Gloves should be worn to clean up any animal excreta (urine, vomitus, or feces), which should be disposed of securely and reported to health-care staff so the area can be properly disinfected.

Handlers should take care to prevent animals from coming into contact with sites of invasive devices, open or bandaged wounds, surgical incisions or other breaches in the skin, as well as any special equipment.

Patients should be approached from the side that does not have such invasive devices as intravenous catheters, because animals may disturb these devices or potentially contaminate them. Patients may request that an animal be placed on the bed. Handlers should make sure that the existing bed linens are clean and then place a disposable impermeable barrier between the animal and the bed. Instead of a disposable barrier, a pillowcase, towel, or extra bed sheet could also be used and then sent for laundering immediately after a single use.

If the animal becomes ill (e.g., vomiting or diarrhea), urinates, or defecates, or there is an injury or adverse event, the visit should end. Afterward, the handler, AAI agency, and health-care setting representatives should assess what happened and the contributing factors. If reasonable changes cannot be made to prevent recurrence, reassess whether AAI is feasible in the current setting, with the current animal or patient or handler.

All patients, visitors, and health-care setting staff should practice hand washing both before and after animal contact. Because access to sinks might not be available, animal handlers should carry a waterless hand sanitizer product with them to offer to anyone who wishes to touch the animal. With concerns for other communicable diseases, many health-care settings now have readily available public dispensers of hand sanitizers mounted throughout the facility, which increases the likelihood and ease of practicing hand hygiene when sinks are not always available.

Facilities should develop a system of recording the areas and/or room numbers where the animal has interacted with patients. AAI organizations may want to keep a record of their visits, but records maintained by the organization need to take care not to violate confidentiality issues related to the policies of the health-care setting. Infection preventionists might also want to document the specifics of visits in patients' medical charts.

Visit Locations

The infection preventionist or other infection control program staff are best able to determine which locations are appropriate for animals interacting with patients in their particular facility. Choosing the site for a visit requires thoughtful consideration. Factors that need to be weighed include the patient's degree of mobility, sensitivities of other patients or staff to animals, and ease of cleaning. In general, suitable areas for patient visits include those that contain surfaces that are easily cleaned, where the animal can be contained if it is not on a leash, are not crowded, and are large enough to permit ease of movement. Such areas should not have loud noises or contain people who are afraid of or are allergic to animals. Such areas may include patients' rooms, common areas such as waiting rooms, lounges, or rehabilitation areas, or specially designated rooms for animal visits. If the area is carpeted, vacuuming of carpeted areas after the visit is highly recommended to address allergy concerns.

Conducting AAI in a common area allows for limiting the degree of contamination by animals to specific areas as opposed to dispersal throughout the facility. In addition, meeting in a common area facilitates social interaction between participants and gets them out of their rooms, which may be a desired outcome for some situations or settings. However, such common areas are more likely to have unannounced patients or other visitors who might be fearful of animals or have allergies. A regular schedule with posted signs can help avoid some of these issues. In long-term care settings, the staff could schedule a group meeting to make sure that everyone approves of the visits and understands the bounds of the program ahead of time so that residents could make a reasoned choice about participation and those with fears or allergies could adapt their schedule to avoid any encounters.

Figure 2.1
Tanner, registered Pet Partner, visits Jessica at Providence Alaska Medical Center, 2009

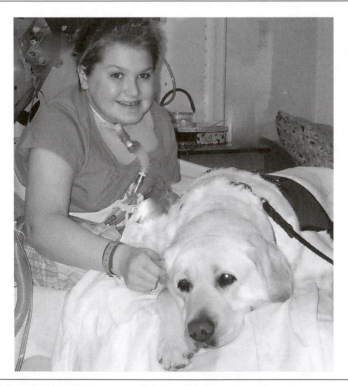

Source: © 2009 Child Life Department, Children's Hospital at Providence, Providence Alaska Medical Center. Photo by Bonnie Hiers. Reprinted with permission.

The other most common place for a visit is the patient's room. The main benefit of visiting patients in their rooms is that this permits animals to interact with those who are nonambulatory and whose ability to socialize with others may be limited. In addition, a private patient's room provides an opportunity for animals to be directed to specific people rather than being exposed to the general population. In some cases, such as in long-term care facilities, room visits may be preferred to establish both the bond between animal and patient and between handler and patient in privacy. It also may be less tiring for an animal to have a smaller crowd and less stressful for the handler to worry about patients or residents taking turns.

Visits are not without challenges. Many patients share rooms with other patients who may not want to interact with an animal either because of allergies, fears, or a dislike of animals.

CASE REPORTS AND STUDIES OF POTENTIAL ZOONOSES IN HEALTH-CARE SETTINGS

Although there are numerous case reports of owners getting zoonotic infections from their pets in less formal settings, few comprehensive studies have been published that focus specifically on AAI programs in health-care settings and the risks of transmission of infectious agents between animals and people.[10–12] A 2005 study of active hospital visitation dogs in Ontario found that 80 percent of 102 animals were shedding at least one potentially zoonotic pathogen including *Clostridium difficile* (58% of dogs), *Pasteurella spp.* (29%), and multidrug resistant *Escherichia coli* (6%).[10] A subsequent study that sampled 200 AAI dogs from Ontario and Alberta every two months for one year revealed that dogs that visited health-care facilities were significantly more likely to acquire MRSA and *C. difficile* than dogs that performed other types of AAIs.[11] Dogs that licked patients in health-care settings were more likely to acquire these hospital-associated pathogens than dogs that did not. All dogs were clinically healthy at the time of testing positive, and although not prescribed medication to clear the bacteria, the majority tested negative in subsequent samples, indicating transient carriage of pathogens.

Because some pathogens like MRSA are often in the community, it would be nearly impossible to say if a newly diagnosed MRSA infection in the dog was from a source in the health-care setting, from anyone in the dog's household, or from another animal or person with whom the animal might have interacted. In extraordinary situations, DNA testing of bacterial culture isolates can be performed to possibly determine the direction of transmission.

For animals that are residents in a long-term care facility, one study showed that, over time, the animals became colonized with strains of MRSA that were also present among some of the residents.[12] With serial testing of the animals, it was also demonstrated that colonization of the animals with the bacteria was transient. A health-care setting where patients live is somewhat of a different situation than a hospital in which visits would typically be short-lived. In a residential setting with a resident animal, there is usually more informal contact, and it may be harder to control interactions and contacts like feeding snacks to the pet and licking. Essentially, these situations become like an extended household where, over time, the humans and animals may share bacteria, and changes in bacterial carriage might be expected mostly with the introduction of new residents or animals.

Case reports of illnesses subsequently being documented in AAI animals or patients after an interaction are hard to find, which is reassuring. Some reasons may be that AAI animals are not a random selection of animals and can be assumed to have above average veterinary care; also, people might be applying common sense and good hygiene to the interactions. The corollary is that there is documentation that animals have picked up human pathogens and not become ill, which is fortunate, but serves as a reminder that AAI may not always be a benign activity for an animal.

Guidelines designed to mitigate the risk of adverse health effects should also include suggestions for minimizing the risk of noninfectious conditions, such as injuries or allergies. Published reports of injuries to people exposed to animals in health-care settings are again rare, although that might be partially a result of underreporting. More subtle adverse health effects may occur and be more incidental—perhaps a staff person, patient, or other visitor to the health-care setting might be startled by the presence of an animal and trip, or have a mild allergic reaction. These risks are not necessarily specific to a health-care setting and could happen anywhere. The concern in health-care settings is that you may have more medically fragile people for whom a small incident or injury could have larger implications. With an established AAI program, these issues can be anticipated and minimized by ensuring controls or protocols are in place and by making sure that people are informed and aware. Any incident or injury, and even a near miss, should always be reviewed by the AAI agency and the infection prevention or administrative staff at the health-care settings to determine if policies and procedures need to be altered to prevent recurrence.

CONCLUSION

Pets are very much a part of people's lives, and animals in homes and health-care settings have been shown to elicit both qualitative and quantitative health benefits to humans. There will always be concerns for potential disease transmission or adverse health impacts between humans and animals; however, with careful forethought and established policies,

Table 2.1

Animal-Assisted Interventions Resources

Resource Name	Type of Information Presented	URL
AKC American Kennel Club	Canine Good Citizen Program	http://www.akc.org/events/cgc/index.cfm
C-BARQ Canine Behavioral and Research Questionnaire	Behavior evaluation tool developed by researchers at the University of Pennsylvania	http://vetapps.vet.upenn.edu/cbarq/
CDC Centers for Disease Control and Prevention Healthy Pets	Website that lists animals and possible diseases of public health concern • Links to AAI organizations	http://www.cdc.gov/healthypets/resources/local_organizations.htm
Delta Society	Organization dedicated to creating positive interactions with animals, particularly through therapy • Information about standards of AAI • Templates for creating a program • References about AAI	http://www.deltasociety.org/
Eden Alternative Homes	Information about group living situations for elders that regularly incorporate animals	http://www.edenalt.org/

these concerns can be managed in health-care settings. Pets are, if not savings lives, at the very least improving the lives of hospital and long-term care facility residents now, and can be expected to do so in the future in greater numbers. As the research increases and diversifies about the possible health benefits of AAI in health-care settings, demand for AAI services may increase, and there will need to be thoughtful and appropriate development of policies to ensure that neither the patients, residents, or animals experience increases in adverse health effects.

FURTHER READING

Becker M, Morton D. *The Healing Power of Pets: Harnessing the Amazing Ability of Pets to Make and Keep People Happy and Healthy*. New York: Hyperion; 2002.

Fine AH, ed. *Handbook on Animal-Assisted Therapy: Theoretical Foundations and Guidelines for Practice*. 3rd ed. San Diego, CA: Academic Press; 2010.

Nightingale F. *Notes on Nursing: What It Is and What It Is Not* (1860). Toronto, ON: Dover Publishing; 1969.

REFERENCES

1. Hooker SD, Freeman LH, Stewart P. Pet therapy research: A historical review. *Holistic Nursing Practice* 2002;16:17–23.
2. Jorgenson J. Therapeutic use of companion animals in health care. *Image Journal of Nursing Scholarship* 1997;29:249–54.
3. Lefebvre SL, Golab GC, Christensen E, et al. Guidelines for animal-assisted interventions in health care settings. *American Journal of Infection Control* 2008;36:78–85.
4. Friedmann E, Son H. The human-companion animal bond: How humans benefit. *Veterinary Clinics of North America* 2009;39:293–326.
5. Johnson RA, Meadows RL, Haubner JS, Sevedge K. Animal-assisted activity among patients with cancer: Effects on mood, fatigue, self-perceived health, and sense of coherence. *Oncology Nursing Forum* 2008;35:225–32.
6. Chu CI, Liu CY, Sun CT, Lin J. The effect of animal-assisted activity on inpatients with schizophrenia. *Journal of Psychosocial Nursing* 2009;47:42–8.
7. Marx MS, Cohen-Mansfield J, Regier NG, Dakheel-Ali M, Srihari A, Thein K. The impact of different dog-related stimuli on engagement of people with dementia. *American Journal of Alzheimer's Disease and Other Dementias* 2010; 25:37–45.
8. Banks MR, Banks WA. The effects of animals-assisted therapy on loneliness in an elderly population in long-term care facilities. *Journal of Gerontology* 2002;57:M428–32.
9. Lefebvre SL, Peregrine AS, Golab GC, Gumley NR, Walter-Toews D, Weese JS. A veterinary perspective on the recently published guidelines for animal-assisted interventions in health-care facilities. *Journal of the American Veterinary Medical Association* 2008;233:394–402.
10. Lefebvre SL, Walter-Toews D, Peregrine AS, et al. Prevalence of zoonotic agents in dogs visiting hospitalized people in Ontario: Implications for infection control. *Journal of Hospital Infection* 2006;62:458–66.
11. Lefebvre SL, Reid-Smith RJ, Walter-Toews D, Weese JS. Incidence of acquisition of methicillin-resistant *Staphylococcus aureus, Clostridium difficile,* and other health-care-associated pathogens by dogs that participate in animals-assisted intervention. *Journal of the American Veterinary Medical Association* 2009; 234:1404–17.
12. Coughlan K, Olsen K, Boxrud D, Bender J. Methicillin-resistant *Staphylococcus aureus* in resident animals of a long-term care facility. *Zoonoses Public Health* 2010;57:220–6.

Chapter 3

Dog Bites and Dangerous Pets

Kira A. Christian, DVM, MPH, DACVPM

INTRODUCTION

Domesticated animals, particularly dogs, can inflict serious injury or illness. Dog bites, for example, cause more than 800,000 Americans to receive medical attention each year, and many more bite injuries go untreated and unreported. On average, approximately a dozen people die each year from dog bite injuries in the United States.

In the first part of this chapter, we will focus on dog bites and the injuries and illnesses that can occur from them. In the last part of this chapter, we will discuss dangerous pets. Pet owners used to keeping domesticated animals might also be drawn to keeping exotic animals as pets; however, exotic animals kept as pets are unpredictable, can cause serious injury, illness, or even death, and can often be destructive. Although it might seem novel and exciting to keep an exotic animal as a pet, most, if not all of these species, do not make safe household pets. We will explore different types of wildlife species typically sought by people to be kept as pets and the dangers associated with this practice.

DOG BITES

Injuries from Dog Bites

A dog bite is a serious matter. Not only can it be frightening to think about being bitten by a dog, but the bite of a dog can have serious repercussions, including injury, illness—for example, being infected with the virus that causes rabies—and even death. Furthermore, being bitten by a dog can cause psychological injury, thereby potentially making the victim fearful of dogs for years to come, perhaps for his or her entire life. The number of recorded dog bite injuries is significantly higher in children than adults. Why? First, children have higher numbers of dog bite injuries recorded compared with adults because children are more likely to seek out interactions with dogs, for example, petting or otherwise showing dogs attention. Second, dogs sometimes see children as more threatening than adults—in other words, a dog might be more likely to try to display dominance over a similarly sized human, such as a child, and as a result intentionally or unintentionally hurt the child. Third, children are also more likely than adults to be presented for care at a health-care facility after a dog bite, thereby increasing the numbers of children counted as having dog bite injuries. In addition, elderly persons and utility workers, such as mail carriers and meter readers, are also frequently bitten by dogs. Unfortunately, sometimes owners are the recipients of their own dog's bite, such as when breaking up a dogfight.

Despite media reports and other rumors, there is no credible scientific evidence that any one breed of dog is more likely to bite than another. All breeds and sizes of dogs have the potential to bite—from American pit bull terriers and rottweilers to Chihuahuas and Yorkshire terriers. Despite this, large dogs are capable of delivering more than 450 pounds of pressure per square inch in a single bite—enough to penetrate light sheet metal—making the bite of a large dog more capable of delivering injury, compared with the bite of a small dog.[1] But it is important to remember that all dog bites are capable of inoculating bacteria to the bite victim, creating infection, and in fact certain bacteria (e.g., *Staphylococcus intermedius*) are more likely to be associated with a bite from dogs weighing less than 40 pounds.[1]

According to the American Pet Association, there are approximately 150 million dogs and cats living in the United States, and animal bites account for 1 percent of annual emergency department visits. For all animal bites, approximately 10 percent require medical attention and 1–2 percent require hospitalization; furthermore, it is estimated that 10–20 people die each year following an animal bite. The vast majority of animal bites to people involve dogs (85–90%), followed by cats (5–10%). Additionally, complications, such as with bacterial infections like *Capnocytophaga canimorsus*, discussed later in this chapter, occur in approximately 15–20 percent of dog-related bites.[2]

Trauma-associated complications can occur after a person receives a dog bite, including wounds that might need surgical correction. One study conducted at the Los Angeles County–University of Southern California Medical Center found that of 86 patients admitted to the hospital for a dog bite, the most common serious injury was an upper extremity (i.e., arm) fracture and/or dislocation (26 patients, or 30.2% of the 86), followed by vascular injury (12 patients, 11.6%). Also, 44 of the 86 patients (51.2%) needed surgery as a result of the injuries, including 28 (32.6%) who needed wound debridement (surgical excision of dead, devitalized, or contaminated tissue), and 22 (25.6%) required orthopedic interventions. It was concluded from this study that many patients admitted after dog attacks will require surgery.

Animal bites can also lead to costly expenditures. The estimated cost in health-care expenditures attributable to animal bites has been estimated at $30 million per year, and surgical costs can accumulate quickly, even when the surgery is an outpatient procedure. Furthermore, not only are the health-care associated costs expensive, but indirect costs associated with missing school or work because of injury or illness increase as well.[3]

Unfortunately, a number of deaths do occur each year in the United States as the result of receiving dog bites. One study conducted by the Centers for Disease Control and Prevention (CDC) in 1996 found that of 109 dog bite-related fatalities identified between 1989 and 1994 in the United States, 57 percent of the victims were less than 10 years of age.[4] Furthermore, the death rate for neonates (i.e., an infant four weeks old or less) was two orders of magnitude higher compared with adults, and the rate for children (aged between one and nine years) one order of magnitude higher. Of deaths with available data, 22 percent involved an unrestrained (e.g., untethered or unleashed) dog off the owner's property, 18 percent involved a restrained (e.g., tethered or leashed) dog on the owner's property, and 59 percent involved an unrestrained dog on the owner's property. In addition, 11 attacks involved a sleeping infant, 19 dogs involved in fatal attacks had a prior history of aggression, and 19 of 20 deaths with this type of data available involved an unneutered dog. One conclusion of this study was that breed-specific approaches (i.e., breed-specific citywide bans such as pit bull bans) to the control of dog bites do not address the issue that many breeds are involved in the dog-bite problem, and that most of the factors contributing to dog bites are related to the level of responsibility exercised by dog owners. In other words, a responsible dog owner will be more likely to have a well-behaved, and less likely to bite, dog.

Another study also conducted by the CDC identified at least 25 breeds of dog involved in 238 dog-bite related fatalities from 1979 to 1998, and although pit bull–type dogs and rottweilers were involved in more than half of these deaths, the authors of the study found that other breeds also may bite and actually cause fatalities at higher rates, meaning fatal attacks inflicted by pit bull–type dogs and rottweilers represent a small proportion of dog bite injuries to humans. One reason for this is the registration of certain types of dog breeds might be biased. Owners of smaller, more fashionable dogs might be more likely to register their dog as a certain breed, compared with owners of larger dogs, who might not be as likely to claim that their dog is of one breed or another, which means that these smaller, more fashionable breeds are more likely to be counted as causing harm compared with larger breeds, which could also be counted as mixed breeds. For example, in 2001 a Pomeranian breed of dog (ranges from 4 to 8 pounds and stands 5 to 11 inches tall), which is regarded as a toy size dog, reportedly killed a six-week-old baby while the caretaker momentarily left the child alone. This incident reinforces the fact that all breeds of dogs have the propensity to bite, not just dogs that are typically identified as being aggressive.[5]

To summarize, dog bites cannot be predicted from breed of dog alone, and the scientific evidence discussed earlier supports this. Two additional takeaway messages are, first, although unneutered dogs may be more frequently counted as inflictors of dog bites, as in the first CDC study mentioned, neutering a dog does not mean a dog will never bite again, and second, never leave an unattended child alone with any breed of dog, and teach children how to respect all animals, including and especially those animals with which the child will be spending time. Overall, the best way to prevent a dog bite is to learn why a dog might bite, recognize common causes of bites, and take steps to prevent them.

3.1.   DID YOU KNOW?

Dog bites can be emergencies. If you are bitten by a dog and the dog's owner is present, request proof of rabies vaccination and get the owner's name and contact information. Clean the bite wound thoroughly with soap and water as soon as possible and consult your doctor, or go to the emergency room if it's after office hours. You should also contact your community's animal control authorities and report the incident.

Why Does a Dog Bite?

A dog can bite for a variety of reasons: fear, defense, training, illness, or pain. A bite sometimes occurs because it was provoked by another animal or a human. We will discuss some warning signs of an impending bite and what dog aggression looks like in order to better help prevent someone from being bitten.

Sometimes a dog will let you know when he might bite. Growling, baring teeth, snarling, and snapping are all behaviors that dogs might display prior to biting. Additionally, nervous-type behaviors such as yawning, licking lips, pacing, and stretching also might indicate that the dog is agitated and could bite. Also, the fur between the dog's shoulders might stand up (also called raising the withers, similar to a person having goose bumps). The dog might pin his ears back and lean forward so all of his weight is centered over the front legs, which makes him look more powerful. Other signs, including panting and drooling, tucking the tail, lowering the ears, gazing away, lowering the body, or vocalizing could also be indicative of an impending bite. Understanding different types of dog aggression might help one also discern whether a dog might bite.

There are different types of aggression exhibited by dogs, some more subtle than others, and it is important to understand these different types in order to learn how to prevent being bitten. The Humane Society of the United States has categorized different types of dog aggression in an easy to understand manner, which we will touch on here,[6] but a veterinary behaviorist can provide you with a much more thorough understanding of this behavior issue and help you in dealing with it.

Fear-motivated aggression is a defensive reaction and occurs when a dog believes he is in danger of being harmed. Similar to such nervous-type behaviors as yawning, licking lips, pacing, and stretching, fear-motivated aggression can be the most difficult type of aggression to recognize. A dog may also be fearfully aggressive when approached by other dogs. This type of aggression is challenging to understand and difficult to break.

Protective, territorial, and possessive aggression are all very similar. Territorial aggression is usually associated with defense of property, and the territory may extend well past the boundaries of your yard. For example, if you regularly walk your dog around the neighborhood and allow him to urine-mark, he may think his territory includes the entire block. Protective aggression usually refers to aggression directed toward people or animals that a dog perceives as threats to his family or pack. Dogs become possessively aggressive when defending their food, toys, or other valued objects.

Another category of aggression recognized by the Humane Society of the United States is redirected aggression, a relatively common type of aggression, but one that is also often misunderstood, in addition to fear-motivated aggression. If a dog is somehow provoked by a person or animal the dog is unable to attack, it may redirect this aggression onto someone else. For example, two family dogs may become excited and bark and growl in response to another dog passing through the front yard, or two dogs confined behind a fence may turn and attack each other because they cannot attack an intruder.

DOG BITE PREVENTION: PERSONAL RESPONSIBILITY

Dog owners have a responsibility to prevent their dog from biting other animals or people, and several tips are presented below and which are available from the American Veterinary Medical Association (AVMA) and the CDC on how dog owners can educate themselves on preventing their own dogs from biting.

Before bringing a dog into your home, consult with a professional (e.g., a veterinarian) to learn what breeds of dogs are the best fit for your household. Do not adopt or buy a puppy on impulse. Before and after selection, your veterinarian is your best source for information about behavior and health. Be sensitive to cues that a child is fearful or apprehensive about a dog. If a child seems frightened by dogs, wait before bringing a dog into your household. Dogs with histories of aggression are not suitable for households with children. Spend time with a dog before adopting or buying him. Use caution when bringing a dog into a household with an infant or toddler, or consider waiting until the child is older.

If you decide to bring a dog into your home, be a responsible pet owner. License your dog with your community as required. Obey leash laws. If you have a fenced yard, make sure the gates are secure. Dogs are social animals; spending time with your pet is important. Dogs that are frequently left alone have a greater chance of developing behavioral problems, such as biting. Remember, a responsible dog owner will be more likely to have a well-behaved dog. Walk and exercise your dog regularly to keep him healthy and provide mental stimulation. Keep your dog healthy and provide training for him in the form of organized classes. Do not play aggressive games with your dog, but socialize your dog well as a puppy and expose him to various stimuli, including animate (other animals and people, belly rubs, touching the muzzle and paws), and inanimate (sounds and objects) stimuli. These activities are most important when a dog is young, but can also be introduced with adult dogs to reinforce these positive behaviors.

Keeping your dog healthy includes neutering your dog—both males and females. As stated earlier in the chapter, unneutered dogs might be more frequently counted as biters, but remember neutering a dog does not mean he will never bite again. Neutering your dog also helps prevent other health problems in the future. Be alert and learn what signs your dog will demonstrate when it is not feeling well or is in pain, both of which can be predisposing factors to a bite. Immediately seek professional advice from your veterinarian if the dog develops aggressive or undesirable behaviors. And finally, never leave infants, young children, or anyone unable to take care of himself or herself alone with a dog—this cannot be emphasized enough.

DOG BITE PREVENTION: COMMUNITY RESPONSIBILITY

The American Veterinary Medical Association's Task Force on Canine Aggression and Human-Canine Interactions recognizes that dog bites are a serious public health problem that can inflict considerable physical and emotional damage on victims and be extremely costly to communities. Decreasing the number of dog bites requires active and ongoing community involvement; passive or periodic attention will not solve this problem. A report was prepared by the Task Force to help state and local leaders find effective ways to reduce the dog bite problem in their communities.[7]

Dog bites are a preventable public health problem. On a community level, many programs are currently in place or being planned to obtain an accurate assessment of how many dog bites occur each year in a particular area in order to develop effective prevention strategies to reduce the number of dog bites. For example, in Georgia, the Department of Community Health developed a dog bite prevention program to decrease the number and severity of dog bite-related injuries, establish further collaboration among individuals and groups (e.g., community-awareness organizations, schools, local business or neighborhood districts, or perhaps those who have been bitten by a dog in the past, or anyone with an interest in preventing these injuries), and provide education and opportunities for behavior change among at-risk populations.[8]

DOG BITE LAWS

Laws with regard to dog bites vary from state to state. The Georgia dog bite law (Title 51, Section 51-2-7) addresses animal bites and states that any "person who owns or keeps a vicious or dangerous animal of any kind and who, by careless management or by allowing the animal to go at liberty, causes injury to another person who does not provoke the injury by his own act may be liable in damages to the person so injured." What this means is that owners of dogs who bite can be held liable for such expenses as medical and legal fees if a court can prove that the owner was negligent in restraining the dog, thus facilitating the bite. For the most part, laws, although they vary, carry the common theme of placing the responsibility on the dog owner.

BREED-SPECIFIC LEGISLATION

Breed-specific legislation has also come to the forefront in the media in recent years. Breed-specific legislation can be defined as laws that either regulate or ban certain breeds in an effort to reduce dog attacks. One notable example is the breed-specific legislation with regard to pit bull–type dogs in the cities of Denver and Aurora, Colorado. The ban was originally enacted by the city of Denver in 1989 and targets pit bull–type dogs; Aurora's ban targets such pit bulls as well as seven other breeds of dogs. Several media reports and popular press articles estimate that more than 3,000 pit bulls in Denver alone have been killed in compliance with this ban. In the study previously discussed, which was conducted by the CDC reviewing dog-bite related fatalities during 1979–1998, specific breeds were not identified as most likely to bite or kill, and thus is not appropriate for policy-making decisions related to reducing dog bites. Despite this, community jurisdictions continue to create breed-based legislation, which is costly to the community.

MAKING PETS DANGEROUS: DOG FIGHTING

Dog fighting has gained incredible amounts of media attention in the past few years with the exposure of people, including celebrities, who fight dogs. Dog fighting is illegal in all 50 states, the District of Columbia, Puerto Rico, and the Virgin Islands, and as of 2008, dog fighting is now classified as a felony throughout the United States. Because of this, dog fighting has become somewhat clandestine, or underground—participants not only want to evade animal cruelty charges, but the other illegal activities that come along with dog fighting, such as gambling. People who fight dogs also find other ways to profit from fights, including charging admission fees and selling the offspring of fighting dogs to other people. In 2007, the U.S. Congress passed the Animal Fighting Prohibition Enforcement Act, which provides felony penalties for interstate commerce, import and export relating to commerce in fighting dogs, fighting cocks, and cockfighting paraphernalia. Each violation can result in up to three years in jail and a $250,000 fine.

Although certain breeds of dog are more commonly associated with fighting, just as with bites, any dog can be used for fighting. According to the American Society for the Prevention of Cruelty to Animals, in the United States, the dog most commonly used for fighting is the American pit bull terrier. Fila Brasileiros, Dog Argentinos, and Presa Canarios have also been used, among others. It must be noted that any type of dog—or for that matter, animal—can be used as a bait animal, which are used to train dogs to attack and kill. Submissive dogs of any breed are often used for this, in addition to other animals such as cats or rabbits, many of whom have been stolen from their homes or from "free to good home" advertisements.

DISEASES FROM DOG BITES

In addition to injury, several diseases, including those caused by viruses and bacteria, can be transmitted to people from bites of dogs (diseases that are transmitted from animals to people are termed zoonotic diseases). Here, we will discuss two diseases caused by a bacteria and one caused by a virus.

Capnocytophaga Canimorsus

Capnocytophaga canimorsus is an organism that has been found in the saliva of healthy dogs and cats as part of the normal flora, or bacterial makeup, of the mouth. Reports of people being infected by C. *canimorsus* have been reported from many countries, including the United States. One study[9] found C. *canimorsus* in the mouths of 21 of 130 (16%) dogs sampled and 28 of 158 (17.7%) cats. These bacteria can be transmitted to people by bite, scratch, or other unknown exposures, but transmission by bite is most common. Although C. *canimorsus* grows in a dog or cat's mouth and may not cause disease in that animal, it can cause disease in a person if an animal carrying these bacteria bites someone.

C. *canimorsus* causes disease by infecting the bite wound itself. Disease in people can range from a mild-appearing local infection at the site of the bite to life-threatening illness, which can include septicemia (infection has entered the bloodstream and has spread throughout the body), and a usually fatal condition called disseminated intravascular coagulation (DIC), which occurs when the body depletes itself of factors that allow blood to clot and is usually fatal. Approximately 25 percent of people who develop severe infection with C. *canimorsus* eventually die from it. However, some studies have shown that people with underlying conditions such as a suppressed immune system (immunosuppression), having had their spleen removed (asplenia), liver disease, current treatment with corticosteroids, or a history of alcoholism might have a worse course of disease and could be more likely to die.

Infection with C. *canimorsus* is usually evident two to three days after the bacteria contaminate the wound, but symptoms could take as long as four weeks to appear. One study revealed that infection with C. *canimorsus* more likely occurs in men (74%), but this does not necessarily mean that men are more vulnerable to infection; this could simply mean that men might have more exposures to animal bites, could be more likely to have an underlying condition that could lead to the development of severe infection, or might be more likely to seek treatment for illness.

There are several examples of unfortunate consequences of infection with C. *canimorsus* in the medical literature. One case of infection[10] occurred in a previously healthy woman aged 45 years who worked in an animal shelter and was bitten by a dog. She began feeling ill with a cough, weakness, and fatigue and presented herself for treatment at a hospital after three days of illness. Life support was withdrawn after seven days in the hospital, having endured a severe course of infection with *C. canimorsus*, including debilitating gangrene, DIC, and subsequent multiple organ failure. This woman did not have any of the typical risk factors described earlier, and it was never discovered why her infection was so severe and resulted in death.

People who work around or with animals, including employees of animal shelters like the woman described above, need to be very cognizant of any type of exposure to animal saliva, and *C. canimorsus* is a good example of why this is very important. A person who suffers an animal bite should always be seen by a health-care provider for evaluation.

Pasteurellosis

Another example of a bacterial infection that people can get from the bite of a dog is the disease pasteurellosis, caused by different species of the bacteria genus *Pasteurella*, a type of bacteria that lives in the upper respiratory tract of animals, including dogs, and is isolated in 50 percent of dog bites. *Pasteurella*, with several species of these bacteria, are the most common organism that causes infection from bite wounds. Other types of animals in which *Pasteurella* frequently are found include cats, livestock, and poultry. Animals with these bacteria living in their upper respiratory tracts are not necessarily ill from the bacteria, but the bacteria can still be passed to a human via a bite, or, less often, a scratch or lick. When a person is infected with these bacteria, infection is apparent within 24 hours and can quickly spread deeper into the tissues, such as joints and bones near where the bite occurred. Worse, it can spread systemically throughout the body and cause damage to other systems, such as the cardiovascular or central nervous systems.[12]

Rabies

Another example of a disease transmitted through animal saliva is rabies, which is a preventable viral disease of mammals most often transmitted through the bite of a rabid animal. Most rabies cases reported to the CDC each year occur in wild animals, like raccoons, skunks, bats, and foxes (known rabies reservoirs). The rabies virus infects the central nervous system, ultimately causing disease in the brain and death. The early symptoms of rabies in people are similar to that of many other illnesses, including fever, headache, and general weakness or discomfort. As the disease progresses, more specific symptoms appear and may include insomnia, anxiety, confusion, slight or partial paralysis, excitation, hallucinations, agitation, hypersalivation (i.e., increase in saliva production), difficulty swallowing, and hydrophobia (fear of water). Death usually occurs within days of the onset of these symptoms, and rabies post-exposure prophylaxis is effective only before the person shows clinical signs of illness. Animal rabies-control programs, including extensive vaccination campaigns implemented during the 1940s and 1950s, resulted in a substantial decline of rabies in domesticated animals in the United States.[11] In 2009, 81 dogs, or 1.2 percent of all cases of rabies in animals, were reported to the CDC.

For more information on diseases that humans can acquire from dogs and cats, see chapters 8 and 9.

DANGEROUS PETS—EXOTIC PETS

Exotic pets, as stated at the beginning of the chapter, are generally considered to be any species other than a dog, cat, fish, or livestock, but definitions may vary by local jurisdiction. Exotic pets, in addition to being challenging to provide adequate care for, are heavily regulated. In addition, there are many rules for importing exotic animals into the United States. In this part of the chapter, we will explore the challenges and dangers of three of the many different types of wild animals that are oftentimes kept as exotic pets. The common theme to these types of animals is that for most exotic animals, as juveniles, they are small and appealing, but often mature into dangerous animals that can injure or kill people. It must also be noted that, as with all animals, zoonotic disease transmission is a risk with these exotic animals, including, but not limited to, the diseases of rabies, pasteurellosis, and a multitude of other pathogens, including internal and external parasites.

Large Cats

The first group of exotic pets we will discuss are large cats. According to the U.S. Department of Agriculture (USDA) Animal and Plant Health Inspection Service (APHIS), large, wild, and exotic cats such as lions, tigers, cougars, and leopards are dangerous animals and should only be kept by qualified, trained professionals. The Animal Care Program, housed within APHIS, is responsible for enforcing the Animal Welfare Act, which includes regulating and inspecting exhibitors of wild and exotic animals, but APHIS does not regulate ownership of these large cats as pets. Oftentimes, the laws in local jurisdictions apply to large cat ownership. Usually, keeping a large cat as a pet is illegal or requires expensive permits, bonds, and proof of insurance. For example, Florida Statutes 379.374 Bond states that a $10,000 bond must be guaranteed to exhibit any Class I wildlife (examples of Class I wildlife in Florida are large cats, large mammals such as rhinoceroses, elephants, and bears, and other large nonmammals such as crocodiles and Komodo dragons), otherwise, the exhibitor must "maintain comprehensive general liability insurance with minimum limits of $2 million per occurrence and $2 million annual aggregate" in order to protect from claims for damages for personal injury, accidental death, or property damage. In other words, it is extremely cost-prohibitive to stay within the limits of the law when in possession of a large cat. As such, small exhibitors, such as roadside circuses, often do get penalized, but such exhibitors oftentimes simply just relocate outside the jurisdiction where they were fined and continue operations.

Large cats can kill or severely injure other animals and people, and the average pet owner, or even a pet owner with previous exotic animal experience, cannot handle a large cat safely. Because of the novelty of these cats, it oftentimes is the predilection of owners to show these animals off. However, these cats are not domesticated, and an animal that seems to be friendly can severely injure or kill someone, especially a child, even when the animals are seemingly being playful. As stated earlier, rabies is a concern in all mammals, including large cats. If one of these large cats is placed in an environment that involves close contact with people and the cat bites or scratches a person, rabies post-exposure prophylaxis might be necessary for the person who was bitten—that is, if the cat is either euthanized and tests positive for rabies or if the cat is no longer available for testing—which is neither benign nor inexpensive.

In addition to the harm that these large cats can inflict on people, the large cat's well-being is usually jeopardized when kept as a pet. A typical pet owner does not have the facilities or access to specialized veterinary care; moreover, local veterinarians that treat domesticated animals are neither qualified nor willing to care for large, exotic animals. The APHIS document referenced at the beginning of this section goes on to state that while juvenile large cats are usually acquired as little cubs, they quickly overcome the owner's ability to provide adequate care. As a result, the animals may be abandoned because many times zoos are unwilling to take these cats, and few sanctuary facilities that can accommodate these large felines remain; subsequently, they will be killed. In summary, keeping an exotic large cat as a pet is dangerous, and often inhumane.

Nonhuman Primates

The second group of exotic pets we will discuss are nonhuman primates. There are about 180 different species of nonhuman primates. Generally speaking, nonhuman primates include prosimians (e.g., simians and tarsiers) and simians (monkeys and apes). Nonhuman primate ownership can be regulated at the local, state, or national level. Even if legal at the state level, numerous local jurisdictions have made it illegal to own a primate as a pet, similar to large cats, and illegal possession can result in fines and confiscation of the animal.

Similar to cubs of the large cats, juvenile nonhuman primates can be visually appealing and appear to be friendly. And again like big cats, nonhuman primates quickly outgrow the ability of their owners to care for them. Nonhuman primates are similar to caring for a human child, meaning they cannot be left alone, nor can they be placed in a crate like a dog or cat—they will oftentimes try to escape to the point of hurting themselves. And, if the owner does attempt to leave a nonhuman primate unattended, the animal could potentially become very destructive inside the owner's dwelling.

One unfortunate example of nonhuman primate ownership is the case of a woman in Connecticut, who was mauled by her friend's 200-pound pet chimpanzee. The chimpanzee had reportedly known the woman for many years, yet when the woman arrived at the chimpanzee owner's place of residence for a visit one day in February 2009, the chimpanzee attacked the woman. The chimpanzee was subsequently fatally shot when emergency responders arrived after a 911 call was placed. Several theories as to why the chimpanzee attacked the woman have circulated, including that the woman had changed her appearance since the last time the chimpanzee saw her, perhaps mistaking her for an intruder, or that the chimpanzee had been suffering from some type of illness, resulting in a behavior change, leading him to suddenly become aggressive. The mauling was so severe that the woman was close to death, and needed multiple surgeries to save her life. She remains severely disfigured. The chimpanzee was well-known in the community and had even gained a bit of fame, having appeared in several television commercials, but turned on a person he had reportedly known for a very long time. An example such as this is a reminder that nonhuman primates such as chimpanzees are truly wild animals, and their behavior cannot be predicted, regardless of their prior history.

Also similar to large cats, caregiving for nonhuman primates, particularly expert veterinary care, is challenging—again, most veterinarians do not want to take on the extra training to be able to care for nonhuman primates, and these animals also present a unique challenge: transmission of diseases to humans particular to primates. Zoonotic disease transmission is a concern with all animals. Nonhuman primates, however, pose a special concern with the risk of zoonotic disease transmission between themselves and humans.

Tuberculosis

Tuberculosis is a zoonotic disease and is marked by infection with bacteria of the genus *Mycobacterium*, of which there are several different species. The bacteria primarily cause disease in the lungs of affected people or animals, but they are capable of infecting any part of the body, including the central nervous system. Animals that are infected with tuberculosis can easily transmit the pathogen to humans. Tuberculosis can be fatal and many different kinds of animals can be infected with the bacteria that cause tuberculosis, including humans, cattle, deer, birds, elephants, and nonhuman primates.

Of nonhuman primates, Old World monkeys such as macaques are highly susceptible to infection with mycobacteria, Old World apes such as baboons and the great apes are considered to have intermediate resistance, while New World monkeys such as tamarins, capuchins, and marmosets are resistant to infection and resultant tuberculosis disease.

Although tuberculosis among nonhuman primates in the wild is uncommon, nonhuman primates kept in close contact with one another are at higher risk of spreading and acquiring infection. Dealers of nonhuman primates often keep these animals in close proximity to one another prior to purchase, thereby putting the buyer of a nonhuman primate at risk for this deadly disease. Signs of infection in a nonhuman primate can vary from such vague signs as weight loss and lethargy to more obvious signs of tuberculosis such as a persistent cough. Because of the wide spectrum of signs of physical illness, it can be very difficult for the buyer of a nonhuman primate to determine on first sight whether the animal has this potentially fatal disease. Institutions that purchase nonhuman primates for scientific purposes have complex standard operating procedures by which they abide, including quarantine and tuberculosis testing. However, the typical private purchaser (it is often an illegal purchase) of a nonhuman primate with the intent on keeping the animal as a pet is likely unaware of the many steps institutions take to ensure their colonies remain free of tuberculosis—which serve to protect the animals, but, most important, to protect the human workers who handle them. Of note, people who work with nonhuman primates in institutional settings are routinely tested for tuberculosis to prevent transmission to the animal population.

Herpes B Virus

Perhaps one of the most notable diseases of nonhuman primates is what is commonly referred to as monkey B virus because of the acute and sometimes fatal encephalitis it can cause when it is transmitted to humans. Macacine herpesvirus-1 (formerly Cercopithecine herpesvirus 1) is a member of the herpes group of viruses that occurs naturally in macaque monkeys and could possibly be found in other Old World monkeys (i.e., nonhuman primates from Africa, Asia, Eurasia, and India). Infection with B virus produces very mild disease in macaque monkeys. Most have no obvious evidence of infection, but some monkeys may have vesicles that progress to ulcers in the mouth, on the face, lips, or genitals, or the eye. These lesions spontaneously heal after a few days, but the virus resides permanently in the nerves of the monkey and may reactivate, causing ulcerative lesions periodically. These relapses are especially likely to occur when the monkey is stressed. (Similar to cold sores in people, Macacine herpesvirus-1 is closely related to the herpes simplex virus of humans.) During these periods, the virus is shed by the monkey into the environment. The virus may also be shed by monkeys without visible lesions or symptoms.

Those at risk for acquiring B virus include animal caretakers, laboratory personnel, zookeepers, or anyone who is exposed to macaques or the fluids and tissues of macaques. The most likely routes of transmission to humans are through bites and scratches or splashes of contaminated animal fluids or secretions (urine, feces). People who are immune-suppressed because of medication or underlying medical conditions, such as those with human immunodeficiency virus, may be at higher risk for infection. The risk of acquiring B virus infections from macaques is probably very low. Although thousands of people have handled macaques since human infection with B virus infection was first reported more than 50 years ago, only about 15 deaths have occurred as a result of infection. Despite these seemingly low numbers, any person who handles a nonhuman primate could potentially be at risk from B virus infection.

Wolf Hybrids

The third group of exotic pets we will discuss are wolf hybrids, or wolf-dog hybrids, which are the offspring of a breeding between a wolf (*Canis lupus*) and a domesticated dog (*Canis lupus familiaris*). These animals, despite their blend with dogs, are still considered to be wildlife and must be treated as such. Wolf hybrids will exhibit physical characteristics of both the wolf and dog in differing combinations and proportions. The proportions are largely guessed at by breeders, and puppies are priced and sold by how much wolf is guessed to make up their genetic background. Once again, wolf hybrid puppies are visually appealing and similar to large cats and nonhuman primates; they will mature to dangerous and destructive wildlife living amongst people.

Although wolves in the wild are for the most part nonaggressive and avoid people whenever possible, and promoters of the wolf hybrid could posit that the more wolf the less aggressive, behavioral traits associated with wildlife could be exhibited by an owned wolf hybrid, thus posing a danger to people.

There is little formally collected data on injuries attributable to wolf hybrids; the study referenced earlier in the chapter that studied dog-bite related fatalities found that of 238 dog bite-related fatalities in the United States between 1979 and 1998, 14, or 5.9 percent, were attributable to wolf hybrids. Additional anecdotal evidence suggests that many aspects of hybrid behavior can be extrapolated from the known behaviors of dogs and wolves. According to the USDA, most attacks by wolf hybrids have been on small children, and many occurred when the animal's predatory instincts were triggered unknowingly by the child, causing the wolf hybrid to regard the child as prey.

One of the most challenging issues with wolf hybrids is the subject of rabies. Along with the exotic pets mentioned earlier, there is no rabies vaccine for use in these species. With wolf hybrids, owners could be tempted to ask their veterinarian to vaccinate the animal against rabies because of the shared genetics of these animals with dogs, for which there are several licensed rabies vaccines. However, just as with wildlife, rabies vaccine is not labeled for use in wolf hybrids. Furthermore, if a veterinarian administers a rabies vaccine to a wolf hybrid in a jurisdiction where it is illegal to keep one of these animals, this could be considered a criminal act.

Despite the fact that no rabies vaccine exists for wolf hybrids, many of these animals have been vaccinated with canine rabies vaccine. Such vaccinations are not officially recommended or recognized, and can be illegal. Consequently, wolf hybrids (vaccinated or unvaccinated) that have bitten a person are treated as wildlife, for which there are no licensed rabies vaccines (the exception is the oral vaccine for raccoons, foxes, and coyotes). It should be noted that zoos do vaccinate their captive mammal collections against rabies, but this is done only to protect the animal from the disease and is not done as a public health prevention measure to protect humans that work with these captive animals. A previously vaccinated healthy dog or cat or ferret that bites a person should be confined and observed daily for 10 days. Any illness that develops during this time should be reported to the local health department and the animal examined by a veterinarian. If signs are consistent with rabies, the animal should be euthanized and submitted for testing (rabies testing is performed on an animal's brain, for which an animal must be euthanized). Alternatively, a wild animal that bites a person should immediately be euthanized and tested for rabies.

In September 2000, the AVMA House of Delegates supported a recommendation by the Council on Biologic and Therapeutic Agents opposing a 1999 proposed rule that would have amended the Virus-Serum-Toxin Act regulations by adding a definition of the term dog. In short, this would have allowed wolf hybrids to be vaccinated against rabies as if they were dogs. The AVMA stated that this proposal could have a significant, negative effect on public health by eliminating the USDA's own requirement of proving rabies vaccine efficacy through direct virus challenge, and this rule would have simply changed the label without any rabies vaccine studies done in a laboratory to see if the vaccine would actually protect wolf hybrids from rabies.

CONCLUSION

Dogs and other animals can be very rewarding pets, especially with proper selection of a pet along with subsequent training and socialization. There are also numerous examples, both scientific and anecdotal, of the noted increases in the well-being of people who own pets. This chapter serves as a reminder that the bite of a dog can be dangerous, as is owning an exotic pet. The very best prevention is to talk to a local veterinarian before considering adopting or buying any pet in order to promote the health and safety of both people and animals.

FURTHER READING

American Society for the Prevention of Cruelty to Animals. Dog fighting frequently asked questions. Available at: http://www.aspca.org/fight-animal-cruelty/dog-fighting/dog-fighting-faq.html.

Green, A. *Animal Underworld: Inside America's Black Market for Rare and Exotic Species*. New York: Public Affairs; 1999.

United States Code. Title 7: Agriculture. Chapter 54—Transportation, Sale, and Handling of Certain Animals. Available at: http://www.gpoaccess.gov/uscode/browse.html.

REFERENCES

1. Goldstein EJC. Bite wounds and infection. *Clinical Infectious Diseases* 1992; 14:633–40.
2. Centers for Disease Control and Prevention. Nonfatal dog bite-related injuries treated in hospital emergency departments—United States, 2001. *Morbidity and Mortality Weekly Report* 2003;52:605–10.
3. Benfield R, Plurad DS, Lam L, et al. The epidemiology of dog attacks in an urban environment and the risk of vascular injury. *American Journal of Surgery* Feb. 2010;76:203–5.
4. Sacks JJ, Lockwood R, Hornreich J, et al. Fatal dog attacks, 1989–1994. *Pediatrics* 1996;97(6 pt 1):891–5.
5. Sacks JJ, Sinclair L, Gilchrist J, et al. Breeds of dogs involved in fatal human attacks in the United States between 1979 and 1998. *Journal of the American Veterinary Medical Association* 2000;217:836–40.
6. Humane Society of the United States. Dog aggression. Available at: http://www.humanesociety.org/animals/dogs/tips/aggression.html.
7. American Veterinary Medical Association Task Force on Canine Aggression and Human-Canine Interactions. A community approach to dog bite prevention. *Journal of the American Veterinary Medical Association* 2001;218:1732–49.
8. Westwell AJ, Spencer MB, Kerr KG. DF-2 bacteremia following cat bites. *American Journal of Medicine* 1987;83:1170.
9. Deshmukh PM, et al. *Capnocytophaga canimorsus* sepsis with purpura fulminans and symmetrical gangrene following a dog bite in a shelter employee. *American Journal of Medical Science* 2004;327:369–72

10. Blanton JD, Palmer D, Rupprecht CE. Rabies surveillance in the United States during 2009. *Journal of the American Veterinary Medical Association* 2010;237: 646–57.
11. Talan DA, Citron DM, Abrahamian FM, et al. Bacteriologic analysis of infected dog and cat bites. Emergency Medicine Animal Bite Infection Study Group. *New England Journal of Medicine* 1999;340:85–92.
12. Willis, J, et al. An overview of tuberculosis in Macaques. Department of Pathology and Department of Infectious Diseases, College of Veterinary Medicine, University of Georgia, Athens, GA, 30602. Available at: www.vet. uga.edu/VPP/CLERK/willis/index.php

Chapter 4

Animal Abuse, Cruelty, Neglect (and the Connection to Human Violence)

Miranda Spindel, DVM, MS, and Lila Miller, BS, DVM

Please note: A glossary is provided at the end of this chapter to describe several words that may be unfamiliar to the reader. Words bolded within the text, except for headings, are included in the glossary.

One of the earliest indicators of society's awareness of the relationship between violence to animals and to humans was a woodcut by Thomas Hogarth in the 18th century depicting the cruelty of unsupervised boys with animals (known as the *First Stage of Cruelty*). Since that time, much has been learned about the connection between animal **abuse** and human violence. In the 1990s, the American Humane Association introduced the phrase **"The Link"** to help raise awareness of the concept that animal abuse is often only one part of a constellation of family and community behaviors that include violence. The recognition that an animal is being abused may provide the first point of intervention in breaking a continuum of violence that includes child, domestic, spousal, or elder abuse and other violent crime that may extend outside a family unit and affect the community. This concept continues to gain acceptance, as evidenced by requirements in some jurisdictions for law enforcement and child abuse investigators to note the presence and conditions of animals in the household to support concerns that they may be dealing with an abusive situation. In addition, to protect pets from abuse, courts in at least 19 states are now adding animals to orders of protection that are granted to victims fleeing domestic violence situations. A better understanding of the relationships between animal abuse, cruelty, and **neglect** and human and animal welfare can help to protect *both* human and animal victims and build positive bridges among community groups. The goal of this chapter is to provide an overview of the topic of animal abuse, cruelty, and neglect so that all community members can play a proactive role in addressing it as a critical factor related to human and animal health and well-being in a community.

UNDERSTANDING CRUELTY TO ANIMALS

Despite their legal status as property, surveys indicate that pets are increasingly identified as family members and are thus at risk for abuse like any other vulnerable family member. Unfortunately, there is no single profile that describes the animal abuser; like family violence, animal abuse crosses all socioeconomic and cultural lines. In order to both treat animal abusers and prevent animal cruelty, it is important to understand that animals may be abused by people for a variety of reasons. Animals may be abused to hurt or control family members. Additional reasons cited by Kellert and Felthous[1] include: "1) to control the animal, possibly to eliminate undesirable characteristics (improper training), 2) to retaliate against the animal for a presumed wrong (punishment), 3) to satisfy a prejudice against a breed or species, 4) to instill aggressive tendencies in the animal, 5) to enhance one's own aggression, 6) to shock people and gain attention (raise one's self esteem), 7) to retaliate or get revenge against another person, 8) displaced hostility, 9) nonspecific **sadism**, including sexual assault." Children may perform acts of animal cruelty or even kill their pets to protect them from further abuse if they are living in abusive situations. They may also carry out such offenses to act out aggression against a more vulnerable household member, to act on aggressive feelings toward abusive adults, or because they are imitating the behavior they have observed. Other reasons cited include doing it "just for fun," or they may be unaware they are causing suffering.[2] Whatever the reason, animal abuse raises cause for concern and requires a response.

THE LINK BETWEEN VIOLENCE AGAINST ANIMALS AND HUMANS

There is an ongoing societal concern about overall violence in communities throughout the United States. In a United Nations survey of murders (per capita) by country, from 1998 to 2000, the United States was ranked first amongst industrialized countries and 24th among all countries that submitted data.[3] Violence in the United States has been deemed a public health emergency and has an impact that costs society billions of dollars.

Researchers believe that animal abuse may serve as a predictor of, precursor to, or rehearsal for future violence against humans in many societies, not just the United States. For example, a 2002 unpublished study from New South Wales, Australia, concluded that animal abuse was a better predictor of sexual assault than many other types of violent criminal behavior.[4] Studies on "The Link" have been undertaken in other countries such as Japan. As communities work to reduce their incidence of violence, recognition is increasingly being paid to animal cruelty as a possible early indicator of future violent crimes. "The Link" should not be misconstrued to imply that all people who abuse animals will escalate to violence against humans or criminal activity. However, research studies yield sobering statistics associating the mistreatment of animals and many different forms of family and societal violence, including child physical and sexual abuse, partner battering, and a link to future violence in children who either witness or commit animal abuses. In one study, 71 percent of women seeking shelter from an abusive situation reported that their partner had hurt, threatened, or killed their pet.[2] In other research, animals were found to have been abused in 88 percent of homes where physical child abuse occurred.[5] A study of men who were prosecuted for animal cruelty revealed that men who abused animals were five times more likely to have been arrested for crimes of violence against humans, four times more likely to have committed property crimes, and three times more likely to have committed drug and disorderly conduct offenses.[6]

Some of the evidence of a relationship between childhood offenses against animals and later violence against humans is compelling. Violent offenders in a maximum security prison have been found to be significantly more likely to have a history of acts of animal cruelty than nonviolent offenders.[7] Several of the young men responsible for recent, highly publicized school yard shootings had histories of animal cruelty. Kip Kinkel (Oregon school shooting) decapitated cats and blew up cows, Andrew Golden (Jonesboro school murderer) shot dogs, Luke Woodham (Pearl High School shooting) beat and torched his dog Sparkle, Eric Harris and Dylan Klebold (Columbine High massacre) mutilated animals, and Michael Carneal, another high school killer, threw a cat into a bonfire. Serial killers Albert DeSalvo, David Berkowitz, and Ted Bundy all committed earlier acts of animal cruelty. Jeffrey Dahmer displayed the heads of dead animals on stakes in his neighborhood. One can only speculate if an early intervention with these young men might have prevented the violence that followed. Margaret Mead, the prominent anthropologist, stated in 1964, "The very worst thing that can happen to a child is to be cruel to an animal and get away with it." The societal implications for intervening in animal abuse cases among children at the earliest stage possible are clear, yet there is still much room for improving efforts to report, comprehensively investigate, and intervene when abuse is suspected.

HISTORY AND DEFINITIONS

Animal Cruelty, Abuse, and Neglect

In the United States, acts that cause harm to people and disrupt society are considered to be criminal acts and are classified as either a misdemeanor offense or a felony offense, depending on their severity. All of the states have anticruelty misdemeanor laws, and 47 currently treat some forms of abuse as felony offenses. Animal welfare activists advocate for felony cruelty statutes not just because of stiffer penalties, but because prosecutors are more likely to file charges and commit resources to investigate felony charges.

Cases of cruelty against animals have been investigated since the earliest days of the animal protection movement. The American Society for the Prevention of Cruelty to Animals (ASPCA), the oldest animal protection organization in North America, was founded by Henry Bergh in 1866 in response to the founder's concern about the abuse of horses. This concern is reflected in the earliest animal cruelty laws that defined cruelty as overdriving or overworking an animal. Historically, however, weak anticruelty laws have hindered attempts to address animal abuse effectively. Animal abuse, neglect, or cruelty often has gone unreported or unsuccessfully addressed through the legal system. Unfortunately, there is no requirement for tracking animal cruelty crimes, although there have been several calls for such a mandate. It is only recently that the rising importance of the human-animal bond, the growing acceptance of animals as family members, or at least as sentient creatures that feel pain and other emotions, is leading society to be less tolerant of animal abuse and more willing to speak out about practices that were acceptable just a few years ago. The media today is much more likely to carry stories about animal abuse, and there is often a widespread public outcry in response to these stories. "Animal cops" programs on television that follow the efforts of animal control agencies to rescue animal victims of cruelty have been very popular with the public and have raised awareness about animal abuse.

Cruelty to animals is complex. Many people and professionals are uncomfortable dealing with animal cruelty because of uncertainty about how it is defined and erratic handling of such cases by the courts. Societal or cultural attitudes may affect the conceptualization of cruelty. Ultimately, it is the legal system that defines cruelty, a term that is often used interchangeably with abuse and neglect, adding to the confusion. In most cases animal cruelty is referred to as animal abuse because this model already exists in child protection.

Investigations of crimes against animals are based on laws that vary from state to state and sometimes from one jurisdiction to another. Therefore, even within the legal system, there is not one clear definition that can be applied for cruelty, abuse, or neglect. Some anticruelty laws are located in statutes that deal with moral conduct and behavior. Most statutory definitions of cruelty include acts of commission as well as omission. In general, animal cruelty is usually defined as causing unjustified injury, needless pain or suffering, or death to an animal, or a failure to provide adequate and necessary care and sustenance. Cruelty may refer to many offenses against animals, including active abuse, passive neglect, animal fighting, abandonment, certain veterinary practices, and so on. Some states clearly exempt certain practices from their animal cruelty laws such as common animal agricultural practices, standard veterinary procedures, hunting, fishing, trapping, animal experimentation, and even rodeos.

The definition of some of these offenses can vary from one area to another. In some states, language may still use wording that dates back to original laws developed over 100 years ago referring to overdriving, overworking, and so on. In other states, a list of acts that define animal cruelty can be found and may include such things as selling baby chicks, offering animals as prizes, docking tails, soring (intentionally causing a horse's feet to be painful to enhance their gait), failing to alleviate painful conditions, and so on.

Each state may or may not also further define what is meant by an "animal" in its anticruelty statutes. Many state laws define animals in their misdemeanor provisions with wording such as "every living or dumb creature except a human being." Some states may leave this open to interpretation, while other statutes are more specific in application of the law, making reference to, for example, mammals, birds, reptiles, and amphibians. In states with felony animal cruelty statutes, some apply the felony cruelty definition to any animal, while others may restrict its application to companion animals, domesticated animals, only to dogs and cats, or to animals acting in certain capacities such as police or service animals. In some cases, felony cruelty requires a consideration of motive, such as depraved or intentional, or may require it to be a second or third offense.

Many statutes define the word "cruelty" to include both intentionally harming an animal, such as staging an organized dog fight, as well as harm that arises from neglect; however, the majority of cruelty cases are likely to arise from neglect. Neglect can be described as a failure to provide adequate food, water, shelter, veterinary care, or other basic sustenance that either endangers an animal's health or causes physical injury or death. Although neglect may seem benign, it can be either willful or unintentional, and if it is part of the state's legal definition of cruelty, it can be prosecuted. The intent or mental state of the person causing animal abuse is taken into account by many prosecutors and statutes when determining whether a crime is a misdemeanor or a felony offense.

Because statutory language is so varied, familiarization with one's own state laws is recommended. One excellent resource is www.animallaw.info (see table of websites at the end of the chapter), and many state animal welfare federations or animal control associations publish reference handbooks that contain state animal laws. Although the legal and medical investigation and prosecution of animal abuse falls to veterinarians, humane officers, and legal professionals, it behooves every citizen who wishes to participate in addressing animal abuse to understand what federal, state, county, and municipal laws apply to animals in their community.

Bestiality and Zoophilia

No thorough discussion of animal cruelty would be complete without addressing sexual contact with and assault on animals, or **bestiality**. Historically, bestiality has been handled by different cultures in a wide variety of ways, ranging from severe punishment in the form of death to no punishment at all. Bestiality is believed to be one of the oldest and rarest forms of animal abuse. Kinsey found in his landmark study of human sexuality in the United States in 1948 that, overall, 8 percent of the U.S. male population surveyed admitted to having had sexual contact with animals.[8] Some researchers believe this estimate may be inaccurate because of a variety of reasons, including reluctance to report this activity, and it is difficult to find more recent estimates. Bestiality was illegal in all states in 1953, but today it is illegal in over half of the states and a felony in at least 16. Enforcement varies widely. It is considered cruelty by many because animals can never give consent, and in many cases the animal is injured or dies as a result of the encounter. In states where bestiality is not illegal, the definition of animal cruelty must be met to prosecute cases.

Sexual assault of animals may occur in a variety of settings. It may be used to satisfy adolescent curiosity about sex, as a substitute for a human sexual partner, or to control more vulnerable family members or children. Female victims of domestic violence (battered women) have reported being forced to have sex with an animal. **Zoophilia**, which is also sexual contact with an animal, is broadly defined as the affinity or sexual attraction by a human to a nonhuman animal. It is used to describe situations in which the person claims to have an emotional attachment to the animal. According to the American Psychiatric Association, zoophilia is defined as a disorder of sexual preference. However, in states where bestiality is illegal, the law does not differentiate between zoophilia and bestiality; zoophilia is also a crime.[9]

Hoarding

Animal **hoarding** was first described in 1981 and more formally defined in 1999. Hoarders are individuals who have so many animals that they are unable to provide the minimal standards of nutrition, shelter, sanitation, and veterinary care, and they deny or seem unaware of the deteriorating conditions of the animals, the environment, and the negative consequences on the health and well-being of themselves or other household members. Animals are often found dead or in such deplorable health that animal cruelty charges are justifiable. It is not unusual for individuals to hoard objects in addition to animals, and hoarders often end up being investigated in response to complaints to the health department by neighbors about filthy conditions or foul odors emanating from the hoarder's home. The Hoarding of Animals Research Consortium (HARC) (http://www.tufts.edu/vet/cfa/hoarding/) that is studying this problem has provided some warning signs to veterinarians that an individual may be a hoarder: (1) perfuming or bathing dirty pets to conceal odors, (2) using a surrogate pet to get medications for other unseen animals, (3) showing an unwillingness to say how many pets are owned, (4) claiming to have just found an animal in deplorable condition, (5) having a constantly changing parade of pets, (6) office visits for problems related to poor preventive health, filth, overcrowding, and stress (fleas, ear mites, intestinal parasites, upper respiratory infections, scald of skin due to prolonged contact with urine), or (7) demonstrating an interest in acquiring more animals. Although hoarders often do actually fit a stereotype of an older single woman with many cats, hoarding can be found in most socioeconomic groups and professions. There are veterinarians and schoolteachers who are hoarders, and any species may be hoarded, including farm animals. Even animal shelters, foster care providers, and rescue groups are increasingly being identified as hoarders and prosecuted for animal cruelty. Hoarding is a behavior that has complex psychological roots and for which there is no simple or universal solution. Hoarders often suffer from a variety of mental health issues and intervention approaches often require multiple community agencies and must be tailored for each case.

RECOGNIZING ANIMAL ABUSE

The often vague wording of anticruelty laws has contributed to a discomfort for professionals as well as community members regarding when to speak out about suspected abuse cases. A specific, defined set of criteria for professionals to use to determine when or how to appropriately intervene has not yet been developed, but there are some key warning signs that may arouse suspicions for both the layperson and professional that an animal has been abused. When recognized, these warning signs can help lead to reporting to the proper authorities and an effective response. The behavior of the animal owner (evasive, indifferent, or annoyed), friends or other family members whose accounts of the problem all differ, or the animal's condition itself may all evoke suspicions. Particular injuries or patterns of injury or aspects of an animal's history that do not make sense are indicators that additional information should be gathered. Multiple physical injuries or clinical signs in one animal, the same animal being brought to a veterinarian several times with suspicious problems, ongoing problems that never resolve despite veterinary treatment and reported owner compliance, or the presence of several animals with suspicious problems are grounds for concern. Malnourishment to the point of emaciation without any known underlying cause also presents cause for concern. Animals with severely matted hair, overgrown hooves or nails (especially to the point of ingrown nails), various wounds, injuries, or skin lesions that are untreated, unhealed, or in various stages of healing, collars that are embedded in the neck, heavy flea, tick, or other ectoparasite infestations, overall filth, or untreated illness are victims of neglect that may meet the statutory definition of animal cruelty.

Other warning signs that animals may be abused include injuries such as burns in unusual or suspicious patterns, multiple fractures in various stages of healing, indicating multiple assaults over a prolonged period of time (the battered pet syndrome), and bruising. Suspicions of illegal dog fighting should be aroused by multiple bite wounds in various stages of healing that are found in locations that are uncommon for normal dog scuffles, such as the head, face, neck, throat, legs, and abdomen. Discrepancies, changes, or contradictions in what an owner or family member says, especially when provided by children who are primarily concerned about their pet, or repeated instances of injury may also raise suspicions of abuse. Abuse cases also may be signaled by indifference about the cause of an injury, refusal to acknowledge the seriousness of a condition or to provide treatment or follow-up care of painful conditions that cause **suffering**, or use of several veterinarians. Animals who are more likely to be abused include young and vulnerable puppies and kittens and those with behavior problems such as loud, incessant barking, digging, aggression, destructiveness, inappropriate house soiling, and so on. Breeds used as guard dogs, such as Rottweilers, pit bulls, German shepherds, and Dobermans, may be abused in an attempt to make them more aggressive. The American pit bull terrier is used most commonly in dog fighting in the United States, but Presa Canarios, Fila Brasileiros, Dogo Argentino, and mixed breeds are also used. Many national humane organizations like the American Humane Association, the Humane Society of the United States, and the ASPCA all have training programs and online resources for individuals who wish to learn more about how to recognize and respond to animal abuse.

WHOSE RESPONSIBILITY IS IT TO REPORT?

When signs of animal abuse or concern for an animal's welfare are recognized, action should be taken. Reporting these suspicions to the proper law enforcement agency is the correct thing to do. However, many cases of animal abuse go unreported due to doubt about what should be reported and to whom, and speculation about an unwanted or inadequate response and outcome. Nonetheless, *any* concern that an animal may be in a dangerous situation should be reported to the appropriate law-enforcement authorities as soon as possible to facilitate an investigation. Even if there is some uncertainty about the situation, it is best to err on the side of caution and report a suspicion. This allows the investigating authority to gather enough information to make the proper determination about the next steps to take. In many cases, no prosecution will occur, but a report may be filed and an opportunity for other appropriate interventions and follow-up is provided. This may simply be owner education. In some cases, medical or social service agencies may be called to provide an intervention to help a troubled family. Reporting animal abuse should not be viewed merely as a way to rescue animals and punish people, but as a way to hold people accountable for their actions and to help them receive services that may benefit the entire family and prevent further violence.

Each community handles animal cruelty complaints differently. In many cases the local police department or animal control agency will be responsible for investigating complaints or will be able to direct concerned citizens to an alternate agency. In some areas, agents working for humane societies, societies for the prevention of cruelty to animals (SPCAs) or other animal welfare organizations will have authority to conduct these investigations. Some of these agents may be empowered to make arrests. Some areas have task forces or federations that are dedicated to preventing cruelty to animals. Suspected cruelty to livestock, wildlife, exotic species, or commercial businesses such as breeders and pet shops may involve the U.S. Department of Agriculture, U.S. Fish and Wildlife Service, or a state's Game and Fish Department. In any situation that is an emergency, dialing 911 is appropriate. Emergency response agencies may only be able to assist if humans are endangered, but should be able to provide proper direction in emergencies. Familiarizing oneself with and identifying resources beforehand, establishing personal contacts with one's local agency structure, and keeping nonemergency contact numbers readily available is one component of building more effective community response plans to animal abuse. If there is uncertainty about the proper agency to contact, the local police department should be able to direct citizens to the proper authority.

Concern about being identified as the person who reported an abuse sometimes outweighs concern about the situation and also can lead to nonreporting. Reports can often be made anonymously, but anonymity cannot always be guaranteed long-term. In addition, law enforcement may be best able to follow up when a credible witness is willing to provide information or even testify if needed. Providing a written, factual statement of what was observed, photographs if available, and names or contacts of others who may be aware of or witness to the situation is most valuable.

It is interesting to note that while anyone can report cases of suspected child abuse, certain health-care professionals, teachers, and individuals are required by law to report suspicions that a child has been abused. Furthermore, in some cases they can be held liable for prosecution if they are aware of abusive situations and fail to report them. Mandated reporting legislation was passed shortly after Dr. Henry Kempe published the "Battered Child Syndrome" in the *Journal of the American Medical Association* in 1962. There was an increase in reporting once physicians and other health-care professionals were legally mandated to do so and provided with training materials and immunity for filing **good faith** reports. A good faith report of a suspicion of abuse should be based on the history and physical examination of the patient. The report launches an investigation by law enforcement to uncover the facts surrounding the patient's condition or injury. In some cases the investigation may not lead to a substantiation of the suspicion, but if the report was filed in good faith, it should have no negative repercussions for the person reporting.

A concern for many individuals who wish to report crimes against animals is fear for one's personal safety, especially in small communities where retaliation may be a real possibility, but if one believes an animal abuser may be violent, that is even more reason to file a report. Reports should be filed so that other members of the team handling abuse, including investigators, prosecutors, and judges may play their parts in the process.

The Veterinarian

One might expect a parallel mandatory situation to exist for veterinarians to report cases of suspected abuse in good faith. Like physicians, veterinarians occupy a unique niche in the community for identifying cruelty. Veterinarians routinely examine and treat sick and injured animals and certainly are considered the best qualified to determine whether an animal is suffering or has been the victim of inappropriate or substandard care. In fact, according to a recent Canadian study, the veterinary profession is linked with animal welfare protection in the eye of the public.[10] In this same survey of 400 Manitoba residents, the top three places where citizens would report animal abuse or neglect were the local veterinarian (42%), local humane society (38%), and uniformed police (24%). Veterinarians may also become aware of welfare concerns for the humans in a household. However, despite opportunities for veterinarians to assume a public health role in the prevention of animal and family violence, awareness and mandatory actions within the veterinary profession have historically lagged behind the field of human medicine in this regard.

Veterinarians may be reluctant to report cruelty for a number of reasons, including a lack of formal training on how to recognize animal abuse, the absence of widely accepted standards for identifying and responding to animal abuse, fear of litigation, negative repercussions and retaliations against the veterinary practice, and concerns about the confidentiality of medical records. Among the unique ethical concerns of veterinarians regarding reporting, many are conflicted when they feel the best interest of the patient may conflict with the desires of the client. Although reporting suspicions about animal abuse may help society and some families, it may also have serious legal consequences for owners who are guilty of the charges.

Veterinarians are mandated in a few states to report cases of suspected abuse or animal fighting and may suffer penalties for failure to do so. But not only do the definitions of cruelty vary from state to state, the language regarding reporting also varies from state to state, ranging from calling for reporting of suspected cases to reporting those based upon reasonable or direct knowledge or known cases. Mandated reporting of animal abuse cases is a controversial and yet evolving subject within the veterinary profession, and there is no state at this time where an average citizen is legally mandated to report animal abuse. In most cases, reporting remains a voluntary decision.

4.1. DID YOU KNOW?

- 25–40 percent of battered women do not leave an abuser because of worry about their animals.[11]

- 75 percent of the time pets are abused by family members in the presence of women or children.[2]

- 31 percent of Chicago inner-city youth have been to a dog fight. The Chicago Police Department has made enforcement of dog fighting part of their antiviolence strategy because "82% of offenders arrested for animal abuse had priors for battery, weapons, or drugs."[1]

[1] Chicago Crime Commission (2004, August). RAV2: Reduce Animal Violence, reduce all violence: A program to amplify human and animal violence prevention and reduction by targeting dog fighting and animal cruelty. *Action Alert*, 1–5.

INVESTIGATION AND PROSECUTION OF CRUELTY—WHY SOME CASES ARE NOT PURSUED UNDER THE LAW

Despite the fact that in many ways society is taking animal cruelty cases more seriously, relatively few people are convicted of animal cruelty each year. There are a number of reasons why cases may not be pursued or are dealt with by means other than criminal charges. First and foremost, it is the state law that ultimately will define cruelty. While a citizen may believe an animal is being cruelly treated, if the situation does not meet the state's legal definition of cruelty, regardless of the animal's quality of life, a crime has not been committed. For the most part, animal control agencies will first attempt to educate owners in situations of benign neglect. Animal control officers may issue an order to comply that requires the correction of violations within a specified period of time, including seeking veterinary care for medical problems, improving shelter, and so on. Some owners may opt to surrender an animal to a shelter if they are unable or unwilling to provide adequate care, and, in some cases, no charges will be filed.

Even when owners opt not to surrender an animal, and conditions do not immediately improve, law enforcement may not immediately investigate or file charges. They may believe these are low priority crimes without a true victim, or they may lack the expertise or resources to investigate. Regardless of whether care has been omitted or deliberate cruelty committed, it can be equally difficult to prove cruelty in a courtroom case. Either way, successful prosecution of cruelty requires strong evidence or an eyewitness account to help link the evidence to the perpetrator. Some cases are dismissed due to insufficient or mishandling of evidence. In cases where a conviction is obtained, remediation and punishment may include a prison term, monetary fine, an order for counseling, or a prohibition from owning animals in the future, or probation. Unfortunately, the animal control or law enforcement agency that is expected to uphold this punishment may not have the resources to monitor the person convicted, and recidivism can be high, especially in animal hoarding cases. Most agencies must conserve their resources and turn to education as the most effective response to mild to moderate neglect. Investigating and trying cases of animal cruelty can be emotionally and financially draining for the agencies involved, especially in cases involving multiple animals, and cases may not be fully pursued if the drain on the agency's resources would be too great. Many agencies are reluctant to prosecute if they feel a conviction is unlikely, as would be the case if the evidence is not strong enough or the suspect appears too sympathetic.

Veterinary forensic science is fairly new and lags behind human medicine. Comparisons and models are often drawn from human forensics, which may not always be admissible in court. While great advances have recently been made in the field of veterinary forensics to develop techniques and collection methods for handling and interpreting evidence, further research is needed before it can be fully accepted and integrated into established, mainstream veterinary science. Information about the link between animal abuse and human violence also needs to gain wider exposure and acceptance. Some law enforcement agencies may simply not yet understand the relationship of animal well-being to human well-being and thus fail to fully investigate crimes against animals. While it is true that some animal abuse cases may receive widespread media coverage and outrage the public, that reaction is often reserved for the most heinous crimes. It is not uncommon to still hear the opinion that it is "just an animal" and that it is not worth using valuable resources to penalize, ruin, or disrupt human lives. Understanding some of these attitudes and reasons why cases are not processed through the legal system can help a community find solutions to effectively decrease animal cruelty.

BREAKING THE CYCLE OF VIOLENCE

Managing cases of animal cruelty requires the work of a cohesive community team that includes citizens, veterinarians, law enforcement, animal control agencies, social services, and the legal system. Increasingly, there are excellent training opportunities available for law enforcement officers and cross-training experiences. The Law Enforcement Training Institute, National Cruelty Investigations School program, and Humane Society University have offered one such training program across the country for more than a decade. There are three levels to the training in order to be certified as a humane investigator, and the programs are geared toward animal control officers, police officers, sheriff's deputies, humane society investigators, or other individuals interested in learning a systematic approach to cruelty investigation. Perhaps equal in importance to knowledge of how to recognize and report these cases is the design and implementation of strategies to prevent them from occurring at all. There are many models for violence prevention that can have positive effects on the welfare of animals and humans in a community. Creative and collaborative approaches are necessary to bring about change.

One of the most accepted keys to prevention of animal cruelty is education. With the clear evidence of the effects of violence in childhood on adult behavior, intervention and education must begin as early as possible. Venues include classroom education, health clinics, church, social and youth groups, Internet and e-mail education, newsletter articles, seminars, counseling services, library meetings, and media campaigns. There are few limits on educational opportunities for teaching about animal abuse in a community. Humane education should not be limited to children. Humane concepts should be incorporated into all aspects of classroom curricula and mainstream media and community events, instead of focusing on just a few days each year or special events.

Animal abuse education can foster formation or expansion of an antiviolence coalition, group, or task force in a community. These groups bring together a wide variety of agencies and individuals in a region that desires to decrease community and animal related violence. Important representatives to include in a coalition might include law enforcement, courts (judges and prosecutors/attorneys), veterinarians, animal protection agencies, health professionals and organizations, child and family services, community programs (Boy Scouts, Girl Scouts), education, legislation, religious representatives, and medical and emergency services (Red Cross, Salvation Army). In communities that have formed antiviolence groups, the opportunity to identify and cross-train professionals at the local level from different agencies to identify and report violence has proven valuable. For example, those performing intake at a shelter for battered women should be trained in the proper questions to ask about animal abuse also occurring in the home. Community antiviolence task forces may help people leave these situations by providing temporary shelters for pets of battered families. Veterinary clinics, humane societies, and private homes have formed effective foster networks to house animals temporarily for families living in shelters. Some communities have formed cruelty response systems involving public, private, and municipal agencies in order to better respond to the public when concerns about animal cruelty arise. Here, people with concerns about animal cruelty are directed to a central number and a lead agency takes the first steps in investigating complaints to streamline processes. This can facilitate reporting for the public, as well as improve a community's ability to follow through and statistically track violence reports in a streamlined fashion. There also may be opportunities for strengthening or introducing new anticruelty legislation that a coalition can actively lobby for.

CONCLUSION

This chapter focused mainly on cruelty, abuse and neglect as defined by our legal system, but it should be acknowledged that the absence of cruelty as legally defined certainly does not equate to an animal having a good quality of life, free from fear, suffering, distress, or anxiety. While some people believe strongly that animals are family members, have rights, and must be protected, others still see animals in very utilitarian terms, as property to be used and discarded at will. Most people probably see animals somewhere in between, as sentient creatures capable of suffering and thus deserving of attention to their welfare. Animal welfare can be defined as a human responsibility that encompasses all aspects of animal well-being, including proper housing, management, nutrition, disease prevention, responsible care, humane handling, and when necessary, humane euthanasia. Well-being has both a physical and behavioral component that allows animals to exhibit behaviors that are considered normal for the species. The increase in animal rights classes at law schools, increasing penalties for cruelty, expansion of cruelty definitions to include such novel ideas as antitethering and antideclawing indicate an increasing societal awareness of, and sensitivity to, animal welfare issues, and perhaps even a burgeoning acceptance of the notion that suffering extends beyond physical pain to include emotional pain and should be legally addressed. Family and community violence, including animal abuse, are critical public health issues that affect everyone, whether one owns animals or not. Without adherence to humane principles for humans and animals, thoughtful intervention and creative approaches, the cycle of violence will undoubtedly continue.

GLOSSARY

Abuse: To treat in a harmful, injurious or offensive way.

Battered: Victim of domestic abuse or violence—typically beaten or physically abused.

Bestiality: Sexual intercourse, contact, or relations between a human and an animal.

Child abuse: Physical, emotional, or sexual mistreatment of children.

Cruelty to animals: Defined by state statute, generally refers to infliction of suffering or harm upon animals for purposes other than self-defense or failure to provide necessary care.

Domestic abuse/violence: Behaviors used by one person in a relationship to control another. May include physical, sexual, emotional, spousal, elder abuse and intimidation.

Elder abuse: Physical, sexual or emotional abuse of an elderly person, usually one who is disabled or frail. The World Health Organization defines elder abuse as "a single or repeated act or lack of appropriate action, occurring within any relationship where there is an expectation of trust which causes harm or distress to an older person."

Good faith: The sincere effort and purpose of performing an action (in this case reporting abuse/neglect/cruelty) with an aim or objective to achieve good results or outcomes.

Hoarding (of animals): Keeping more than usual numbers of animals without the ability to properly care for them, denying this inability, and failing to recognize its negative impact on the animals.

"The Link": Used to refer to the established connection between animal abuse and human violence.

Neglect: Failure to meet basic needs, including nourishment, medical care, shelter, or other needs for which the victim is unable to provide itself.

Physical abuse: Abuse involving contact that is intended to cause feelings of intimidation, pain, injury, or other physical suffering or bodily harm.

Sadism: Derivation of pleasure as a result of inflicting pain or watching pain inflicted upon others.

Sexual abuse: The forcing of undesired sexual behavior upon another.

Spousal abuse: A form of domestic violence, also known as intimate partner violence, where the abuser or victim can be the husband or wife.

Suffering: The bearing of pain or distress.

Zoophilia: Sexual attraction to animals.

FURTHER READING

Arluke A, ed. *Just a Dog: Understanding Animal Cruelty and Ourselves (Animals, Culture and Society)*. Philadelphia: Temple University Press, 2006.

Ascione FR, and Lockwood R, eds. *Cruelty to Animals and Interpersonal Violence: Readings in Research and Application*. West Lafayette, IN: Purdue University Press, 1998.

Heide, KM, and Merz-Perez, L, eds. *Animal Cruelty: Pathway to Violence Against People*. Walnut Creek, CA: AltaMira Press, 2004.

Table 4.1

Selected Web Resources to Understand Cruelty

Name of site	URL	What reader can find here
American Humane Association	http://www.americanhumane.org/	Founded in 1877, the only national organization dedicated to protecting both children and animals.
Humane Society of the United States	http://www.humanesociety.org/ http://www.hsus2.org/firststrike/	The nation's largest animal protection organization.
Animals and Society Institute	http://www.animalsandsociety.org/	Nonprofit, independent research and educational organization that advances the status of animals in public policy and promotes the study of human-animal relationships.

The Latham Foundation	http://www.latham.org/	Publications, videos, etc., focusing on humane education.
ASPCA anti-cruelty glossary	http://www.aspca.org/fight-animal-cruelty/cruelty-glossary.html	Common words and definitions related to animal cruelty.
Florida State University Institute for Family Violence Studies	http://familyvio.csw.fsu.edu/?page_id=25	On-line tutorials on a variety of domestic violence issues.
Animal Legal Defense Fund	http://www.aldf.org/	Animal rights law organization. Information about anti-cruelty law, cases, subjects.
ASPCA/Michigan Animal Legal and Historical Center list of state anti-cruelty laws	http://www.aspca.org/fight-animal-cruelty/advocacy-center/state-animal-cruelty-laws/ http://www.animallaw.org	Quick sites for looking up the laws relating to animal cruelty by state.
ASPCA animal cruelty site	http://www.aspca.org/fight-animal-cruelty/	Resources for the public on fighting animal cruelty.
Hoarding of Animals Research Consortium (HARC)	http://www.tufts.edu/vet/hoarding/	Information on animal hoarding.
American Humane Association Pets and Women's Shelters Listing	http://www.americanhumane.org/human-animal-bond/programs/pets-and-womens-shelters/domestic-family-violence-shelters.html	List of domestic violence shelters that allow pets on site.
Ahimsa House Safe Havens Directory	http://www.ahimsahouse.org/directory/	List of domestic violence shelters that allow pets on site.
Pet Abuse.com	http://www.pet-abuse.com/pages/animal_cruelty.php	Information about animal cruelty and database of cruelty cases.

(Continued)

Table 4.1   (Continued)

Name of site	URL	What reader can find here
Humane Society of the United States' First Strike Campaign PDF	http://files.hsus.org/web-files/HSI/E_Library_PDFs/eng_develop_first_strike_campaign.pdf	How to develop a coalition against violence—step by step instructions.
Colorado Bar Association	http://www.cobar.org/index.cfm/ID/20121/DPDVP/Domestic-Violence:-Make-It-Your-Business/ http://www.cobar.org/index.cfm/ID/20130/DPWCP/Colorado-Alliance-for-Cruelty-Prevention-Committee/	Colorado-based information on domestic violence and cruelty prevention.

REFERENCES

1. Kellert SR, Felthous S. Childhood cruelty toward animals among criminals and non-criminals. *Human Relations* 1985;38:1113–29.
2. Ascione F, ed. *The International Handbook of Animal Abuse and Cruelty, Theory, Research, and Application*. West Lafayette, IN: Purdue University Press, 2008.
3. Seventh United Nations survey of crime trends and operations of criminal justice systems, covering the period 1998–2000. United Nations Office on Drugs and Crime, Centre for International Crime Prevention. Available at: http://www.unodc.org/pdf/crime/seventh_survey/7sc.pdf.
4. Clarke, JP. New South Wales police animal cruelty research project (unpublished report). Sydney, Australia: New South Wales Police Service, 2002.
5. DeViney E, Dickert J, Lockwood R. The Care of Pets Within Child Abusing Families. *International Journal for the Study of Animal Problems,* 1983; 4:321–9.
6. Arluke A, Levin J, Luke C, Ascione F. The relationship of animal abuse to violence and other forms of antisocial behavior. *Journal of Interpersonal Violence* 1999;14:963–75.
7. Merz-Perez L, Heide KM, Silverman IJ. Childhood cruelty to animals and subsequent violence against humans. *International Journal of Offender Therapy and Comparative Criminology,* 2001;45:556–73.
8. Kinsey, AC. *Sexual Behavior in the Human Male*. Philadelphia, PA: WB Saunders, 1948.

9. Munro HMC, Thrusfield MV. Battered pets: Sexual abuse. *Journal of Small Animal Practice,* 2001;42:333–7.

10. Enns A. MVMA public awareness and attitude survey, final report. Enrg Research Group, Manitoba Veterinary Medical Association, 2006:27.

11. Arkow, P. Animal abuse and domestic violence: Intake statistics tell a sad story. *Latham Letter,* 1994;15:17.

Chapter 5

Emerging Diseases

Tegwin K. Taylor, DVM, MPH, DACVPM

Please note: A glossary is provided at the end of this chapter to describe several words that may be unfamiliar to the reader. Words bolded within the text, except for headings, are included in the glossary.

INTRODUCTION

Not too long ago, many health experts believed that infectious diseases were a thing of the past. In fact, in 1969, the U.S. Surgeon General reported, "the time had come to 'close the book on infectious diseases.'"[1] Several books were written regarding the eradication of infectious diseases during the 1950s and 1960s, years before smallpox became the first disease to be eradicated.[1] The great advancements in public health up to that time, such as improved sanitation and the advent of vaccines and antibiotics, certainly contributed to this false sense of security. However, not only did infectious diseases avoid being eliminated, they flourished into the 21st century.

Infectious diseases today account for 15 million (26%) of the 57 million annual deaths around the world.[2] An emerging disease is a newly recognized infectious disease, or a known infectious disease whose reported **incidence** is increasing among a specific population. Human immunodeficiency virus (HIV), which causes acquired immunodeficiency syndrome (AIDS), is perhaps the most significant emerging disease of our time. AIDS was first recognized in 1981. In 2008 alone, 2.7 million people were newly infected with HIV, and over 2 million deaths were associated with AIDS.[3] In addition, more than 33 million people worldwide were living with AIDS at that time, including over 2 million children.[3] It is believed that deaths from HIV/AIDS will soon surpass the 1918 influenza **pandemic** and become the deadliest disease in recorded history.[2] Although recent progress has been made through the prevention of new HIV infections and a decrease in the number deaths related to AIDS, HIV/AIDS will remain a major global health issue for years to come.

In recent years, the World Health Organization (WHO) has referred to HIV/AIDS as the world's most urgent public health challenge, and yet it is just one of hundreds of emerging diseases impacting populations globally. A study published by Jones in 2008 identified the emergence of 335 diseases between 1940 and 2004.[4] This study was the first to analytically support the general belief that emerging diseases were increasing in incidence. These findings confirm that infectious diseases are not only a present concern, but a threat to the future of public health.

FACTORS THAT IMPACT EMERGING DISEASES

In 1992, the **Institute of Medicine (IOM)** published *Emerging Infections: Microbial Threats to Health in the United States,* which assessed the impact of emerging diseases up to that time. In that initial report, the following six factors affecting emergence were identified:

1. Microbial adaptation and change.
2. Economic development and land use.
3. Human demographics and behavior.
4. International travel and commerce.
5. Technology and industry.
6. Breakdown of public health measures.[5]

About a decade later in 2001, the IOM Committee on Emerging Microbial Threats to Health in the 21st Century convened to accomplish several objectives, including the reassessment of factors affecting emergence. The committee's efforts produced *Microbial Threats to Health: Emergence, Detection, and Response,* published in 2003. Identified in this report were seven additional factors impacting the emergence of infectious diseases:

1. Human susceptibility to infection.
2. Climate and weather.
3. Changing ecosystems.
4. Poverty and social inequality.
5. War and famine.
6. Lack of political will.
7. Intent to harm.[5]

In anticipation that future discoveries would continue to add to the list, the authors categorized these 13 factors into 4 broad areas:

1. Genetic and biological factors.
2. Physical environmental factors.
3. Ecological factors.
4. Social, political, and economic factors.[5]

Several subsequent articles have supported these findings, and the analysis by Jones in 2008 found that emerging diseases are significantly associated with socioeconomic, environmental, and ecological factors.[4] This study also concluded that the highest proportion of emerging diseases (~26%) from 1980 to 1990 were attributable to increased susceptibility to infection, suggesting that the increase in emerging infectious disease events in the 1980s is largely associated with the HIV/AIDS pandemic.[4]

In 2008, the IOM's Board of Global Health and the National Research Council's Board on Agriculture and Natural Resources of the National Academies convened a committee to review global responses to **zoonotic** diseases and assess zoonotic disease surveillance systems. Their report, *Sustaining Global Surveillance and Response to Emerging Zoonotic Diseases,* was published in 2009, on the heels of the 2009 H1N1 pandemic. This report also highlights several specific drivers impacting emergence of zoonotic diseases, including the following:

Human-animal interface

Human population growth and mobility

Global food systems and food safety

Wildlife trade

Deforestation

Climate change

Figure 5.1
Selected Emerging and Reemerging Diseases, 1980–2010

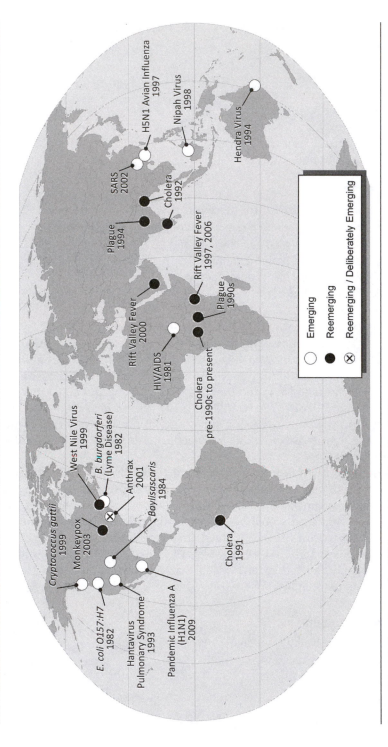

Source: Elaine J. Hallisey, Geographer/GIS Analyst. Adapted from Fauci, 2001.

Biotechnology and lack of **biosecurity**

Inadequate governance

Impacts of technology[6]

While a thorough description of these drivers is outside the scope of this chapter, the committee concluded that a review is needed to increase understanding of these factors, specifically to address the significant gaps in detection and response to zoonotic diseases.[6]

> The emergence and spread of microbial threats are driven by a complex set of factors, the convergence of which can lead to consequences of disease much greater than any single factor might suggest. Genetic and biological factors allow microbes to adapt and change, and can make humans more or less susceptible to infections. Changes in the physical environment can impact on the ecology of vectors and animal reservoirs, the transmissibility of microbes, and the activities of humans that expose them to certain threats. Human behavior, both individual and collective, is perhaps the most complex factor in the emergence of disease.
>
> Emergence is especially complicated by social, political, and economic factors—including the development of megacities, the disruption of global ecosystems, the expansion of international travel and commerce, and poverty—which ensure that infectious diseases will continue to plague us.[5]

REEMERGENCE OF HISTORICAL DISEASES

In addition to the detection of novel infectious diseases, many previously recognized diseases have reemerged from history. These "old" diseases have required significant attention from public health experts in recent years, and some of them are described here.

Anthrax

Anthrax is caused by *Bacillus anthracis*, a spore-forming bacterium that is found worldwide. Anthrax is probably best known for its use as a **bioterrorism** agent following the September 11, 2001, attacks in the United States. Prior to 2001, the use of anthrax as a biological agent had been documented several times. In consideration of these applications, anthrax has received the distinction of a "deliberately emerging" disease. However, anthrax has caused natural infections in animals and people for thousands of years.

Anthrax spores survive easily in the environment, and the disease is **enzootic** in several areas. Sporadic outbreaks also occur elsewhere, including North America. **Ruminants** are most frequently affected and are often exposed through ingestion of anthrax spores from contaminated soil or plants. Human cases are typically associated with exposure to infected animals or animal products, such as hides, hair, and drums.

Clinical signs in animals include **edema** and respiratory difficulty leading to collapse. However, sudden death often occurs, and a bloody **exudate** from the nostrils or mouth is frequently noted. Human infection manifests in three forms: **cutaneous** (skin), inhalation, and **gastrointestinal.** Cutaneous infections account for over 95 percent of natural anthrax cases.[7] Anthrax spores enter the skin through direct contact, and abrasions and cuts can increase susceptibility to infection. Within several days, a **pustule** develops and becomes a black **eschar,** the hallmark of cutaneous anthrax infections. The eschar usually resolves within several weeks, although it can occasionally result in systemic infection. Without treatment, up to 20 percent of cutaneous cases are fatal.[7] Inhalation anthrax occurs after respiratory exposure to anthrax spores. Signs initially may be nonspecific, but respiratory distress develops within a few days. Gastrointestinal anthrax occurs after consumption of contaminated food, usually meat from infected animals. This form of anthrax is most commonly seen in developing countries, where food safety systems may not prevent exposure. Inhalation and gastrointestinal forms of anthrax are severe and often fatal. While antibiotics are available and effective, the recognition of anthrax exposure and illness does not typically occur early enough for successful treatment.

5.1. DID YOU KNOW?

A zoonotic disease, or zoonosis, is a disease that can be transmitted between animals and humans. Approximately 60 percent of emerging diseases are zoonotic, and among emerging zoonotic diseases, over 70 percent originate in wildlife.[4]

Cholera

Cholera is caused by the bacteria *Vibrio cholera,* of which there are many strains, or serogroups. The O1 serogroup of *V. cholerae* has caused pandemics for centuries, while the O139 serogroup has become a significant public health concern since 1992. Cholera **epidemics** are typically associated with unsafe drinking water, inadequate sanitation, and poor hygiene and often occur in developing countries where basic public health infrastructure is lacking. In 1991, an epidemic of *V. cholerae* O1 erupted in coastal Peru and spread to 16 other countries. Within a year, 400,000 cases including more than 4,000 deaths occurred.[8] The first and only epidemic due to *V. cholerae* O139 started in 1992 in southern India and Bangladesh. By 1994, the O139 serogroup had caused outbreaks in more than 11 Asian countries. In 2006, Word Health Organization (WHO) recorded more than 250,000 cases and 6,000 deaths associated with the O1 serogroup.[7] Approximately 99 percent of these cases occurred in sub-Saharan Africa, and they are part of the ongoing "seventh pandemic" of cholera, which began in 1961.

During epidemics, humans are the primary **reservoir** for *V. cholerae*. **Transmission** of cholera occurs through ingestion of food or water containing toxigenic *Vibrio cholerae* O1 or O139 from a natural environmental source or from the feces of an infected person. Clinical signs include profuse, watery diarrhea, which is often referred to as rice-water stool. In severe cases, death from dehydration may occur within several hours, and **mortality rates** can exceed 50 percent. If cases are identified quickly, treatment with appropriate rehydration can reduce the mortality to less than 1 percent. Prevention of cholera and other diarrheal diseases remains a significant public health challenge, as more than one billion people do not have access to safe water and 2.6 billion people do not have access to proper sanitation, resulting in over 4,500 child deaths every day due to waterborne and other enteric diseases including cholera.[8]

Influenza

Influenza is caused by several influenza viruses, typically referred to influenza types A, B, and C. Influenza A viruses have the most public health significance and include all animal influenza viruses as well as human influenza A viruses. Type A viruses are classified into subtypes and are named based on two surface proteins—hemagglutinin (H) and neuraminidase (N). Sixteen different H proteins and nine different N proteins exist, allowing for 144 possible subtype combinations (e.g., H1N1, H3N2, H5N1, etc.). Influenza viruses are constantly changing, and new subtypes can develop through direct transmission of a virus from an animal to a person, or through the formation of a **reassortant virus**. Reassortment is possible when two or more influenza viruses simultaneously infect an animal or human. The viruses exchange genetic material, developing into a new, or novel, influenza virus, typically containing genetic material from more than one species. Influenza pandemics, including the 2009 H1N1 pandemic, are often the result of novel reassortant viruses. The 2009 H1N1 influenza virus contains human, swine, and avian genes.

Transmission of influenza viruses occurs through inhalation of the virus following close or direct contact with infected people or animals, or through direct contact with surfaces contaminated with influenza virus. Clinical signs can include fever, cough, sore throat, headache, and muscle or body aches. Gastrointestinal signs are sometimes noted and develop more frequently in children. Most healthy individuals recover from illness within several days, but severe disease and death can occur. In an average year, seasonal influenza affects 5–20 percent of the U.S. population[7] and causes an estimated 3–5 million severe infections worldwide.[8] Young children, the elderly, and people with suppressed immune systems are typically most susceptible, and more than 90 percent of seasonal influenza deaths occur in people over 65 years of age.[7]

On June 11, 2009, WHO declared its first influenza pandemic in more than 40 years. Three other influenza pandemics have occurred within the last century: 1918, 1957, and 1968. The 1918 pandemic was the most devastating, killing more than 50 million people worldwide.[2] Within a few months, this influenza virus was more deadly than the entire four-year span of World War I.[5] The pandemic that occurred in 1957–1958 produced

Figure 5.2
Highly magnified transmission electron micrograph (TEM) of 2009 pandemic influenza A (HINI)

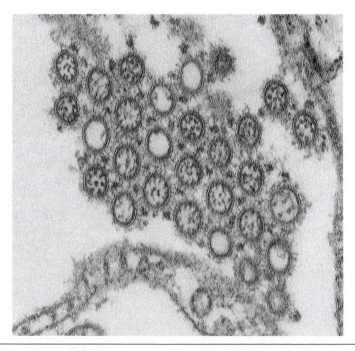

Source: CDC Public Health Image Library; photo by Cynthia Goldsmith.

an estimated 70 million U.S. cases in two months and 70,000 American deaths overall. The third pandemic started in 1968 and was the mildest of the three, causing about 34,000 American deaths. Although thousands of infections and deaths have occurred worldwide, the **morbidity** and mortality produced by the 2009 H1N1 pandemic has been comparatively mild. However, the time and resources invested by the world's health-care systems and public health agencies in response to this new virus was substantial. In addition, the early naming of the virus as "swine flu," unnecessarily cost the U.S. pork industry approximately $28 million per week, including the loss of exports to at least 15 different countries.[6]

Before the 2009 H1N1 influenza virus emerged, most attention was focused on the highly **pathogenic** strain of avian influenza (H5N1), also a type A strain. The first human case of H5N1 was detected in Hong Kong in 1997. Since then, sporadic cases and outbreaks have continued to occur in several countries. Hundreds of people have been infected with H5N1, and approximately 60 percent of them have died.[7] A majority of infections have been among people exposed to sick poultry, although limited person-to-person transmission has been documented. Given the more **virulent** capacity of the H5N1 virus, scientists are concerned about it becoming readily transmissible to people. Also, because sustained person-to-person transmission of the 2009 H1N1 virus is occurring in areas where H5N1 cases are occurring, the potential for emergence of another novel reassortant influenza virus is feasible.

Plague

Plague is caused by the bacterium *Yersinia pestis*, which is found in several parts of the world. Plague is also known as the Black Death, which killed approximately 50 million people,[2] including 25 percent of Europe's population during the 14th century.[1] Since the 1990s, there has been an increase in the overall annual incidence of plague, and the disease has been reported in countries where plague had not been detected for decades.[7] In 2007, more than 2,000 cases of plague with over 150 deaths were reported from seven countries, and more than 99 percent of these occurred in Africa.[7] Cases in the United States are typically limited to the western states and often occur following exposure to wildlife or their fleas. However, several cases of plague in people have been the result of transmission from pet cats.

Wild rodents are the natural reservoir for plague, and fleas serve as a vector for infection. Transmission of plague to animals and people usually occurs through the bite of an infected flea, although person-to-person transmission through coughing and inhalation of aerosols has occurred. Infection in animals can range from asymptomatic to acute death. Many wild carnivores, as well as dogs, seem to be relatively resistant to clinical infection, while cats are quite susceptible. Clinical signs in cats include fever, anorexia, dehydration, and enlarged, sometimes draining, lymph nodes.

Human infection occurs in three main forms: **bubonic, septicemic,** and **pneumonic.** Bubonic infection can be nonspecific at first, but people typically develop enlarged, painful, draining lymph nodes (called buboes). Bubonic plague can lead to the septicemic form, and in rare cases can lead to such other complications as meningitis or bleeding disorders. Pneumonic plague can occur after direct inhalation of bacteria or as a sequalae to septicemia. If not treated, 50–60 percent of people with bubonic infection will die, and septicemic and pneumonic cases are typically fatal.[7] Early treatment with antibiotics is effective, but plague infection is often not recognized in time. Minimizing contact with rodent environments and fleas is the best way to prevent exposure to plague in animals and people.

Figure 5.3
A Norway rat in a Kansas City, Missouri, corn storage bin. The Norway rat is a known reservoir for plague

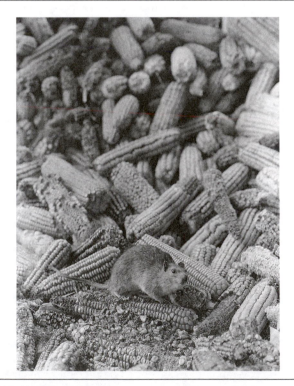

Source: CDC Public Health Image Library.

Tuberculosis

Tuberculosis has been a known cause of global illness for centuries, and several species of *Mycobacteria* exist and can infect mammals. However, the species of most concern to public health is *Mycobacteria tuberculosis*, the primary cause of human tuberculosis. In recent years, more than nine million new cases of tuberculosis have occurred annually worldwide.[7] A vast majority of these cases occur in developing nations, where tuberculosis is a primary cause of morbidity and mortality. Tuberculosis is transmitted through inhalation of bacteria after exposure to an infected individual. Less than 10 percent of people exposed to the *M. tuberculosis* **organism** will actually develop active tuberculosis infection; the majority of people will have a latent infection, where they do not show signs of disease and are not capable of transmitting tuberculosis. These latent infections can last for years. Disease most often develops in those individuals with recent exposure to tuberculosis and those with compromised immune systems. Clinical signs of pulmonary tuberculosis include cough, fever, chills, and weight loss. Eventually, the cough produces purulent sputum. Prompt and appropriate treatment of tuberculosis can eliminate infection, but this is hard to achieve in many parts of the world.

The emergence of HIV has further complicated efforts to eliminate tuberculosis, as co-infection with tuberculosis is fairly common among those with HIV. In fact, in some sub-Saharan African areas, 10–15 percent of the adult population is co-infected with HIV and tuberculosis.[7] During the late 1980s to early 1990s, several highly fatal outbreaks of **multidrug-resistant tuberculosis (MDR-TB)** occurred among HIV-infected individuals in institutional settings in several countries. Transmission to other patients and health-care workers also occurred. Efforts to control the spread of MDR-TB have been fairly effective, although estimates suggest that almost 5 percent of tuberculosis cases worldwide are now due to MDR-TB strains.[7] Of more concern, **extensively drug-resistant tuberculosis (XDR-TB)** has also emerged recently. During an outbreak in South Africa from 2005 to 2006, 52 of 53 (98%) patients diagnosed with XDR-TB died.[7]

"Emergence of XDR-TB is a good example of the need for strong health systems to improve public health security, because it is essentially a manmade problem. It is created primarily by inadequate health systems and the resulting failures in programme management, especially poor supervision of health staff and of patients' treatment regimens, disruptions in drug supplies, and poor clinical management, all of which can prevent patients [from] completing courses of treatment."[9]

Yellow Fever

Yellow fever is caused by the yellow fever virus and was responsible for the American Plague of 1793–1798. It impacted several major U.S. cities and killed an estimated 25,000 people overall, including approximately

10 percent of Philadelphia's population.[2] The yellow fever epidemic was so profound it was the stimulus for establishing what eventually became the U.S. Public Health Service.

Yellow fever has three transmission cycles: **sylvatic**, intermediate, and urban. The sylvatic cycle occurs between mosquitoes and nonhuman primates in tropical regions of Africa and South America. The intermediate cycle of yellow fever occurs between mosquitoes and humans in parts of Africa, and the urban cycle occurs between mosquitoes and humans historically in the Americas. A significant urban yellow fever outbreak has not occurred in more than 50 years in the Americas, although sporadic cases and outbreaks continue to occur in South America and parts of Africa.[7]

The reservoir for yellow fever is *Aedes* mosquitoes, primarily *Aedes aegypti*, as well as nonhuman primates; transmission is vector-borne through the bite of a mosquito. Clinical signs in nonhuman primates are similar to those in humans. Many infections appear to be asymptomatic, but mild infections may produce fever, headache, muscle aches, nausea, vomiting, and diarrhea. Approximately 15 percent of cases do not resolve on their own, and death can occur in up to 50 percent of those with severe illness.[7] WHO estimates that yellow fever accounts for approximately 200,000 infections and 30,000 deaths worldwide each year, with the vast majority of infections occurring in Africa. Prevention of disease is achieved by minimizing exposure to *Aedes* mosquitoes. A yellow fever vaccine is recommended for people traveling to Africa, and the vaccine is part of the national vaccine schedule in 33 of 44 countries where yellow fever is **endemic**.[7]

RECENTLY EMERGING ZOONOTIC DISEASES

Antimicrobial-Resistant Infections

The introduction of antimicrobial agents into human and veterinary medicine is considered one of the most significant achievements of the 20th century. Despite the life-saving effects of antimicrobial agents, the development of antimicrobial resistance has occurred over time and resistant organisms now comprise a considerable proportion of emerging diseases. Compounded with the fact that, today, new antimicrobial agents are rarely developed, antimicrobial-resistant infections have become one of public health's biggest challenges. While it is outside the scope of this chapter to thoroughly review antimicrobial resistance, briefly described here are two examples of significant antimicrobial-resistant infections with zoonotic concerns that have emerged in recent years.

Fluoroquinolone-Resistant *Campylobacter* Species

Campylobacter jejuni and *Campylobacter coli* are bacteria found worldwide and are a common cause of diarrhea in humans (primarily *C. jejuni*).

An estimated 2.4 million cases occur in the United States every year, with approximately 12 percent of these resulting from international travel.[10] Many animals serve as the reservoir **host** for *Campylobacter* species and shed the bacteria in their feces. Transmission to humans often occurs through consumption of contaminated food or water, or through direct contact with infected animals. Food-borne infections in the United States are often associated with the consumption of contaminated poultry products. Many infections of *Campylobacter* appear to be asymptomatic; however, clinical signs can include fever, nausea, vomiting, diarrhea (possibly bloody), and abdominal pain. Occasionally, more severe symptoms may result and patients with *Campylobacter* infections that are resistant to fluoroquinolones (a class of antibiotics) are at greater risk of severe infection and death. A fluoroquinolone is often the antibiotic of choice for treatment of severe *Campylobacter* infections in adults. Therefore, when an adult patient presents with a fluoroquinolone-resistant infection, the treatment options are limited.

Fluoroquinolone-resistant *Campylobacter* infections in people were first noted in the late 1980s. In the late 1990s, an increase in prevalence of fluoroquinolone-resistance among U.S. human *Campylobacter* isolates was detected. Two fluoroquinolones were approved by the U.S. Food and Drug Administration (FDA) for use in poultry in 1995 and 1996. Following the detected increase in fluoroquinolone-resistant infections in humans, the FDA conducted a risk assessment regarding fluoroquinolone use in poultry. This risk assessment estimated that more than 150,000 people acquired fluoroquinolone-resistant *Campylobacter* infections through consumption of contaminated poultry in one year.[10] Based on this risk assessment, and after a lengthy public hearing, the FDA withdrew the approval of fluoroquinolone use in poultry, effective in 2005. This is the first time an animal drug has been taken off the market due to the emergence of antimicrobial resistant infections in people.[9]

MRSA

Methicillin-resistant *Staphylococcus aureus* (MRSA) is a bacterium that is resistant to the antibiotic methicillin, as well as several other similar antibiotics known as beta-lactams. MRSA was first detected in 1961 and now comprises 30–40 percent of hospital-acquired infections worldwide.[10] Since the 1990s, a separate strain of MRSA has developed outside the hospital setting and is referred to as community-acquired MRSA. From 1999 to 2008, the incidence of community-acquired MRSA among children admitted to hospitals increased by 10 times.[11]

MRSA can cause infection in animals, but the main reservoir is believed to be humans. Transmission of MRSA primarily occurs through direct contact with a person who is colonized or infected with MRSA.

Individuals who are colonized with or carry MRSA harbor the bacteria without becoming sick. It is estimated that between 25 and 50 percent of the human population carries *S. aureus,* while approximately 1 percent of the U.S. population is colonized with MRSA.[9] Generally, only individuals suspected of having MRSA infection (not colonization) need to be tested and treated. Clinical signs of MRSA in people typically include skin and soft tissue infections. Severe illness is more common with hospital-acquired MRSA infections and can include pneumonia, septicemia, or death. Hospital-acquired infections more commonly occur in people with underlying health conditions, while community-acquired infections typically occur in otherwise healthy people. Clinical signs in animals also primarily include skin and soft tissue infections, and severe infections are less frequent. The currently available evidence suggests that most MRSA infections in animals, primarily dogs and cats, are secondary to MRSA infections in humans; however, infected animals can serve as a source of infection for other animals and humans.

The Healthcare Infection Control Practices Advisory Committee provides guidance for health-care professionals on the prevention and control of MRSA infections in health-care settings. Practicing good hygiene, such as covering skin wounds with bandages, avoiding contact with visibly infected areas of skin, and washing hands and showering after exercise is recommended to prevent exposure to MRSA in non-health-care settings.

Baylisascaris

Baylisascaris is a disease caused by *Baylisascaris procyonis,* the raccoon roundworm, and was first recognized in humans in 1984. As of 2003, 25 infections of *B. procyonis* had been documented in people, with 20 percent of these resulting in death.[9] Raccoons are the main reservoir for *B. procyonis* and dogs can also serve as hosts. Transmission from raccoons occurs when other animals or people accidentally ingest *B. procyonis* eggs, often in contaminated soil. *Baylisascaris* infections have been documented in nearly 100 animal species, and clinical signs can range from asymptomatic to severe. Adult raccoons and dogs typically show no signs of infection, although young animals infected with a large number of worms may develop intestinal obstructions. Most cases of *Baylisascaris* in other animal species have been associated with neurological signs.

Clinical signs in people are associated with the migration of *B. procyonis* **larvae** to various organs, including the central nervous system and eyes. Severity of signs is associated with the number and location of migrating larvae, and it is possible that nonclinical infections occur when small numbers of larvae exist. Raccoons tend to urinate and defecate in "latrines," located at the base of trees or on fallen logs, woodpiles, and rooftops, and *Baylisascaris* eggs easily survive in feces and in the

Figure 5.4
Raccoons are the natural reservoir for Baylisascaris

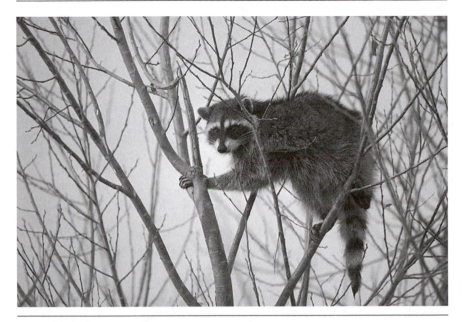

Source: U.S. Fish and Wildlife Service; photo by Dave Menke.

environment. Minimizing exposure to raccoons and their droppings is the best way to prevent baylisascaris infection, as most human cases have been associated with regular contact or observation of raccoons around homes or property.[10]

Cryptococcus Gattii

Cryptococcus gattii is a fungus typically found in tropical and subtropical areas of the world. In 1999, *C. gattii* emerged from Vancouver Island, British Columbia, and in 2004, it was first detected in the Pacific Northwest region of the United States. *C. gattii* has continued to cause sporadic cases and outbreaks in these areas. The reservoir for *C. gattii* appears to be soil and bark of trees, and transmission of *C. gattii* to animals and people occurs through inhalation of infectious spores from the environment. Infection can occur in both healthy and immune-compromised individuals. Respiratory signs are often associated with illness and may include fever, coughing, and difficulty breathing. Severe infections can occur and may lead to central nervous system involvement or death. While medication is available and can be effective against infection, the recognition of *C. gattii* exposure and subsequent illness is often not early enough for successful treatment. Although the incidence of *C. gattii* infection is increasing in the Pacific Northwest region, it is still a rare occurrence overall, and currently, there are no specific recommendations to prevent infection.

Escherichia Coli O157:H7

E. coli O157:H7 is one of several *E. coli* bacterial strains that produce Shiga toxins, and these are collectively known as **Shiga toxin**-producing *E. coli* (STEC). STEC is the primary cause of diarrhea-associated **hemolytic uremic syndrome (HUS),** a life-threatening illness in people. *E. coli* O157:H7 was first recognized following an outbreak associated with hamburger in the United States in 1982 and it is now thought to cause more than 90 percent of diarrhea-associated HUS cases in North America.[7]

The reservoir for *E. coli* O157:H7 is ruminant animals, primarily cattle, which shed the organism in their feces. Transmission to people typically occurs through ingestion of the bacteria, commonly through consumption of contaminated food products, such as hamburger, produce, and unpasteurized milk. Exposure to *E. coli* O157:H7 also occurs through direct contact with animals, and this type of exposure has been associated with petting zoos. Person-to-person transmission can occur and has been documented among family members as well as in daycare settings. *E. coli* O157:H7 does not appear to cause disease in animals.

Bloody diarrhea is the most prominent clinical sign in humans. Serious complications occur in a small percentage of cases, including the development of HUS, which occurs most commonly in children and can be fatal. Prevention of infection is best achieved by practicing good food safety techniques, such as thoroughly cooking hamburger to 160 degrees Fahrenheit and avoiding consumption of unpasteurized dairy products and some juices. Washing hands thoroughly with soap and water, especially before eating and after contact with animals, is also important. Scientists are researching techniques to minimize the transmission of *E. coli* O157:H7 to people, and are also exploring a vaccine that would decrease the shedding of the organism in cattle.

Hendra Virus

Hendra is caused by the Hendra virus, which is closely related to the Nipah virus. The first cases of Hendra were detected in horses and people in Hendra, Australia, in 1994. Since then, sporadic cases of Hendra have occurred in Australia, with the most recent case occurring in a horse in 2010. Fruit bats (flying foxes) are the reservoir for Hendra, and transmission to horses is believed to occur through inhalation or ingestion of the virus from the contaminated environment. Clinical signs in horses generally appear as either a respiratory or neurological illness. Although rare, the disease onset is usually quick and severe, often resulting in death. As of July 1, 2010, four of the seven people known to be infected with Hendra virus have died. Human infections have occurred in people who had close contact with sick horses. Like horses, reported symptoms in people have ranged from nonspecific to progressive **encephalitis**.

Lyme Disease

Lyme disease is caused by the bacterium *Borellia burgdorferi*. The first cases of Lyme disease were recognized in 1975, following an outbreak of arthritis near Lyme, Connecticut; however, *B. burgdorferi* was not identified as the causative agent until 1982. Now, cases of Lyme disease have been reported in other countries and almost all states. Within the United States, tens of thousands of infections are detected every year, with the majority of infections occurring in the Northeast, the upper Midwest, and along the northern Pacific coast. These areas coincide with the distribution of *Ixodes* ticks, the primary vector of Lyme disease. Wild animals, such as mice and gray squirrels serve as reservoirs for the organism, and deer play an important role as hosts for *Ixodes* ticks. Ticks feed off these animals and become a carrier of *B. burgdorferi*.

Transmission of *B. burgdorferi* to domestic animals and people is vector-borne, through bites from various life stages of *Ixodes* ticks. Many infections in animals appear to be asymptomatic, but fever and arthritis are reported frequently in dogs and horses. A characteristic skin rash, **erythema migrans** (also referred to as the "bull's eye"), is the first symptom identified in 70–80 percent of infections in people.[7] Other signs, including fever, headache, muscle aches, and enlarged lymph nodes may be present early on. If not treated, up to 60 percent of people infected with *B. burgdorferi* will develop arthritis,[7] and a small percentage of infections may lead to severe or chronic conditions, such as neurological abnormalities or arthritis. Treatment is most effective when symptoms are recognized early and a diagnosis is confirmed, but minimizing exposure to tick habitats is the best means of preventing infection with Lyme disease. Therefore, when venturing into tick habitats, wearing appropriate clothing (such as long-sleeved shirts, pants, and boots), applying an insect repellent with DEET, and inspecting for attached ticks will minimize an individual's risk of exposure.

Monkeypox

Monkeypox is caused by the monkeypox virus, which somewhat clinically resembles smallpox infection (though smallpox was eradicated in the late 1970s). Monkeypox was first discovered in 1970 in Africa, in what is now the Democratic Republic of the Congo. Monkeypox is endemic only to parts of Africa, and outbreaks have sporadically occurred there since monkeypox was first recognized. However, in 2003, a multistate outbreak occurred in the United States as a result of the importation of infected wild animals from Africa. The imported animals, intended to be sold as pets, subsequently infected American prairie dogs. The prairie dogs were sold as pets and subsequently infected people, leading to an outbreak of more than 70 cases, many of which required hospitalization.

Although many animal species can become infected, the reservoir for monkeypox is thought to be African rodents. Transmission of monkeypox can occur through bites from infected animals or inhalation of the virus from the air but typically occurs after direct contact with infected animals. Person-to-person transmission also occurs, but is rare. A self-limiting rash is the typical clinical sign in animals. This rash eventually develops into **pocks** and can persist for several weeks, and the pocks eventually form scabs. Clinical signs in people may be nonspecific at first, including fever, headache, and sore throat. Respiratory signs can also appear. Enlarged lymph nodes are often seen, and a skin rash typically occurs within 10 days. The skin lesions, most commonly seen on the extremities, usually resolve within 2–3 weeks. Severe illness and death from monkeypox rarely occurs, although mortality rates in Africa range from 1 to 10 percent, and children are more susceptible.[11] While the smallpox vaccine is cross-protective, WHO does not routinely recommend **prophylactic** vaccination. To prevent transmission of the monkeypox virus in endemic areas, minimizing exposure to potentially infected animals and humans is recommended. In the United States, the importation and sale of six species of African rodents has been prohibited since the outbreak to prevent reintroduction of the monkeypox virus.

Nipah Virus

Nipah is caused by the Nipah virus, which is closely related to the Hendra virus. Nipah emerged in swine and people in Malaysia and Singapore during an epidemic in 1998–1999. Fruit bats (flying foxes) are the reservoir for Nipah, and transmission to swine is believed to occur through contact with the contaminated environment. In Malaysia, human cases occurred after close contact with infected pigs, and Singapore cases were identified among people with close contact to pigs imported from Malaysia. In 2001, a single outbreak affected people in India, and from 2001 to 2005, several outbreaks occurred among people in Bangladesh. No swine exposures were associated with the outbreaks in India and Bangladesh. Clinical signs in pigs can range from asymptomatic to sudden death, with most pigs showing no signs of illness. In younger pigs (one to six months old), respiratory signs are more common in comparison to older pigs, in which neurological signs are more frequently reported.[9] Most infections

Figure 5.5
Close-up of monkeypox lesions on the arm and leg of a four-year-old child in Liberia in 1971

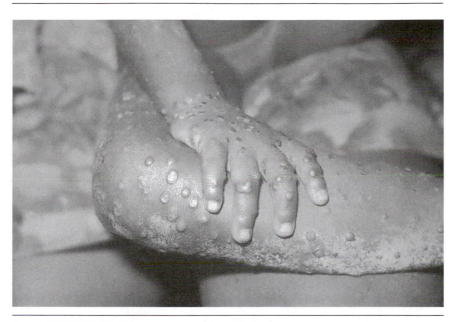

Source: CDC Public Health Image Library.

in people are believed to be asymptomatic. In clinical cases, nonspecific illness may be noted, including fever and headache; however, acute neurological signs are the most frequently reported. Most cases of Nipah infection were observed among people in close contact to pigs, and case fatality rates ranged from 70 to 75 percent.[7]

Rift Valley Fever

Rift Valley fever (RVF) virus was first detected in animals and people in the early 1930s in Kenya. Several outbreaks have occurred in Kenya and other parts of Africa since then, with the most recent taking place in South Africa in 2010. RVF was also detected outside Africa during an outbreak in Saudi Arabia and Yemen in 2000. *Aedes* mosquitoes are thought to be the primary reservoir for RVF and outbreaks are often seen after heavy rainfall. Transmission to animals, primarily ruminants, is through the bite of a mosquito, while transmission to humans can be via mosquito or through exposure to animals or animal tissues infected with RVF. Abortion is the most common clinical sign in animals. Death in young animals is often noted, and fever, anorexia, and weakness may be seen. Frequently reported signs in people include fever, weakness, and headache. **Ocular** lesions, as well as severe disease with bleeding can also occur.[7] Vaccinating livestock for RVF can help control the spread of disease, and minimizing exposure to mosquitoes and potentially infected animals is recommended to prevent RVF infections in people.

SARS

Sudden acute respiratory syndrome (SARS) is caused by a new coronavirus that emerged from China in November 2002. Over the next several months, the disease spread across the globe to 26 countries, causing 8,098 illnesses and 774 deaths.[7] Many infections were hospital associated, and the last documented case was linked to a laboratory worker in China in 2004. The masked palm civet was thought to be the initial source of human infection during this epidemic, although similar SARS-like coronaviruses have been detected in Chinese horseshoe bats and other wild animals in the same region of China.[7] During the outbreak, person-to-person transmission occurred through direct contact with infected people, exposure to respiratory droplets, and through **fomites.** Clinical signs in people range from asymptomatic to severe respiratory distress and death; the overall case fatality rate for this epidemic was approximately 9.6 percent.[7] For SARS to return, the virus would need to reemerge from the human population, an animal reservoir, or be released through a laboratory accident.

Variant Creutzfeldt-Jakob Disease

Variant Creutzfeldt-Jakob Disease (vCJD) is a rare, degenerative brain **neuropathy** first recognized in the United Kingdom in 1996 and is believed to be caused by a **prion.** Infection in people has been linked to the consumption of cattle products contaminated with **bovine spongiform encephalopathy (BSE).** BSE (also known as mad-cow disease) was first detected in cattle in the UK in 1986 and likely emerged as a result of cattle eating meat and bone meal contaminated with scrapie-infected sheep products. The incidence of BSE in cattle in the UK peaked in the early 1990s, shortly before cases of vCJD were recognized in people. Four cases of vCJD in the UK are believed to be associated with blood transfusions, from preclinical vCJD donors. Clinical signs in humans take years to develop, although a specific **incubation** period has not yet been determined for vCJD. Behavioral or psychiatric disturbance is the typical presentation, and the average duration of illness is 14 months. Cases of vCJD are eventually fatal. Avoiding exposure to BSE-infected tissues through the food supply is the primary means of prevention, and many countries have implemented strategies to minimize the risk of BSE in their cattle populations. Genetic factors contribute to the susceptibility to vCJD as well.

Viral Hemorrhagic Fevers

Viral hemorrhagic fevers (VHF) are caused by viruses within four different viral families. A majority of VHFs produce vascular damage, which leads to hemorrhaging, although this symptom alone is typically not life-threatening. Most VHFs are zoonotic and require an animal reservoir or vector for transmission to people. Secondary transmission from person to person also occurs with several VHFs, and severity of disease can range from mild to fatal. Described here are just a few examples of emerging zoonotic VHFs.

Ebola and Marburg

Ebola and Marburg viruses are endemic to Africa, except for Ebola-Reston, which is endemic to the Philippines. Although it is not completely understood, recent evidence suggests that bats are the reservoir for Ebola and Marburg viruses. Most Ebola viruses cause infections in nonhuman primates and people. While Reston can infect people, it does not appear to cause illness in people, and in 2008, Reston was detected in pigs in the Philippines. Clinical signs of Ebola and Marburg viruses in nonhuman primates and people may be nonspecific, including fever, malaise, and vomiting. Bleeding tendencies, such as bruising and intestinal hemorrhaging are common. Severity of infection varies among the viruses, but outbreaks can be severe, with mortality rates reaching up to 90 percent.[7] Transmission to humans has typically occurred after close or direct contact with infected nonhuman primates. Person-to-person transmission occurs through direct contact with infected tissues and often takes place in hospital settings or through contact with victims during burial procedures. Prevention of person-to-person transmission is best achieved by practicing strict infection control protocols, including the use of personal protective equipment, such as gloves, gowns, eye protection, and respirators. However, in areas of Africa where outbreaks of Ebola and Marburg viruses occur, these practices are challenging to accomplish.

Hantavirus Pulmonary Syndrome

At least 25 different hantaviruses exist, with infections in humans ranging from nonexistent to severe illness, depending on the virus. The Sin Nombre virus is the primary cause of hantavirus pulmonary syndrome (HPS) in North America. HPS was first described in the southwestern United States in 1993. Rodents are the reservoir for all hantaviruses, with the deer mouse, a common mouse throughout many parts of the United States, being the primary reservoir for the Sin Nombre virus. Transmission to people occurs primarily through inhalation of the virus, typically in aerosolized dust contaminated with rodent droppings. Clinical signs of HPS may be nonspecific for several days, followed by acute respiratory distress. In severe cases, patients require mechanical ventilation. Although HPS is a relatively rare disease, 35–50 percent of infections can result in death.[7] Minimizing exposure to rodents and their environment, such as rodent-proofing homes and safely cleaning up rodent droppings, is the best way to prevent infection with hantaviruses.

Lassa Fever

Lassa fever was first recognized in 1969 in Lassa, Nigeria. Lassa fever has not been detected outside of West Africa, but it is estimated that hundreds of thousands of infections occur annually. Wild rodents serve as the reservoir for this virus, and transmission primarily occurs through direct contact or aerosolization of virus in rodent droppings. However, Lassa fever can also be sexually transmitted from person to person. Approximately 80 percent of people experience asymptomatic or mild, nonspecific illness, but pregnant women frequently experience severe signs, including death and fetal loss.[7] Minimizing exposure to rodents and their environment, such as rodent-proofing homes and safely cleaning up rodent droppings, is the best way to prevent infections of Lassa fever. However, in developing areas where Lassa fever is endemic, these preventive measures may be challenging.

West Nile Virus

West Nile virus (WNV) is found in many countries, but its first detection in the western hemisphere occurred in the summer of 1999 in New York. WNV has continued to spread westward across the nation, infecting thousands of people. WNV is transmitted primarily through the *Culex* genus of mosquitoes, and birds act as the main reservoir. Many animals species naturally infected with WNV do not develop clinical signs, but signs in birds and horses can be severe, including encephalitis and death. Human infection can also range from mild to severe. Approximately 80 percent of human infections are asymptomatic,[8] but severe illness and death can occur, especially in older individuals. Decreasing exposure to mosquitoes, by minimizing time outdoors when mosquitoes are most active (dawn and dusk), wearing appropriate clothing (such as long-sleeved shirts, pants, and boots), and applying an insect repellent with DEET, is the most effective way to decrease the risk of infection from WNV and other mosquito-borne diseases.

In addition to the **arboviruses** briefly described in this chapter, many other important arboviruses exist and including dengue fever, Japanese encephalitis, LaCrosse encephalitis, Crimean-Congo hemorrhagic fever,

St. Louis encephalitis, Murray Valley encephalitis, and Eastern, Western, and Venezuelan equine encephalitis viruses.

CONCLUSION

Described in this chapter are just a few selected examples of the hundreds of emerging diseases identified globally. Infectious diseases are traveling faster around the world than any time in history, with over 1,100 epidemics occurring between 2002 and 2007.[8] These events confirm that infectious diseases, particularly zoonotic diseases, remain a threat to the future of public health. Most recent zoonotic diseases have emerged from developing nations, yet the majority of resources available to detect and respond to these diseases are in developed nations, where pathogens are least likely to originate.[4] The annual cost of a global surveillance system is estimated to be $800 million, while economic losses from emerging zoonotic diseases have exceeded $200 billion in the past 10 years.[6] Obviously, the impact of emerging diseases on the international community is profound, and the issues surrounding emerging diseases cannot be resolved by individual countries.[6] Therefore, collaboration across borders and disciplines is imperative for tackling the infectious diseases of tomorrow.

This belief is perhaps best exemplified by Dr. Gerald T. Keusch and Dr. Marguerite Pappaioanou, cochairs, IOM Committee on Achieving Sustainable Global Capacity for Surveillance and Response to Emerging Diseases of Zoonotic Origin. In the preface to *Sustaining Global Surveillance and Response to Emerging Zoonotic Diseases*, they state the following:

Although the time from the detection of a cluster of severe pneumonia cases in Mexico to the identification of the cause as influenza A (H1N1) 2009 and global awareness and a patchwork global response was shorter than that experienced in previous outbreaks, we believe that the urgency will only grow to create an even more effective system for sustained, integrated, early human and animal disease detection that is immediately followed by and intimately linked to a timely and appropriately targeted response. Achieving such a system is not easy: If it were, it would have been accomplished decades ago. But given the inevitability of disease emergence occurring again and again, the solution requires strong leadership and commitment to ensure that multiple disciplines from different sectors will work closely together to address the myriad complex and sophisticated challenges they will pose . . . the committee believes it is high time for national and international public health leadership . . . to address how global and effectively integrated zoonotic disease surveillance can be achieved.[6]

GLOSSARY

Arbovirus: any virus that is transmitted through an arthropod vector, such as a mosquito or tick.

Biosecurity: refers to preventive measures put in place to protect against the introduction of an infectious disease.

Bioterrorism: the use of biological agents, such as infectious pathogens, for terrorist purposes.

Bovine spongiform encephalopathy (BSE): also known as mad-cow disease, is a transmissible spongiform encephalopathy of adult cattle.

Bubonic: refers to buboes, which are enlarged, inflamed lymph nodes.

Cutaneous: refers to or involves the skin.

Edema: an abnormal collection of fluid in tissues, which causes swelling.

Encephalitis: an acute inflammation of the brain.

Endemic: a status given to a disease or condition when it persists within a population in a specific area.

Enzootic: a status given to a disease or condition when it persists within an animal population in a specific area.

Epidemic: the occurrence of more cases of a disease than would be expected for an area during a given time period.

Erythema migrans: refers to the skin rash often seen in the early stages of Lyme disease.

Eschar: a scab of the skin.

Exudate: a fluid that has oozed out of a tissue or its vessels due to injury or inflammation.

Fomite: refers to any inanimate object that can transmit disease.

Gastrointestinal: relates to the stomach and intestinal tract.

Hemolytic uremic syndrome: an illness characterized by the abrupt onset of decreased urine production, loss of kidney function, and anemia; it may be accompanied by edema, hypertension, blood-clotting disorders, and seizures.

Host: an organism that harbors or nourishes another organism.

Incidence: the number of new cases of disease that develop during a given time period, such as a year.

Incubation: the time between exposure to an infectious agent and the appearance of clinical signs or symptoms.

Institute of Medicine of the National Academy of Sciences: established in 1970 to be an adviser to the federal government to identify issues of medical care, research, and education.

Larva: an immature stage of development for an animal, such as a worm; larvae is the plural of larva.

MDR-TB: multidrug-resistant tuberculosis; MDR-TB is defined as resistance to at least isoniazid and rifampin, common first-line antimicrobial agents used to treat tuberculosis.

Morbidity: refers to the state of being diseased, while the **morbidity rate** is the ratio of the number of diseased individuals to the total population of an area.

Mortality: refers to death, while the **mortality rate** is the ratio of the number of deaths from a given disease to the total number of cases of that disease.

Neuropathy: a functional disturbance or pathological change in the peripheral nervous system.

Ocular: refers to or involves the eyes.

Organism: an individual form of life, such as a plant, animal, bacteria, fungus, virus, or parasite.

Pandemic: an epidemic that spreads over a very wide area, throughout an entire region, or even the world.

Pathogenic: refers to the ability to cause disease.

Pneumonic: refers to the lungs or pneumonia.

Pock: refers to the characteristic pustular lesion of pox viruses.

Prion: refers to a small protein particle that can self-replicate; prions are believed to be responsible for degenerative neurological diseases, such as scrapie in sheep, BSE in cattle, and variant Creutzfeldt-Jakob disease in people. Because prions lack detectable nucleic acid, they are not inactivated by the usual procedures for destroying viruses.

Prophylactic: refers to an agent, often a vaccine or drug, that prevents disease.

Pustule: a small inflamed swelling that is filled with pus; a pimple.

Reassortant virus: a virus that contains genetic material from more than one species.

Reservoir: any person, animal, plant, soil, or substance in which an infectious agent normally lives, multiplies, and depends on for survival; the reservoir typically harbors the infectious agent without harming itself but serves as a source of infection for others.

Ruminants: animals with four stomach compartments (rumen, reticulum, omasum, and abomasums); cattle, sheep, and goats are examples of ruminants.

Septicemia: a clinical syndrome in which infection is disseminated throughout the body in the bloodstream; **septicemic** refers to the condition of having septicemia.

Shiga toxins: a family of related toxins with two major groups, Stx1 and Stx2. The most common sources for Shiga toxin are the bacteria *S. dysenteriae* and Shiga toxin-producing *Eschericia coli* (STEC), which includes serotype O157:H7 and other enterohemorrhagic *E. coli.*

Sylvatic: refers to diseases associated with wild animals.

Transmission: the transfer of a disease from one animal/person to another.

Virulent: the ability of any pathogen to produce disease.

XDR-TB: extensively drug-resistant tuberculosis; XDR-TB is defined as MDR-TB plus resistance to any fluoroquinolone (a type of antimicrobial agent) and any of the three injectable antimicrobial agents: amikacin, kanamycin, and capreomyocin.

Zoonotic: refers to diseases that can be transmitted between animals and people.

FURTHER READING

Books

Acha PN, Szyfres B. *Zoonoses and Communicable Diseases Common to Man and Animals.* 3rd ed. 3 vols. Washington, DC: Pan American Health Organization; 2003.

Rabinowitz PM, Conti LA. *Human-Animal Medicine: Clinical Approaches to Zoonoses, Toxicants, and other Shared Health Risks.* Maryland Heights, MO: Saunders; 2010.

Spickler AR, Roth JA, Galyon J, Lofstedt J. *Emerging and Exotic Diseases of Animals.* 4th ed. Ames, IA: Iowa State University College of Veterinary Medicine; 2009.

Articles

Cutler SJ, Rooks AR, van der Poel WHM. Public health threat of new, reemerging, and neglected zoonoses in the industrialized world. *Emerging Infectious Diseases* 2010;16(1)l:1–7.

Taylor LH, Latham SM, Woolhouse MEJ. Risk factors for human disease emergence. *Philosophical Transactions of the Royal Society of London* 2001;B356:983–9.

Woolhouse MEJ, Gowtage-Sequeria S. Host range and emerging and reemerging pathogens. *Emerging Infectious Diseases* 2005;11(12):1842–6.

REFERENCES

1. Snowden FM. Emerging and reemerging diseases: A historical perspective. *Immunological Reviews* 2008;225:9–26.
2. Morens DM, Folkers GK, Fauci AS. Emerging infections: A perpetual challenge. *The Lancet Infectious Diseases* 2008;8:710–19.
3. Joint United Nations Programme on HIV/AIDS. AIDS epidemic update, December 2009. Available at: http://data.unaids.org/pub/Report/2009/JC1700_Epi_Update_2009_en.pdf.
4. Jones KE, Patel NG, Levy MA, et al. Global trends in emerging infectious diseases. *Nature* 2008;451:990–94.
5. Smolinski MS, Hamburg MA, Lederberg J. *Microbial threats to health: Emergence, detection, and response.* Washington, DC: National Academy Press; 2003.
6. Keusch GT, Pappaioanou M, Gonzalez MC, et al. *Sustaining Global Surveillance and Response to Emerging Zoonotic Diseases.* Washington, DC: National Academy Press; 2009.

7. Heymann DL. *Control of Communicable Diseases*.19th ed. Washington, DC: American Public Health Association; 2008.

8. World Health Organization. The world health report 2007: A safer future, global public health security in the 21st century. Available at: http://www. who.int/whr/2007/en/index.html.

9. Nelson JM, Chiller TM, Powers JH, et al. Fluoroquinolone-resistant *Campylobacter* species and the withdrawal of fluoroquinolones from use in poultry: A public health success story. *Clinical Infectious Diseases* 2007;44:977–80.

10. Dvorak GD, Spickler AR, Roth JA. *Handbook for Zoonotic Diseases of Companion Animals*. Ames, IA: Iowa State University College of Veterinary Medicine; 2008.

11. Herigon JC, Hersh AL, Gerber JS, et al. Antibiotic Management of Staphylococcus aureus infections in U.S. Children's Hospitals, 1999–2008. *Pediatrics* 2010;125(06):e1294–1300. Available at: http://pediatrics.aappublications.org/content/125/6/e1294.long.

12. Fauci AS. Infectious diseases: Considerations for the 21st century. *Clinical Infectious Diseases* 2001;32:675–85.

Chapter 6

Wildlife Trade, Demand, and Health

Kristine M. Smith, DVM, DACZM

Humans have always shared their environment with animals. Fascination with and hunting of wild animals has been reflected as far back as early cave art. Although the life of the individual animal or human was often inherently at risk during such interactions, at what point did similar encounters become a potential threat to entire populations of animals and humans? Scientists approximate that with the domestication of animals, alteration of the environment for agricultural use, and broader movement of animals and goods there entered a new era of infectious disease resulting from enhanced pathogen exchange among animals and between humans and animals. It is these advances to which scientists attribute the manifestation of diseases such as pertussis, measles, mumps, tuberculosis, and even the common influenza and cold viruses.[1] In fact, from the plague to the Spanish flu, most of our historic pandemics have stemmed from contact with animals.

More recently, attention has turned toward pathogen emergence from the wild animal kingdom. Many diseases of livestock and other domestic animals are fairly well recognized and often, although not always adequately, managed. Diseases of wildlife, however, pertaining to their ability to affect domestic animals and humans, are not as well understood. Largely the knowledge we do have is not acted upon in the form of risk assessment or preventative measures. In the past decade alone we have witnessed several novel disease events (while continuing to experience the ongoing impacts of more familiar pathogens) that have threatened global health, food security, and economies, stemming from and spreading through the manipulation and trade of wild animals. This chapter will explore the anthropogenic drivers behind disease transmission between species as they relate to wildlife extraction and trade and touch upon the options available to mitigate similar future events.

HUMAN-ANIMAL INTERFACE

As the population of humans on the planet continues to rise, the natural boundaries between people and wildlife are fading. People are expanding into wild lands to live, grow crops, and create access to natural resources. Along with population growth has been an exponential rise in livestock numbers and agricultural use of land, even further decreasing the divide between humans, their domesticated animals, and wildlife. The loss of these natural geographical buffers between humans or their domestic animals and wildlife have allowed for increased pathogen transfer from wildlife into naïve human and domestic animal hosts (and vice versa) through both direct contact and indirect contact via disease vectors (e.g., mosquitoes, ticks, and fleas) and sharing of natural resources such as soil and water.

Typically, human populations living along the edges of remaining wildlife habitat in developing countries are among the poorest in the world. These populations are remote and have little access to health care. It is these people who are most likely to suffer from disease and to depend on direct natural resource extraction for their livelihood and subsistence. Likewise, the domestic animals belonging to these populations are less likely to have veterinary medical care and frequently suffer from infectious diseases such as bacterial and parasitic infections, which are much less common in developed countries with adequate agricultural disease control (biosecurity) practices. Wildlife living along this interface with humans and domestic animals may also experience amplified stress and illness due to habitat loss and hunting pressure. This combination of direct and indirect contact along with heightened pathogen loads allows for elevated risk of disease exchange between wildlife, livestock, and humans.

Transmission of diseases from wildlife to humans can occur through vectors, as in the cases of yellow fever, plague, and West Nile virus; through the environment (e.g., water, soil, and air), as in the case of anthrax and cholera; or through direct contact (e.g., respiratory or body fluids), as in the case of psittacosis or Ebola virus. Similar transmission events occur from wildlife to domestic animals along analogous means. Conversely, livestock and other domestic animals have served as a source of disease to wildlife, threatening naïve populations, as in the case of rinderpest virus. Upon becoming infected with pathogens from livestock, wildlife populations can at times maintain and become an ongoing source of disease reintroduction to livestock, as in the case of bovine tuberculosis or brucellosis. These diseases not only threaten food security, but many also infect humans. For example, bovine tuberculosis (*Mycobacterium bovis*), the bovine equivalent of human *Mycobacterium tuberculosis,* has spilled over from cattle into wildlife in many places around the world. The disease has made its way into free-ranging African buffalos (*Syncerus caffer*) of South Africa's Kruger National Park. The buffalo spread the disease amongst themselves, transmit it to their wildlife predators (such as lion and cheetah), and serve as a continual source of the disease to naïve cattle populations, making the likelihood of eradication of the disease in cattle a difficult one. Humans become infected by drinking the unpasteurized milk of infected cattle. Such infections have proven especially dangerous to immunosuppressed people already suffering from human immunodeficiency virus (up to one-sixth of the area population).

The potential for humans to serve as disease reservoirs to wildlife is also increasingly becoming recognized. Examples include historic introductions of polio, measles, scabies, and intestinal parasites from area inhabitants and extractive industry personnel to vulnerable great ape populations, and the more recent transfer of *Mycobacterium tuberculosis* from humans to wild populations of banded mongooses (*Mungos mungo*) through exposure to human waste dumps.

Increased exposure to wildlife through intensification of natural resource extraction and trade is altering the complexity of this human-animal interface and the inherent pathogen exchange that accompanies it. Scientists are struggling to evaluate and mitigate the risks to human and animal health associated with these activities, while trying to better understand the drivers behind such behaviors so that comprehensive solutions may be found.

NATURAL RESOURCE EXTRACTION

Humans fundamentally rely upon intact ecosystem services such as clean water, air purification, and environmental detoxification for basic survival. In addition, natural environments supply many services to human well-being, from shelter to the more tangential spiritual benefits.

Even advances in technology are challenged to adequately replace such services. For example, the cost of building a water filtration plant to filter the increasing sewage from New York City was estimated at $5–$8 billion, with an additional $300–$500 million in annual operating costs. This compares to a one-time cost of $1.5 billion (including landowner compensation) to halt development in part of the Catskill Mountains and restore the integrity of the watershed's natural purification services.[2]

Among the impacts on health and well-being, alteration of ecosystems such as clearing forests and building roads can disrupt natural balances to favor opportunistic pathogen emergence or spread. Kyanasur forest disease was historically very restricted to a small area of undisturbed forest in India. Once forests were cleared, the ticks carrying this virus proliferated by feeding on grazing cattle and promoted disease spread causing thousands of potentially deadly human infections.[3] Scientists have observed similar patterns with malaria epidemics following deforestation in sub-Saharan Africa. Such examples of the complex interactions between environmental change and alterations in disease ecology are only recently becoming recognized and appreciated.

Hunting of wild animals for subsistence has always taken place in local communities worldwide, and often in a sustainable way. However, changing dynamics have tipped the scales on wildlife harvesting in many areas. Shrinking wildlife habitat, increased accessibility, human migration into once wild lands via commercial logging roads, and ease of transportation of goods between rural villages and urban markets are just a few factors eliminating the sustainability of wildlife harvesting. Hunting of wild animals to put food on the tables of local villages is being superseded by a livelihood geared toward providing exotic products and food choices to the urban wealthy. The desire for rural "fresh" food by rising city populations has enhanced the wet market trade, providing access to live or recently slaughtered wild animals from local, regional, or even distant forests. Thus, while historically disease transfer from a wild animal to a hunter would have likely remained restricted to that hunter or his family, or even local village, today such exposures are rarely isolated events. Animals, their products, and the people who encounter them are easily transported from remote locations to urban cities, contacting humans and animals along the way. The health impacts of these trade chains go beyond disease transmission; forest wildlife populations that have historically provided a crucial source of protein to rural families are now dwindling.

The traditional use of wildlife species for cultural or medicinal purposes has also been ongoing around the world for centuries. The World Health Organization (WHO) reports that more than three-quarters of the world's 6 billion people rely primarily on animal and plant-based medicines, including many of the advanced medications available in developed countries. In this light, the use of wild animals for medicinal purposes has greatly contributed to the health of humans. Yet most of the indigenous populations that supply this knowledge benefit relatively little from the profit. Further, harvesters supplying the global demand for wildlife used in traditional Chinese medicines have lost perception on sustainability in exchange for the monetary gain in providing for the mass market. Today, the use of rare animal parts, such as those from rhinos and tigers, has become a luxury market, as diminishing wildlife populations fail to support the unforgiving demand.

The utilization of wild animals as pets has been responsible for the majority of live animal demand in the Western Hemisphere. This market involves billions of individual live animals ranging from corals to nonhuman primates, originating from all over the globe.

GLOBAL WILDLIFE TRADE AND THE UNITED STATES

Globalization of today's society has transformed human travel, trade of plants and animals from local to everyday international practices. On the global scale, wildlife trade is one of the largest trade operations in the world, with the illegal aspect alone representing a multi-billion-dollar industry that has been compared to the international drug trade. Wildlife and wildlife products are traded as food, trophies, pets, fashion, medicine, and aphrodisiacs. There are no adequate estimates of the full scale of wildlife traded throughout the world given its vastness, scope, and partial underground existence.

In 1973, the Convention on International Trade in Endangered Species of Wild Fauna and Flora (CITES) agreement was signed and today has over 120 member nations. This international wildlife conservation agreement regulates trade in certain species, with a focus on critical and endangered populations. However, despite the relatively successful implementation of this treaty over the past two decades, the illegal trade in wildlife continues to flourish.

Dated estimates of live wildlife traded (primarily as pets) at the global level every year, excluding nonvertebrates, are more than 40,000 primates, 4 million birds, 640,000 reptiles, and 350 million tropical fish.[4] These numbers represent only the tip of the iceberg and do not consider regional and local level trade (which far outweigh the global estimates), trade in bushmeat (meat of wild animals hunted for food) and other wildlife and wildlife products, and likely underestimate the illegal trade in live animals that goes undetected. The total volume of wildlife products (both legal and illegal), such as bushmeat, fashion and decorative items, and medicinal products traded every year is impossible to quantify due to its enormity. Estimated annual harvests for bushmeat is more than 5 million tons of wild mammal meat from Neotropical (0.15 million) and Afrotropical

(4.9 million) forests.[5] Estimates of animals harvested for traditional Chinese medicine every year is nearly unquantifiable. Harvests of seahorses alone for this purpose reportedly exceed several dozen tons per year, placing all species used on the CITES II list.

Although most Americans tend to associate the wildlife trade with Asia and Africa, the United States is one of the world's largest consumers of imported wildlife and wildlife products. The U.S. Fish and Wildlife Service (USFWS) reported importation of wildlife into the United States increased 62 percent within a decade from 1992 to 2003, with declared shipments alone escalating from approximately 74,500 to nearly 120,000 per year. Between 2000 and 2004, USFWS records reflected imports of more than 1 billion individual animals (including aquatic species) and an additional 5 million kilograms of animals (only classified by weight) into the United States. These numbers reflect permitted or intercepted illegal imports only. The United States is one of the largest consumers of the exotic pet trade, with more than 90 percent of its live animal imports destined for commercial purposes.[6]

Not only does the global trade of wildlife threaten source populations, but live animals that are transported to new regions have potential to disrupt the local ecosystem balance, threaten plant and animal agriculture, and damage economies if released.[6] Beyond the environmental impacts, translocation of wildlife can result in the introduction of viruses, bacteria, fungi, and parasites that they carry into new environments, an act that scientists have termed pathogen pollution, with potentially devastating consequences to native wildlife health.

WILDLIFE TRADE AND INFECTIOUS DISEASES

WHO reports that 26 percent of human deaths worldwide are caused by infectious diseases and nearly 75 percent of infectious diseases are considered zoonoses (pathogens transmissible between animals and humans). It is interesting to note that the majority of these zoonoses originate in wildlife. Thus, infectious diseases acquired from contact with wildlife is of substantial concern to global health. Despite advances in medicine, more than 35 new infectious diseases (mostly zoonoses), or about one every eight months, has emerged in humans since 1980.[4] Whereas historically disease spillover events from wildlife to humans were more likely to remain local—perhaps even undetected—today advances in technology have permitted ease of travel, allowing emerging diseases to become a global health threat in a matter of days. A good example of this is the recent H1N1 pandemic (originating from reassortment of human, pig, and wild bird influenza strains in domestic pigs), which spread at four times the rate of previous influenza pandemics, reaching dozens of countries within a little over a month. The virus spread across the United States within a few weeks, resulting in eventual introduction to all 50 states, causing the highest reported death toll of any other country. By the time WHO declared the event a pandemic, more than 70 countries were affected. Numbers reported to WHO included more than 340,000 laboratory confirmed cases and more than 4,100 deaths worldwide, although in most areas where the disease became endemic, such as New York City (believed to have experienced at least 500,000 cases alone), testing was no longer recommended by the Centers for Disease Control and Prevention (CDC) unless severe symptoms were present.

The 2004 WHO/Food and Agriculture Organization (FAO)/The World Organization for Animal Health (OIE) report on drivers of zoonotic emergence reflects upon the anthropogenic movement and manipulation of domestic and wild animals, including globalized trade, as the next big trigger point for emerging disease since the advent of agriculture.[7] The movement and intermingling of wildlife, domestic animals, and humans that occurs during the process of wildlife extraction and trade creates the perfect mixing pot for interface disease emergence and spread. Wildlife are extracted from deep within their habitats, placed in stressful captive situations, and exposed to other species of wildlife from distant locations; domestic animals used for hunting, transport, or sale; and human hunters, traders, sellers, and consumers along the trade chain and in large market hubs. These conditions present unique opportunities for pathogens to meet naïve hosts, infect them, and potentially even evolve and adapt in their new hosts to something potentially more dangerous than before. The risk for disease exchange across species and geographic borders is higher than it has ever been with mere local or regional consumption and movement. The practice of wildlife trade is becoming more and more sophisticated through establishment of major trade hubs across the globe, increasing species mixing from remote regions. The potential for pathogen exposure, exchange, and adaptation are limitless.

The following is a review of several diseases that have threatened human health as a consequence of extraction and trade of wild animals.

Monkeypox Virus

The 2003 outbreak of monkeypox virus in the United States is an excellent example of disease transmission across species and geographical boundaries via the wildlife trade. In December 2003, a shipment of 800 small mammals of nine different species (including six genera of African rodent) from Ghana entered Texas destined for the pet trade. Animals from this shipment were then forwarded to a Midwest pet dealer where they were housed in the vicinity of several prairie dogs. People who purchased the prairie dogs as pets subsequently developed fever,

Figure 6.1
A mix of wild and domestic animals await sale in a market in Vietnam while their cage serves as a resting place for their vendor's lunch

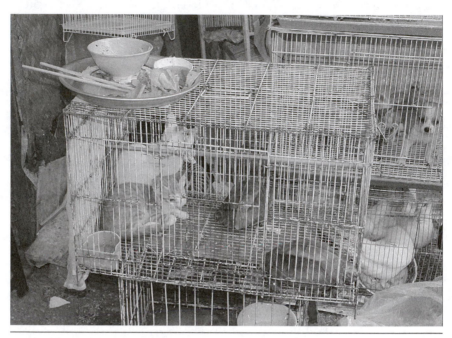

Source: © Martin Gilbert. Used by permission.

respiratory disease, and skin lesions. More than 70 similar cases across six states occurred before the end of the outbreak, 24 percent of which required hospitalization. Some of these cases were thought to be the result of human-to-human transmission. Investigation by the CDC revealed one Gambian giant rat, three dormice, and two rope squirrels that were imported via the shipment from Africa tested positive for monkeypox virus. The rodents had been legally imported for the pet trade. The disease was somehow transmitted to adjacently housed prairie dogs at the dealer.

Monkeypox is one of several viruses in the poxvirus family. Poxviruses have had significant impact on humans, livestock, and wildlife—and some of these highly infectious agents are able to jump from one species to another with deadly consequences. Within the poxvirus family, monkeypox is of the same genus as smallpox. Prior to the report of this disease entering the United States, community acquired monkeypox had never been reported outside of Africa. In Africa, monkeypox disease is typically acquired through the hunting of rodents and nonhuman primates, and previous outbreaks have resulted in mortality rates of 10 percent. Fortunately, in the case of the U.S. outbreak, no deaths occurred.

This chain of events emphasizes the fact that a pathogen does not need to have high prevalence in the trade to have a serious impact on humans in another area of the globe. In response to this outbreak, the CDC and the Food and Drug Administration (FDA) issued a joint order banning the import and interstate transport of the six African rodent species (tree squirrels, rope squirrels, dormice, Gambian giant pouched rats, brush-tailed porcupines, and striped mice). In September 2008, the FDA lifted its portion of the ban, allowing interstate movement to recommence.

SARS

Coronaviruses have long been recognized to occur in a wide range of animals species, including humans, causing anywhere from very mild to severe respiratory and/or gastrointestinal disease. The outbreak of SARS-associated coronavirus illustrates how a relatively little known pathogen of wildlife can become world famous in a matter of days.

The outbreak started with several hundred cases of respiratory disease in Guangdong Province, China, and within a few months had spread internationally, eventually leading to 8,098 known cases and 774 deaths (with a case-fatality rate of 9.6%) in 29 countries around the world. The masked palm civet (*Paguma larvata*), common in the wildlife trade markets of China, was suspected to be the source of the pandemic. However, it is now believed bats are the natural host, likely infecting civets through contact between these species in trade markets in Guangdong Province. These findings were supported by a study showing a zero percent prevalence in wild caught farm civets compared to an 80 percent prevalence in civets exposed to the wildlife trade.[8] The civets in this case served as transmitters of the bat coronavirus, wherein the virus was able to adapt and infect humans.

Bats have been shown to host a variety of coronavirus strains as well as such other zoonoses as rabies, henipaviruses (Nipah and Hendra viruses), and Menangle virus. Despite this, bats remain common in the wildlife trade for a range of purposes. from food to display items at trade shows, the latter being a reason for importation into the United States. Bats are a critical component of their native ecosystems, and for a variety of factors (longevity, low reproductive rate, roosting behavior, and loss of habitat), the conservation of many of their populations are threatened by their lack of ability to sustain current harvests by the wildlife trade.[9]

Highly Pathogenic H5N1 Influenza

Avian influenza viruses have been linked with their natural hosts, wild aquatic birds, for probably hundreds of years. Avian influenzas are made up of various combinations, or subtypes, based on two categories of antigen (proteins) they carry on the outer surface of the virus, abbreviated H (hemagglutinin) and N (neuraminidase). There are 16 different H subtypes and 9 different N subtypes, leading to 144 possible subtype combinations (e.g., H5N1, H1N1, H9N3, etc.), each with numerous strains that are constantly evolving and adapting in their host(s). In the natural host, wild birds, the virus rarely ever causes serious illness. However, when the low pathogenic forms of these viruses spill over into other species, such as chickens or pigs, they have the capacity to change and mutate into high pathogenic forms, deadly to those infected. Transmission of avian influenza viruses from wild water birds to domestic birds and mammals occurs most commonly when animals are not housed in a manner to protect them from contact with wild birds. Once infected, especially if the virus then mutates to a particularly contagious strain, poultry can then spread the disease to other birds and mammals including humans. Numerous particularly dangerous strains have caused human outbreaks in the past, most notably the 1918 Spanish flu pandemic and the currently circulating H5N1 virus. The potential for an avian influenza virus to mix with a human influenza virus in a co-infected human to become a dangerous strain that can easily pass from human to human is of great concern. This did occur with the 1918 virus that killed between 50 and 100 million people worldwide in one year alone, and the fear is that the same will happen with the current H5N1 strain, which has a higher case fatality (60%). The fact that the virus has become endemic in areas of Southeast Asia such as Indonesia is of great concern regarding this potential scenario.

The degree of interspecies mixing (wild birds, domestic birds, mammals, and humans) in live trade markets, particularly in Asia where H5N1 highly pathogenic avian influenza first emerged, is of great concern. The role of these markets in the initial emergence (first transmission event) of H5N1 virus remains unknown, but they are likely to have played a role somewhere along the line. Subsequent spread and eventual permanent establishment in parts of Asia are largely attributed to the trade of domestic waterfowl and poultry in these markets. In 2004, two endangered hawk eagles smuggled into Belgium were intercepted and tested positive for the highly pathogenic H5N1 virus, as did a parrot intercepted at an airport in Great Britain in 2005. Although the wild bird trade itself was not the primary force in the spread of highly pathogenic H5N1, these cases exemplify the ability of the illegal trade to transmit diseases between species and penetrate geographic and legal barriers set by governments to protect their agriculture and citizens. Despite extensive surveillance, the lack of evidence to support a significant role of free-ranging wild birds in disseminating the highly pathogenic form of H5N1 to humans or poultry shows that anthropogenic factors are key drivers of this disease.

Immunodeficiency Viruses

There are two types of human immunodeficiency viruses in circulation today, HIV-1 and HIV-2. HIV-1 has four different subgroups, characterized as M (responsible for the well-known global pandemic), N, O, and P. In 1999, a group of researchers led by Dr. Beatrice Hahn of the Center for AIDS Research at the University of Alabama, Birmingham, discovered that three of these groups (M, N, and O) emerged in humans as result of several spillover events from chimpanzees (*Pan troglodytes troglodytes*) of western equatorial Africa likely within the early part of the 20th century. Researchers believe the most likely route of transmission was contact with chimpanzees infected with simian immunodeficiency virus (SIV) and hunted for bushmeat. More recently, scientists identified HIV-1 group P in a Cameroon woman, linking it to a gorilla strain of SIV, which is also believed to have originated from chimpanzees. HIV-2, another strain found primarily in people from West Africa thus far, is most closely related to the SIV strain of sooty mangabeys (common in the pet and food trade in Africa), and has originated through even more numerous cross-species transmission events, yielding HIV-2 groups A to H.

Although in the past critics speculated perhaps the virus was introduced into humans via contaminated polio vaccinations or at a research laboratory, these theories have been discredited by evidence through Hahn's work that the animal-to-human transmission events occurred prior to vaccination campaigns, that the pathogen host species are different from those used in vaccination development, and the fact that distribution of the various strains and clades of (both HIV-1 and HIV-2) viruses in people reflect that of the corresponding SIV strains in wildlife throughout the area of emergence.

Serosurveillance studies have shown a prevalence of SIV greater than 30 percent in free-ranging chimpanzees, sooty mangabeys, and green monkeys. However, serologic (antibody) evidence exists for numerous SIV strains in a large number of additional species, some of which have only been partially characterized, and the discoveries continue.[10] It is likely we are not aware of all the nonhuman primate-to-human transmission events that have occurred.

Despite the relatively high prevalence of lentiviruses such as SIV, nonhuman primate species such as chimpanzees and mangabeys continue to be hunted for the bushmeat trade. The possibility for novel transmission events and subsequent global dissemination of new HIV strains exists.

6.1. DID YOU KNOW?

- Congressional Reporting Service reported that 25 percent of 212 invasive species established in the wild in the United States were originally imported as pets.

- In 1994, Belgium customs officers were hospitalized with psittacosis after confiscating exotic parakeets smuggled from India.

- In China, early SARS infection was most common in live animal traders.

- A 2009 outbreak of salmonellosis in nearly 70 American children was attributed to an increase in pet frogs, sparked by a popular children's film.

T-Lymphotrophic Viruses

In the same retrovirus family as SIV and HIV is human T-lymphotrophic virus (HTLV), also originating from a simian counterpart in African nonhuman primates, and simian T-lymphotropic virus (STLV). So far, there have been four HTLV viruses found in humans that are very similar to, and are believed to have originated from, corresponding STLV strains in various species of nonhuman primates via multiple transmission events.

HTLV-1 infects 15 million to 20 million people worldwide and is spread from person to person via bodily fluids. It was not until decades after the disease was first discovered that scientists found it could cause cancer disorders (leukemia and lymphoma), neurologic disease (paraparesis), and several other illnesses still being uncovered. It has been directly linked to STLV-1, endemic in many nonhuman primate species from both Africa and Asia. HTLV-2 is rarer and is not as clearly linked to disease, and is believed to have derived from its STLV analog in the distant past. The additional discoveries of HTLV-3 and HTLV-4 and a novel strain similar to STLV-1 were recently made in nonhuman primate hunters in Cameroon. HTLV-3 was found to have emerged from STLV-3, endemic in nonhuman primates in the same region of Africa. A simian analog of HTLV-4 has yet to be found. Scientists are currently investigating the prevalence and health impact of these new strains. One study showed that 89 percent of hunted bushmeat in Cameroon was infected with STLV strains.[1] These findings have strengthened the belief that humans were and remain exposed to these viruses via handling and consuming bushmeat.[11]

Other Retroviruses

Also within the *Retroviridae* family are simian type D retrovirus (SRV) and simian foamy virus (SFV), both endemic in nonhuman primates. SRV has been found in a high number of Asian macaque species, in which it causes a severe immunosuppressive disorder similar to SIV. SFVs have been found in high percentages of Asian and African free-ranging nonhuman primates, as well as captive nonhuman primates in the United States, and do not typically cause illness in the host. Both viruses can infect humans. In fact, a recent study found 5.3 percent of the people tested who work with captive nonhuman primates had antibodies to SFV.[12] The mode of transmission for these viruses is unknown, but many infected claimed never to be bitten by a nonhuman primate, suggesting a less invasive mode of infection. However, evidence indicates these viruses are not easily spread from human to human, although scientists have isolated live virus from carriers decades after infection. Infected humans have yet to exhibit clinical illness definitively attributed to SFV, although suspected links between SFV infection and predisposition to other diseases are being investigated. Retroviruses are known for their potential to cause immunosuppression and their long latency periods, meaning they tend to linger for years in the infected host before causing disease.

Salmonella

The hunting and trade of wildlife can result in an ideal mechanism for not only the emergence of novel pathogens such as HIV and SARS, but also the recurrence and propagation of such well-known pathogens as *Salmonella*. Reptiles are common carriers of *Salmonella* and are more prone to shedding the disease when stressed. The numbers of live reptiles present in the wildlife trade markets around the globe are nearly incalculable. In Asia, live reptiles are commonly sold at wet markets for human consumption—the estimated number of turtles consumed in China alone per year is more than 30 million. According to the Animals Asia Foundation, between 2002 and 2005 more than 30 million native turtles were exported legally from the United States, 70 percent destined for the meat markets of Asia.

In 1975, the FDA banned the importation of turtles with shells less than four inches in length due to the higher capacity for these young reptiles to shed *Salmonella*, the likelihood of small children to handle these pets, and the large number of childhood cases of salmonellosis that were being seen. The ban is reported to have prevented an estimated 100,000 cases of salmonellosis each year in children. However, because of weaknesses in enforcement and exceptions in the law (such as sales for educational purposes), cases of directly and indirectly transmitted salmonellosis in children continue to occur, such as the three-week old infant who died acutely of a *Salmonella* infection that was definitively linked to a pet turtle in the home.

Other reptiles and species of wildlife kept as exotic pets are also capable of transmitting *Salmonella*. Estimates in the early 1990s showed U.S. trade accounted for 80 percent of the total world trade of 70 endangered reptile species. Approximately 1 million pet reptiles are imported into the United States every year, and according to the U.S. Department of Agriculture (USDA), lizards comprise more than 80 percent of all live reptile imports. Iguanas are one of the most common reptile pets, frequently carry salmonella, and are capable of shedding it regardless of their age or size.[3] African pygmy hedgehogs, sugar gliders, and birds have also been implicated in human salmonellosis cases in the United States. Although many animals, including humans are capable of carrying and transmitting *Salmonella*, the strains of the bacteria found in these exotic species are often atypical and potentially more dangerous. In fact, the CDC reports *Salmonella* illness remains a major public health problem, with an estimated 1.4 million human *Salmonella* infections occurring annually in the United States, resulting in approximately 15,000 hospitalizations and 400 deaths. A recently proposed bill in the Louisiana state legislature that would require iguana retailers to inform new owners of the risk of salmonellosis was voted down.

Other Zoonoses

There are many other examples of diseases that have either emerged, been spread, or have the potential to be transmitted via the trade in wildlife. Hantaviruses, leptospirosis, psittacosis, lymphocytic choriomeningitis, ringworm, plague, rabies, yellow fever, tularemia, herpes B, Nipah virus, Lassa fever—the list goes on and on.

Beyond the threat to humans, there are innumerable examples of animal diseases that, through the trade of wildlife and domestic animals, have had detrimental impacts on populations of wildlife as well as agricultural industries. *Batrachochytrium dendrobatidis* (also known as chytridiomycosis or chytrid fungus), responsible for decimation of amphibian populations worldwide, is believed to have been spread by international trade of African frogs decades ago. International spread of reportable fish diseases such as spring viremia of carp and koi herpes virus have been facilitated by the lack of quarantine requirements for fish importation by nations (including the United States) and have threatened both food fish and ornamental fish industries. Foot and mouth disease, a highly contagious viral disease of domestic livestock that can infect any cloven hoofed domestic or wild animal (and a few others such as hedgehogs and elephants), has plagued many nations for centuries, but spread most significantly after

World War II. The disease has resulted in more international trade bans than any other disease, led to the culling of billions of livestock animals, and has had cumulative primary and secondary worldwide economic impacts impossible to imagine. The direct cost of the 2001 outbreak in the UK (believed to have originated from illegally imported meat fed to pigs) alone was estimated at $20 billion.

Furthermore, infectious diseases do not always need direct contact to encounter new hosts. Vector-borne diseases (diseases transmitted by vectors such as mosquitoes, ticks, or fleas) also have potential to be distributed through trade. In 2000, the USDA banned three species of tortoise—leopard tortoise (*Geochelone pardalis*), African spurred tortoise (*Geochelone sulcata*), and Bell's hingeback tortoise (*Kinixys belliana*)—due to their ability to carry the Amblyomma tick, which can transmit heartwater, a disease deadly to cattle. Mosquito-borne West Nile virus suddenly appeared in New York in 1999, a city that receives some of the highest numbers of humans and animals from abroad. Although more difficult to recognize because of the requirement for an adequate host and vector species to be present in the same region of importation, vector-borne diseases in some ways pose an increased risk for disease introduction due to their decreased likelihood of being recognized at the border.

GLOBAL RESPONSE

The movement and intermingling of wildlife, domestic animals, and humans that occurs during the process of wildlife extraction and trade creates the perfect mixing pot for disease emergence and spread. Not only are those who engage in the trade at risk from zoonotic disease, but in today's globalized society a pathogen can become a global pandemic in a matter of days.

In addition to impacts on public health, disease outbreaks destabilize trade, have devastating effects on human livelihoods and food security, and have caused hundreds of billions of dollars of economic damage globally.[4] The economic impact associated with the SARS outbreak alone resulted in a 2 percent loss of the total East Asia and Southeast Asia GDP in 2003. It is clear from such experiences that the cost of implementing disease surveillance surrounding high-risk activities such as the wildlife trade and instituting key preventative measures would likely outweigh the price of the next global pandemic.

With so many complex and evolving factors influencing the health of our planet, we can no longer take unilateral approaches to solve multilateral problems. To adequately address the complexities of behaviorally driven zoonotic disease emergence and spread, closer collaboration among public and wildlife health sectors, social scientists, policy makers, the pet industry, and others is required. The human and animal health sectors must work together before outbreaks occur to investigate risks associated with specific zoonotic pathogens. Governments should support this type of professional cross-pollination through education and working committees, and encourage sharing of wildlife trade data through a global information network, as no one sector can successfully tackle this challenge alone.

Wildlife are a vital component to basic ecosystem functioning, on which humankind depends in so many ways, from basic subsistence, to clean air and water, to spiritual well-being. We should not view wildlife as sources of disease, but rather as cohabitants on this planet that (like humans) naturally carry pathogens with which they have evolved for thousands of years. We cannot (and in most cases should not) eliminate these pathogens in wildlife. Instead, we must reexamine the human behaviors that compromise natural boundaries to interspecies disease transmission and put at risk ecosystem health, and therein our own.

DOMESTIC RESPONSE

Cross-collaboration, legislation and enforcement loopholes, and capacity needs should also be addressed at home. There is currently very little health regulation of wildlife and wildlife products entering the United States, posing an unexamined risk to public health and the U.S. economy. New York is the most frequent port of entry for people and shipments into the United States and together with Los Angeles and Miami accounts for more than half of all known wildlife imports entering the country, with New York and Los Angeles also hosting the highest human populations in the country. According to USFWS, countries of origin of imports into the United States whose shipments were most often refused include China, the Philippines, Hong Kong, Thailand, and Nigeria. Endemism in these countries of diseases of risk to human health are many, including highly pathogenic H5N1, Nipah virus, and simian immunodeficiency virus to name a few.

Regulating agencies include the U.S. Fish and Wildlife Service— tasked to enforce CITES, the Endangered Species Act, and the Lacey Act (and to protect the health of U.S. native wildlife populations although no veterinary capacity exists within the agency); U.S. Department of Agriculture—tasked to protect the health of our livestock and poultry and other agricultural products; and the Centers for Disease Control and Prevention—tasked to protect human health. The USFWS Office of Law Enforcement (OLE) keeps the Law Enforcement Management Information System (LEMIS), a database where legal wildlife shipments and confiscations of illegal wildlife shipments are recorded. However, especially in the case of confiscated illegal shipments, the level of detail regarding species or number of animals entered into the system is often limited. and it is thus difficult to assess potential health risks associated with importations.[6]

Few imported wildlife taxa are regulated from the public health perspective. Imported wild bird species are required by USDA to undergo a mandatory quarantine upon arrival and/or be deemed to be free of poultry diseases, including highly pathogenic H5N1 and psittacosis, which can also infect people. In certain cases, this requirement is limited to a health certificate from a veterinary officer in the country of export and visual inspection upon arrival. Although the Wild Bird Conservation Act of 1992 has greatly restricted the legal importation of many wild bird species, smuggling of these birds across the Mexican border appears to be increasing. USDA also regulates importation of certain exotic ruminant species, some fish, hedgehogs, tenrecs, and brushtail possums from specific areas with foreign animal diseases, such as foot-and-mouth disease, and the few species of tortoises that previously were imported carrying ticks harboring heartwater disease. At present, USDA does not regulate any species from a public health perspective. The CDC regulates nonhuman primate imports, mandating they undergo a one-month quarantine at their destination facility (if permitted). Despite the capacity for these species to harbor numerous zoonotic pathogens, imports are only required to receive standard testing for tuberculosis (unless obvious signs of illness are exhibited).

Some species are banned altogether (unless a permit is acquired) by the CDC from entry into the United States due to public health concerns, largely in response to disease introductions after they have already occurred. These include turtles with shells less than four inches in length, bats, civets, and six genera of West African rodents. Small turtles were banned in 1975 due to salmonellosis outbreaks in children handling them as pets. Civets were banned following the 2002–2003 SARS epidemic. West African rodents were banned following their role in the 2003 monkeypox outbreak, resulting in higher numbers of rodents being imported from other continents.

The agencies do an excellent job of enforcing their regulations with what resources they have, but the limited regulations that exist are based on past mishaps rather than potential risk. Further, there is no agency with the overall task of monitoring potential health risks associated with trade in wildlife.

For the most part, screening for wildlife pathogens is left to the discretion of the importer. Research laboratories and American Zoological Association–accredited facilities maintain a high level of health and disease inspection to protect their staff and animal collections. However, for the bulk of live wildlife destined for the pet trade there are no current health requirements in place. This gap could represent a major health risk to the U.S. public, domestic animals, agricultural industry, and native wildlife populations.

Similarly, although illegal to import, there has historically been no surveillance system in place for pathogens in smuggled animals or animal products. The amount of these items entering the United States every year is likely significant. At U.S. borders, live animals and animal products being smuggled into the country in passenger luggage or mail are subject to inspection and/or confiscation if detected by the Department of Homeland Security's Customs and Border Protection and Customs and Border Protection Agriculture Specialists (CBP). However, CBP is the first, and often only, interception point for drugs, weapons, plants, animals, and all other illegal or smuggled materials entering the country—and the workload is substantial. On a given day, CBP processes more than 1 million passengers and pedestrians and more than 79,000 shipments of approved goods at points of entry. At John F. Kennedy Airport in New York alone, CBP processes millions of international passengers and more than 1 million metric tons of international freight annually. The sophistication and sheer volume of the wildlife trade undermines the ability of CBP to intercept all items of risk. Bushmeat and other illegal trade products from abroad are making their way into U.S. markets on a routine basis. Although state agencies monitor for such items, these markets often operate with a very low profile and thus remain unobserved.

When items are successfully confiscated, CBP routinely notifies the relevant agency when one of their regulated animal or plant items is detected. The agency (e.g., USFWS, CDC, USDA) will then make a record of, confiscate, and place (in the case of live animals) or incinerate (in the case of plants or animal products) high-risk items to alleviate any potential risk of introduction of injurious species or diseases into the country. However, the lack of disease surveillance of confiscated items ignores the potential risk posed by similar items that go undetected, and prohibits research that would inform regulations and public health campaigns. This current gap in knowledge presents an ill-defined risk to human health in the United States and globally.

An interagency working group, calling upon additional expertise where needed (such as in wildlife health) has been recommended to assess risks posed to human, native wildlife, pets, and our agricultural industry by wildlife imported into the United States. Improved record systems, risk analysis based on science rather than past outbreaks, and creation of a safe list of imported species are among the recommendations by scientists that merit consideration. Fundamentally, the regulating agencies are lacking the support necessary to face this growing challenge.

As part of the global community, developed countries must recognize their role in overexploitation of natural resources in developing nations in exchange for helping to preserve these valuable resources while creating sustainable livelihoods and protecting global health. Considerations surrounding these complex issues are many, and it will take a cooperative, multidisciplinary approach to solve the threats posed to conservation and human and animal health.

FURTHER READING

Chomel BB, Belotto A, Meslin F. Wildlife, exotic pets, and emerging zoonoses. *Emerging Infectious Diseases* 2007;13:6–11.

Karesh WB, Cook RA, Gilbert M, et al. Implications of the wildlife trade on the movement of avian influenza and other infectious diseases. *Journal of Wildlife Diseases* 2007;43:55–9.

Marano NM, Galland GG, Blanton JD, et al. Public health impact of global trade in animals. In: Relman DA, Choffnes ER, Mack A, rapporteurs. *Infectious disease movement in a borderless world: Forum on microbial threats.* Washington, DC: National Academies Press; 2010:134–49.

Pavlin BI, Schloegel LM, Daszak P. Risk of importing zoonotic diseases through wildlife trade, United States. *Emerging Infectious Diseases* 2009;15:1721–6.

Wolfe ND, Dunavan CP, Diamond J. Origins of major human infectious diseases. *Nature* 2007;447:279–83.

REFERENCES

1. Pearce-Duvet JMC. The origin of human pathogens: Evaluating the role of agriculture and domestic animals in the evolution of human disease. *Biological Review Cambridge Philosophical Society* 2006;81:369–82.
2. Harvard Medical School Website. *Biodiversity: Its importance to human health: Interim executive summary.* Available at: http://chge.med.harvard.edu/publications/documents/Biodiversity_v2_screen.pdf.
3. Chomel BB, Belotto A, Meslin F. Wildlife, exotic pets, and emerging zoonoses. *Emerging Infectious Diseases* 2007;13:6–11.
4. Karesh WB, Cook RA, Bennett EL, et al. Wildlife trade and global disease emergence. *Emerging Infectious Diseases* 2005;11:1000–2.
5. Fa JE, Peres CA, Meeuwig JE. Bushmeat exploitation in tropical forests: An intercontinental comparison. *Conservation Biology* 2002;16:232–7.
6. Smith K, Behrens M, Schloegel LM, et al. Reducing the risks of the wildlife trade. *Science Policy Forum* 2009;324:594–5.
7. Greger M. The human/animal interface: Emergence and resurgence of zoonotic infectious diseases. *Critical Reviews in Microbiology* 2007;33:243–99.
8. Tu C, Crameri G, Kong X, et al. Antibodies to SARS coronavirus in civets. *Emerging Infectious Diseases* 2004;10:2244–8.
9. Mickleburgh S, Waylen K, Racey P. Bats as bushmeat. *Oryx* 2009;43:217–34.
10. Beer BE, Bailes E, Sharp PM, et al. Diversity and evolution of primate lentiviruses. In: Kuiken CL, Foley B, Hahn B, et al., eds. *Human retro-viruses and AIDS.* Los Alamos: Theoretical Biology and Biophysics Group, 1999: 460–74.

11. Courgnaud V, Van Dooren S, Liegeois F, et al. Simian T-cell leukemia virus (STLV) infection in wild primate populations in Cameroon evidence for dual STLV type 1 and type 3 infection in agile mangabeys (*Cercocebus agilis*). *Journal of Virology* 2004;78(9):4700–9.
12. Switzer WM, Bhullar V, Shanmugam V, et al. Frequent simian foamy virus infection in persons occupationally exposed to nonhuman primates. *Journal of Virology* 2004;78(6):2780–9.

Chapter 7

Immunocompromised, High-Risk Populations and Animals

Radford G. Davis, DVM, MPH, DACVPM

PETS AND OUR HEALTH

In 1988, approximately 56 percent of U.S. households had a pet. By 2008, that figure was up to 62 percent.[1] The animals we have as pets today go beyond dogs and cats and hamsters to include more homes than ever with reptiles, a multitude of "pocket pets," birds, and other exotic species. We have remarkable relationships with our pets, which bring us benefits we are hard-pressed to find elsewhere: nonjudgmental devotion, companionship, entertainment, improvement in our physical and psychological well-being, and much, much more.

For many people, pets are family members. We understand, too, that having an animal companion requires that we provide them with comfort, shelter, veterinary medical care, nutritious food, water, relief of pain, and all of the other things that one should provide a family member and friend. And just like the other family members we share our home with, we can also share diseases with our pets. Some disease agents can be carried by animals and transmitted to people (zoonoses), and there other, far fewer, disease agents that people can transmit to their pets.

For people, like animals, the immune system is vital to keeping invading pathogens at bay, battling them if the pestilential agents do make it into our systems, and ultimately getting rid of them so that we may fully recover our health. Should our immune system be overwhelmed by invading microbes, or perhaps be outwitted by a microbe (HIV is a good example), or if our immune system is compromised or suppressed in some manner, then our chances of winning the fight against disease diminishes, and so does our survival.

OUR IMMUNE SYSTEM

Our immune system is composed of many components, a redundant and sometimes overlapping system, to fight off microbes and keep us healthy. Some aspects of it are quite simple and others highly complex. If our immune system falters or is overwhelmed by microbial invaders, disease and possibly death can result. The first component of our immune system that a pathogen might overcome to gain entry into our bodies is that of our physical barriers: our skin and the linings of our respiratory tract, gastrointestinal tract, and urinary tract, to name the most prominent ones. Wounds to our skin allow for easy access by microbial invaders. Our respiratory tract attempts to expel invaders by stimulating coughing and sneezing, and vomiting and diarrhea are the ways our gastrointestinal tract deals with foreigners. Of course, we have lots of good bacteria in our intestines, which help us process food and extract vitamins and minerals and so forth, so not all bacteria are unwanted. We can also find certain bacteria on our skin quite commonly, some of which are actually beneficial and others that may cause disease if given the right circumstances.

The next layer of defense for a microbe is our innate immune system. Here, enzymes in our bodies kill bacteria. Certain cells such as macrophages and neutrophils (types of white bloods cells) can detect bacteria and move in to destroy them, which can also give us inflammation at the site (think red, tender, and swollen when you have a cut on your finger). These white blood cells try to neutralize the pathogen and keep it from spreading. Additional products are produced by the body at this time, further helping kill the invaders. The innate component of our immune system has no memory, and the response is pretty much the same no matter who the invader is, though the response can be smaller or larger depending on the number of microbes. The innate system is always on, ready to respond.

Our last component of our immune system is more refined, more elaborate, complex and elegant, and it is the acquired immunity we get from an infection. Acquired immunity recognizes something specific about the invaders. This immunity has memory so that the next time it meets the same pathogen the response is quicker and more lethal. Acquired immunity takes days to develop after an exposure, so it is not immediate like the barriers or the innate components of our immune system, but without it we are not likely to live long, which is the unfortunate outcome with AIDS patients. Receptors on T cells and B cells of the acquired immune system can recognize a large number of foreign molecules, helping respond with a sweeping annihilation, and some cells retain memory of that encounter and are quicker to respond in greater numbers in the future—which is the basis for vaccination. Antibodies, produced by the B cells, latch onto structures on the outside of a pathogen and target it for destruction, and this is called the humoral immune response (since antibodies are found in the body's "humors," or fluids).[2] With the cell-mediated immune response, the body's T cells recognize proteins inside pathogens that are presented to them on special structures of a cell. The T cells either kill the infected cell outright or secrete products that help other parts of the immune system kill the pathogen. On top of all of this we have cells that keep our immune response from becoming too exuberant and cells that retain memory for faster response next time the same pathogen dares to appear.

THE IMMUNOCOMPROMISED PERSON

So what does it mean to be immunocompromised? The immunocompromised category includes anyone whose immune system is operating below the normal efficiency of a healthy adult for whatever reason—hence, compromised, leaving them open to more easily developing disease if infected. Broadly, the following groups are considered to be immunocompromised:[3]

- Infants (under one year of age)
- Pregnant women
- Elderly, especially over the age of 65 years
- Those on immunosuppressive medications, such as organ transplant recipients and chemotherapy patients
- Those receiving radiation therapy
- Those suffering from diabetes, kidney failure, liver cirrhosis, and malnutrition
- AIDS patients

Of course, this list is not exhaustive and other conditions that suppress the immune system could be listed. In the next few sections, we will consider some of these populations in more depth as well some situations and some animals that put immunocompromised people at higher risk for disease. It should be noted here that normal, healthy animals can carry and shed microbial pathogens (bacteria, viruses, protozoa, parasites) that can infect people. The risk of acquiring these agents is generally low. Also, just as important, the risk of an immunocompromised person acquiring a zoonotic infection is no greater than the risks faced by the average person; however, if the immunocompromised person does acquire infection, then he or she is more likely to develop severe consequences since the immune system is not as capable of eliminating the infection before disease sets in.

One last point: it is important to discern between those zoonotic infections immunocompromised people can acquire (which could be a very long list) versus those they do acquire. We could fill volumes discussing all the zoonoses that an immunocompromised person might acquire, but it would serve us better to discuss the high-risk populations, situations, animals, and consequent diseases that they are likely to encounter.

CHILDREN

Reptiles and Amphibians

The very young have not seen enough infectious pathogens in their short lives to develop a robust immune response with memory, so when they are infected by a microbe they are at higher risk for developing a more severe outcome—disease or even death. As a general guide, most public health professionals consider children under five years old to be at greater risk of illness from zoonoses, but those less than one year of age are at even greater risk. Objects such as pacifiers can fall to the ground and then placed back in the child's mouth, exposing them to pathogens.

Some animals pose a higher zoonotic risk to all immunocompromised individuals, but children are at somewhat greater risk because they are more likely to handle or encounter certain high-risk animals that other people are not. A good example of this is reptiles and amphibians. *Salmonella* is considered part of the normal flora of the intestinal tract of these animals (that is, they are part of the normal bacteria), yet we are all at risk for contracting salmonella from these animals unless we take proper precautions. Children are at higher risk, however, not only because their immune systems are not as well developed as those of adults, but because they are less likely to wash their hands after handling these animals compared to adults and more likely to do less than ideal things with them, such as put a small turtle in the mouth. There are many case reports of severe illness and even death in children, including infants, from salmonella acquired from the reptile or amphibian in the home. At the time of writing this book chapter, the United States was experiencing an outbreak of salmonella that caused illness in 217 individuals in 41 states and was linked to water frogs, specifically African dwarf frogs. People from 1 year to 73 years old became ill, with 71 percent of illnesses occurring in those less than 10 years old. No deaths have been reported.

While direct contact with the animals creates the highest risk for acquiring *Salmonella*, even indirect contact can pass along this pathogen. In 1996, it was estimated that nearly 400 people contracted salmonellosis from the wooden barrier at a Komodo dragon exhibit at the Denver zoo (ages ranged from three months to 48 years). In 2004, an 80-year-old woman in Wyoming contracted *Salmonella* and became severely ill. It was discovered that her family, whom she visited, owned a turtle and cleaned its bowl in the kitchen sink, where the meals were prepared.

It is the small turtles that kids are most attracted to and from which they are most likely to acquire *Salmonella*. Because of this, in 1975 the Food and Drug Administration (FDA) implemented a ban on the sale of turtles with a carapace diameter of four inches or less. The ban is estimated to prevent 100,000 cases of salmonellosis each year. The enforcement of this ban is left up to the states, so you may occasionally see people breaking the law and selling them since enforcement is difficult. Turtles under four inches can only legally be sold for scientific, educational, or exhibition purposes.

The Centers for Disease Control and Prevention (CDC) and the National Association of State Public Health Veterinarians have put out recommendations to prevent the transmission of *Salmonella* from reptiles and amphibians to humans, which can be found in Table 7.1.

Table 7.1
Recommendations for Preventing the Transmission of Salmonella from Reptiles and Amphibians to Humans[4]

Pet store owners, health-care practitioners, and veterinarians should provide information to owners and potential purchasers of reptiles and amphibians about the risk for acquiring salmonellosis from their pets.

Persons should always wash their hands with soap and water after handling reptiles and amphibians or their cages.

Persons at increased risk for infection with serious complications from salmonellosis (e.g., children aged under 5 years and immunocompromised persons) should avoid contact with reptiles and amphibians.

Reptiles and amphibians should be kept out of households with children aged under 5 years or immunocompromised persons. Families expecting a new child should give away their pet reptiles and amphibians before the infant arrives.

Reptiles and amphibians should not be allowed to roam freely throughout the house.

Reptiles and amphibians should not be kept in child-care centers.

Reptiles and amphibians should be kept out of kitchens and other food-preparation areas to prevent contamination.

Kitchen sinks should not be used to bathe pets or to wash their dishes, cages, or aquariums. If bathtubs are used for these purposes, they should be thoroughly cleaned afterward.

Pets in the Classroom

Which pet is best for a classroom or day care setting is arguable to some degree—no animal is sterile, and some animals are more likely to scratch or bite than others, but that doesn't mean we need to exclude all animals from the classroom. Animal husbandry, animal behavior, and proper handling of animals are important topics for children to learn and carry into adulthood. That said, certain pets should be kept out of classrooms with young children due to their inherent zoonotic risks. In addition to reptiles and amphibians, baby poultry (chicks, ducklings, and goslings) should not be around children under five years of age. Young ruminants, such as goats, sheep, and calves, may appear healthy but still shed zoonotic pathogens such as *Cryptosporidium*, *Campylobacter*, and *Escherichia coli* 0157:H7, so it is best that contact with these animals be limited and supervised to ensure hand washing after each contact. Ferrets, mice, and hamsters may bite, so younger children may be at greater risk of bites because they are less able to handle these types of animals in a prudent, cautious manner. Some children may be allergic to cats or afraid of dogs, so these issues must also be considered when choosing a pet for the classroom. Birds should be tested for *Chlamydophila psittaci* and an avian veterinarian consulted before placing them in the classroom. Some birds can also inflict severe bites.

Children should be supervised at all times in how they interact with an animal, ensuring also that children wash their hands well after touching the animal. A specific area in the classroom should be designated for animal contact (the animal should not be allowed to roam free), and all areas where the animal has been should be cleaned and disinfected afterward, and if children are put in charge of cleaning they should be supervised. No food or drinks should be permitted in the area where children interact with the animal. The chosen pet should have regular veterinary checkups, be in excellent health, free of parasites, and have all necessary vaccinations (including rabies for those animals that can be vaccinated for this). The National Association of State Public Health Veterinarians, in their document *Compendium of Measures to Prevent Disease Associated with Animals in Public Settings, 2009*, has many guidelines for pets in school and child-care settings,[5] most of which are summarized here.

Some states have restrictions on what animals are allowed in schools and/or child-care settings. For example, in Iowa the law specifically states:

Animals kept on site shall be in good health with no evidence of disease, be of such disposition as to not pose a safety threat to children, and be maintained in a clean and sanitary manner. Documentation of current vaccinations shall be available for all cats and dogs. No ferrets, reptiles, including turtles, or birds of the parrot family shall be kept on site. Pets shall not be allowed in kitchen or food preparation areas.

Stray animals, aggressive animals, wild animals, monkeys, rabies reservoir animals (raccoons, bats, skunks, foxes, coyotes), venomous/poisonous animals, and inherently dangerous animals (lions, tigers, bears, etc.) should never be allowed into a school or child-care center.

Choosing a pet for the classroom should be done in consultation with a veterinarian, school officials, and parents so that a suitable pet can be found that is unlikely to transmit a zoonosis and is unlikely to inflict trauma or inflame allergies.

Animal Exhibits—Petting Zoos

Every year there are numerous children, and some adults, who contract illness from attending a petting zoo or other animal exhibit. In fact, from 1996 to 2008, there were approximately 100 documented human outbreaks connected with petting zoos,[5] and very probably there were many more cases that never came to light. *E. coli*, *Salmonella*, and *Cryptosporidium* are three of the most common zoonotic pathogens found in a petting zoo that are responsible for human illness. There are, of course, many other zoonotic diseases that can be contracted in an animal exhibit–petting zoo setting if precautions are not taken. For example, livestock-birthing exhibits can be found at some fairs. Q fever (*Coxiella burnetii*), leptospirosis, listeriosis, brucellosis, and chlamydosis can be acquired if there is contact with birthing materials or fluids, contact with objects contaminated with birthing fluids, or, especially in the case of Q fever, through contaminated dust that becomes airborne. Orf, a virus, is commonly carried by sheep, goats, and such wild ungulates as reindeer and primarily causes lesions on the hands, arms, or faces in people. These agents pose health concerns not just to children, but to healthy adults as well, and they are a particular concern to immunocompromised individuals, especially pregnant women, which we will discuss later in this chapter.

Of course, as you might imagine, many of our recommendations for classroom settings also apply pretty well to animal exhibits–petting zoos. For example, it is recommended to keep raccoons, foxes, and skunks out of petting zoos since they are more likely to carry rabies than other, domestic, animals. In addition to most of the classroom recommendations, toys, pacifiers, sippy cups, and baby bottles should be kept out of a petting zoo as they might become contaminated if touched to a surface or dropped on the ground, subsequently infecting the child. Strollers should be kept out, too. There should be no smoking or eating or drinking, and there should be staff and parental supervision of children at all times. Running water and soap should be out in plain sight at the exit for everyone to wash up before leaving, with attention to making sure children can reach the soap, faucet, and sink on their own. Everyone should wash their hands well for 20 seconds before leaving.

Petting zoos can be a great way to introduce children to animals they are not familiar with—maybe they have only read about goats or only seen sheep in movies—but exhibit owners, staff, and parents all have responsibilities and duties to ensure the experience is a safe and positive one for children.

HIV/AIDS

After HIV enters the body, one of its primary targets to infiltrate is the CD4+ T cells, which help direct the body's immune response to infection. During the final stages of HIV infection, known as AIDS, a person's T cell levels drops dramatically, allowing other microbes to easily infect the person and cause disease, and possibly death. A person does not die from the virus directly, but from the immunocompromised condition that allows other pathogens (or even cancers) to invade, remain unchecked, and cause disease. These microbes are considered to be secondary invaders or opportunistic. In fact, opportunistic infections, including some zoonoses, were responsible for up to 90 percent of deaths of those with AIDS prior to 1998. Today, deaths among those with AIDS due to opportunistic infections have dropped to around 50 percent, thanks to advances in antiviral medications and new approaches to treatment and prevention.

The CDC estimates there are approximately 1.1 million people infected with the HIV virus in the United States, and 1 in 5 of those infected do not know it. A person with HIV can live decades under today's medical care, and more people today are living with AIDS than ever before. This translates into potentially years of being at higher-risk to the severe consequences of zoonoses. AIDS-defining diseases (of which there are 26) that are animal-related include: cryptococcosis, cryptosporidiosis, mycobacteriosis, salmonellosis, and toxoplasmosis.[6] It should be pointed out that food, water, and the environment can serve as sources of infection for all of these agents in addition to animals, and in some cases, such as with *Toxoplasma gondii*, which causes toxoplasmosis, the animal (cat) is very unlikely to be the direct source of infection for people.

People often wonder if a person with HIV or AIDS should own a pet. One study of those living with AIDS found no significant difference between pet owners and non–pet owners in rates of opportunistic infections,[7] indicating that pet ownership does not dramatically increase the risk of AIDS-defining zoonotic opportunistic infections. It has been shown that those with AIDS who owned pets reported less depression than those with AIDS who did not own a pet, especially among those with less social support. Because of societal stigmas and discrimination, perhaps even isolation, those with HIV/AIDS may have a very strong bond with their pets, a bond that is beneficial to that person and their mental and physical well-being.

PREGNANT WOMEN

Pregnancy involves a balance of the mother's immune system that prevents attack against the fetus while at the same time keeping the mother, and therefore the fetus, healthy. This is a highly complicated proposition. While parts of the mother's immune system might be suppressed in order to allow her to carry the child to term, other components will be enhanced. It is believed that during pregnancy, the CD4+ T cells decrease, while the CD8+ T cells increase.[8] It is this suppression of CD4+ T cells that some believe increase the pregnant woman's susceptibility to viruses and to some pathogens that like to live inside cells, like the bacteria *Listeria monocytogenes*. This suppression of CD4+ cells has a benefit of sending women with rheumatoid arthritis and multiple sclerosis, both T cell-mediated diseases, into remission.[8] B cell function and antibody production are normal during pregnancy, and granulocytes, a type of white blood cell that is part of the innate immune system for killing invaders, may increase. Taken as a whole, a pregnant woman is more likely to respond to an infection with an antibody response than a T cell-mediated response.[8] This shift in the immune system is likely regulated by hormones, such as estrogen and progesterone, and serves to down regulate the cell-mediated immune response that would be harmful to the fetus. But again, this is a highly complex system and many other factors are likely play a role in this change in the immune system. In the end, the pregnant woman undergoes a rebalancing of her immune system, leaving maternal defenses intact. Nevertheless, some infections in pregnant women pose a higher risk for the health of the fetus, both in utero and after birth, as well as for the health of the mother.

Given all of this, there are some disease agents that the pregnant woman should be aware of and take precautions to avoid. It cannot be emphasized enough that, due to inherent zoonotic risks, pregnant women should not help pregnant animals in the delivery process or otherwise be around animal birthings.

Toxoplasma Gondii

Many people consider *Toxoplasma gondii* to be of paramount concern to the pregnant cat owner. However, even though cats are the definitive host for this zoonotic protozoa, they only shed this organism in their feces for a short duration (1–2 weeks), and only once in their lifetime. People are more likely to acquire infection with this pathogen from soil that has been contaminated by *Toxoplasma* oocysts (the egglike stage of this pathogen) in cat feces. These oocysts, after about 24 hours, become very hard and can survive for a year or longer in soil. Vegetables and water can sometimes be contaminated with this organism and serve as a medium for infection in people. Herbivores, such as sheep and cattle, can also pick this up while grazing, resulting in muscle cysts that can cause infection in the consumer unless the meat is well cooked. For these reasons, it is important to wear gloves when working with soil or sand, wash vegetables well, and cook your meat properly, and of course wash your hands thoroughly after taking off your gloves or after handling meat. Also, scooping out the litter box daily eliminates the oocysts before they become nearly indestructible. Disinfection of the litter box should be done weekly.

There are many different clinical outcomes for people who are infected with *Toxoplasma gondii,* ranging from no illness to severe illness. The risk to the fetus is mostly limited to the mother acquiring infection during pregnancy. Prior to pregnancy, a women infected with *Toxoplasma gondii* develops an immune response that keeps the cyst stage of this organism in check, where it does not cause illness. Many people are infected and actually do not know it. In this cyst stage, the organism is essentially dormant. At this stage, if the woman's blood were tested we would find that she had antibodies to *Toxoplasma gondii.* It is very unlikely that a woman who has been infected prior to becoming pregnant will go on to infect her fetus. However, a woman who is antibody negative for *Toxoplasma gondii* is at risk for becoming infected during pregnancy and passing on this infection to her fetus, where it can lead to a number of mild or severe outcomes.

Infants born to mothers who acquire their infection in the first or second trimester are more likely to have congenital disease as compared to mothers who are infected during their third trimester. However, it is during the third trimester when the fetus is more likely to become infected. No matter what trimester the mother is infected in, up to 85 percent of children will have some signs if not treated. Manifestations of congenital infection can vary from nonspecific to severe, with children developing rash, anemia, hydrocephalus, encephalitis, chorioretinitis (inflammation of the eye, especially the retina), blindness, epilepsy, or other consequences, with some signs not showing up for years after birth.

Should a woman (or anyone already infected with *Toxoplasma gondii*) become severely immunosuppressed, say due to medications or disease, she is at risk of having her latent or dormant infection reactivate, at which time she could conceivably infect her fetus.

Cats acquire this agent primarily by eating rodents and other animals. Cats that have lived indoors their entire lives are unlikely to become infected. There is no need to test the healthy cat for this disease. Again, cats only shed the oocysts for a short period of time, so veterinarians are not likely to discover this if they perform an analysis on the feces of the cat.

And a cat that is positive for antibodies will not shed this pathogen again in its lifetime unless it becomes severely immunocompromised by disease or medications.

In addition to the steps already mentioned, see the end of this chapter for a more thorough list of recommendations on how you can prevent being infected by *Toxoplasma gondii*.

7.1. DID YOU KNOW?

Conservatively speaking, when we count up everyone who could be classified as immunocompromised, that equates to nearly 20 percent of the U.S. population.

Listeriosis

Listeria monocytogenes is a bacteria that can cause life-threatening illness (listeriosis) in many immunocompromised people, from transplant recipients to the elderly to pregnant women. This agent can be found in the intestines of many species of domestic and wild animals, particularly sheep, goats, and cattle, without showing illness. It can also be found in soil and vegetation. While people might acquire this agent directly from animals, it is food and food products that are most often responsible for human infection. Raw, unpasteurized milk or cheese, meats, and even raw vegetables can be a source. We likely ingest this microbe almost daily. Pregnant women are about 20 times more likely to get listeriosis than healthy adults. There are several different clinical signs a person with listeriosis can show, but the biggest concern is to the unborn fetus. Infection of a pregnant woman can result in miscarriage, stillbirth, premature delivery, or infection of the child. An eight-state outbreak in 2002 in the northeastern United States led to 46 confirmed cases, seven deaths, and three stillbirths or miscarriages.[9]

Q Fever

Coxiella burnetii, the causative agent of Q fever, is shed in birthing fluids and membranes, particularly from sheep, goats, and cattle, but also rarely from other animals, such as cats. It is also shed in the urine, feces, and milk. People usually acquire the infection through inhalation. When livestock give birth outdoors, the fluids containing *Coxiella burnetii* evaporate, leaving behind this very hardy and environmentally resistant pathogen, which can be sent downwind with the next strong gust. Or it can contaminate the indoor barn, where it can be aerosolized in dust. Someone helping in calving, lambing, or kidding can get splashed in the face with birthing fluids, or they might not wash their hands good enough before eating—both good ways to become infected. About half of those infected never show signs, but those who do may experience severe fever, headaches, muscle aches, sore throat, sweats, vomiting, diarrhea, and even pneumonia. Disease in some cases can be severe and prolonged, with some needing heart valve transplants, and with death occurring in as much as two-thirds of those who develop chronic disease. Infection in pregnant women can be asymptomatic or can result in abortions, premature deliveries, and stillbirths, especially when the infection occurs during the first trimester. It also thought possible that the disease can reactivate in later pregnancies.

Chlamydophila Abortus

A major cause of abortions and loss of lambs in most areas of the world that raise sheep, the pregnant woman and her fetus are also at risk if infected with Chlamydophila abortus. Infection may lead to spontaneous abortion if the woman is infected in the first trimester, and later infections may lead to stillbirths or premature birth. Other health effects may include kidney failure, liver disease, and other severe outcomes, including death. Most cases of infection with this agent are linked to exposure to sheep or goats and are associated with helping animals in birthing, handling infected animals, or coming into contact with contaminated clothing. Hand-to-mouth activities, such as eating or smoking, can transmit this pathogen if hands are not washed well. This agent, like the other species of Chlamydophila, is fairly resistant to drying and can remain in the environment for some months.

Brucellosis

There are several different species of the bacteria Brucella, and many of them can infect animals and people. This disease agent has been found in sheep, cattle, goats, pigs, dogs, hares, wild rodents, some marine mammals, bison, elk, reindeer, and perhaps a few other animal species. This agent typically causes reproductive disease in infected animals (abortion, inflammation of testicles). Brucella organisms can be shed in reproductive fluids and tissues (placenta), and milk, which is a very good reason why a person should not drink milk unless it is pasteurized. It has rarely been reported in meat, but this is a much less significant route of human infection. People can acquire Brucella through ingestion in contaminated milk, cheese, or other dairy products, through direct contact with infected birthing fluids and tissues, inhalation (usually while helping deliver a newborn), and splashes of birthing fluids to the face. Much rarer modes of transmission include person to person and mother to unborn fetus. Most infections in people come from contaminated raw dairy products.

Signs in people infected with *Brucella* can be quite varied and include a cyclical fever, night sweats, headaches, joint pain, and malaise. The disease can progress and symptoms worsen: arthritis, inflammation of the heart valves, and disease of various organs, including the gastrointestinal tract and the nervous system. In pregnant women, *Brucella* infection has led to spontaneous abortions.

Leptospirosis

Leptospirosis is the most widespread zoonoses in the world, being more common in tropical areas. There are more than 200 serovar (strains) of *Leptospira interrogans* that are able to cause disease in people and mammals. These bacteria have been found in more than 180 animal species, including animals we might have close contact with, such as cattle, horses, and dogs. The bacteria survives best in moist, wet environments, and infection in an animal may result in illness, depending on many factors, such as which serovar is infecting the animal. Infection often results in the microbe being excreted in the urine, which can find its way into water and spread to other animals or people. Sometimes animals can shed these organisms for years. People usually acquire this infection through contact with contaminated water or directly from the infected urine of animals. Infection in people can result in a very broad range of signs and symptoms, from no signs, a self-limiting illness of flulike symptoms, to such more dramatic signs as severe conjunctival redness, severe muscle pain, severe headache, nausea, vomiting, diarrhea, cough, kidney failure, liver disease, jaundice, meningitis, and even death. Among livestock, this agent can cause abortions and stillbirth. In pregnant women, infection has been reported to result in abortion and fetal death.

Recreational exposures to this agent appear to be on the rise. In 1998, the United States had its biggest outbreak ever when more than 100 triathlon athletes and more than 225 community citizens in Illinois fell ill after swimming in a contaminated lake.

Lymphocytic Choriomeningitis Virus (LCMV)

LCMV is a virus that is most often found in the house mouse (*Mus musculus*), and rarely found in our pet rodents, such as guinea pigs, hamsters, and gerbils. However, these more domesticated rodents can be infected through contact with the droppings or urine of the house mouse even before they enter our homes. LCMV can be a serious concern in the immunocompromised person. In 2005, the CDC reported four cases of LCMV in organ transplant recipients, with three deaths. These cases were traced back to a hamster sold in a pet shop. Two other hamsters and a guinea pig in the same pet shop were found to be infected with LCMV. People can contract LCMV by coming into contact with the urine, feces, saliva, or nesting materials of infected rodents. Signs of illness in people include fever, chills, vomiting, aching, headache, and possibly meningitis. Those who are immunocompromised are more likely to have a more severe outcome, including death.

Pregnant women infected with this agent are at risk for abortion and possible congenital manifestations, such as chorioretinitis, blindness, hydrocephalus, and mental retardation. Because of these risks, the CDC recommends that pregnant women, women planning to become pregnant, and other immunocompromised individuals not have rodents as pets. That said, the risk of one pet rodent harboring LCMV is low, and shedding of LCMV is probably highest just after purchase. Therefore, since exposure to this virus occurs early on when the rodent is brought into the home, continued handling and interaction with the pet is unlikely to increase the risk to the immunocompromised person.

Lyme Disease

More research is needed into the adverse health effects of *Borrelia burgdorferi* infection in pregnant women, but there is some evidence to suggest that there is heightened risk for abortion, stillbirth, preterm birth, and possibly endometriosis. This tick-transmitted disease is not thought to be a common cause of stillbirth.

Other Diseases of Concern to Pregnant Women

Many viruses, bacteria, and protozoa can directly infect the mother, cause placental damage, stillbirth, and severe maternal illness. Roughly 10–25 percent of stillbirths in more developed countries may be due to infections.[10] *Escherichia coli,* group B streptococcus, and *Ureaplasma urealyticum* (all bacteria) are common causes of stillbirth. Syphilis, where common, can be a significant cause of stillbirths. Malaria can also cause stillbirth in those women pregnant for their first time. Parvovirus and Coxsackie's virus are two important viral causes of stillbirth.

THE ELDERLY

With age, the cell-mediated and humoral immune systems decline, what is called immunosenescence,[2] leaving elderly individuals at increased risk. Virtually all of the recommendations we have made for other groups so far apply to the elderly as well. If animals are to be allowed into a nursing home, it is important to work with the health-care staff to meet their guidelines and ensure that the animal is in excellent health and has regular veterinary examinations. Consultation with a veterinarian can help identify a safe, appropriate pet. Some animals that are high risk, such as reptiles, amphibians, chicks, and ferrets, should never be allowed in a nursing home.

PET FOODS AND HUMAN HEALTH RISKS

Something as simple as feeding a pet can pose a health risk to an immunocompromised individual. Some people choose to feed their dogs or cats raw diets containing raw meat and/or raw eggs believing such food provides the animal more energy, improves their health and immunity, or that the diet is more natural and that the body is able to utilize micronutrients or vitamins not found in commercially prepared, cooked pet foods. Raw or not, pet foods do have a public health risk.

The feeding of raw meat does carry some health risks for the pet as well as anyone around the pet. Raw meat is not sterile, no matter whether it is destined for human consumption or for pet food. A common meat contaminant is *Salmonella*, but other microbial pathogens may also contaminate meat, such as *Escherichia coli, Campyloacter, Yersinia, Giardia, Toxoplasma, Neospora, Cryptosporium, Clostridium*, and many others.[11] *Salmonella* can be found in the intestinal tracts of most animals and commonly on raw chicken sold in the supermarket. In one study, 30 percent of dogs fed a homemade raw meat diet shed *Salmonella*.[11] Disease outbreaks in pets fed raw meat have resulted in pet illnesses and deaths from *Salmonella* and other pathogens.

Dogs may or may not show signs of illness when infected with *Salmonella*, depending on many factors, but can still shed this agent in their feces. It has been estimated that *Salmonella* can be found in the feces of 1 to 36 percent of healthy dogs and 1 to 18 percent in healthy cats.[12] In fact, dogs may become subclinical carriers (not showing illness) of *Salmonella* with the potential to shed for weeks to months. This shedding in the pet's feces can result in the accidental transmission to other pets and people, which is a significant concern for immunocompromised individuals, who may unknowingly be exposed to *Salmonella* shed by other people's pets. *Salmonella* can spread person to person, and people also can become subclinical shedders for years—Typhoid Mary, who was a chronic carrier of *Salmonella typhi*, caused a number of illnesses and deaths over a period of many years in her job as a cook.

Transmission of *Salmonella* to people, especially children, can occur if strict hygiene is not followed when picking up or discarding animal feces or in cleaning up after the pet. Food bowls and the area around the bowl can be contaminated and serve as a source of infection. People can also be infected handling the meat during preparation and feeding, which is why hand washing and the thorough cleaning of knives, utensils, and cutting boards is essential. Lastly, even if the meat is not contaminated, eggs can be.

For all of these reasons, feeding raw meat and/or raw eggs to pets in a household where an immunocompromised person lives is not recommended. Though there are no documented instances of raw food diets causing illness in people to date, such cases may not be identifiable because they are sporadic, single, and not associated with large outbreaks, and illness could be thought to be acquired through foods meant for human consumption. No matter, in the end it is simply not worth the risk to the health of the immunocompromised person or their family to feed such a diet to their pet.

While there is a recognized public health risk with raw food diets, and raw meat is much more likely to be contaminated with microorganisms harmful to human health, even ordinary pet foods can lead to human illness under the right conditions. Almost all dog and cat foods and treats are meat-based and therefore run the risk of being contaminated if not heated properly to kill *Salmonella* and other harmful bacteria during manufacture. Human salmonellosis has been linked to feeding dry pets foods and pet treats, but not canned foods. The first documented outbreak of human salmonellosis due to commercial dry dog and cat foods occurred from 2006 to 2008. These dog and cat foods where manufactured at one plant under different brands and were linked to 79 human cases of salmonellosis, with 48 percent of these cases occurring in children under two years of age.[12] Illness was significantly associated with feeding the pet in the kitchen (a place where cross-contamination can occur in areas of eating and food preparation) and with contact with a dog, but not, interestingly enough, associated with children putting pet food in their mouths. Illness was not reported in the dogs or cats from those people who became ill, though this organism was found in the feces of several dogs. Interestingly, the extent of the outbreak was not as severe as it might have been, suggesting that, in addition to kitchen contamination, those infected might have been more susceptible. In this outbreak, it is believed that the flavor enhancers that were applied to the food after it was cooked were contaminated with *Salmonella*.

PREVENTION

Microbial agents capable of causing disease and death can be acquired from many sources, directly from animals, from food (meat and produce), water, other people, soil, insects, and likely a few other places. There are estimated to be more than 1,400 infectious agents that can cause disease in people, and about 61 percent of these come from animals. It should be noted that it can sometimes work the other way, and that humans may pass disease on to animals. The ultimate goal of achieving and maintaining good health, whether we are talking about infectious diseases or chronic diseases, such as heart disease, is prevention. Prevention is priority. If we can implement measures that prevent infection to begin with, then the risk of a person developing a severe illness or dying becomes very small, no matter if the source of the infection is a dog, a hamburger, or a friend.

While one size doesn't fit all, preventing zoonotic disease transmission to immunocompromised individuals is often very practical, utilizing guidelines and common sense. Sometimes, a human health care professional will tell an immunocompromised person that he should not have a pet or that he should get rid of his pet. This is rarely true or necessary and depends on many variables: current health and health history of the animal, level of veterinary care, diet, species of animal, behavior of animal, whether the animal goes outdoors or not, travel exposure, and much more. Such decisions about whether an immunocompromised person should have a pet should be conducted on a case by case basis. Sometimes physicians misunderstand the zoonotic risks, which is why it would be a good idea for the physician of the pet owner to talk with the veterinarian to better understand that risk and make a more informed decision. An immunocompromised pet owner should always consult both his veterinarian and his physician for advice on the risks of pet ownership and the risks of being around animals in general. The psychological and physical benefits of having a pet outweigh the small risk of zoonoses to an educated and careful pet owner,[3] including most immunocompromised individuals. One study of those with AIDS found no significant difference between pet owners and non–pet owners in rates of opportunistic infections,[7] indicating that pet ownership does not dramatically increase the risk of AIDS-defining zoonotic opportunistic infections.

The testing of healthy animals for zoonoses is not recommended since most of these diseases can be avoided and prevented by good veterinary care, good animal and human hygiene, good husbandry, avoidance of high-risk animals, and other measures mentioned in this chapter and listed in Tables 7.1 and 7.2. Above all, washing your hands well for 20 seconds after touching animals, pet foods, food and water bowls, meat, soil, pet feces, pet bedding, and before eating is the best way in which you can avoid acquiring a zoonotic disease. The use of alcohol-based hand sanitizers with a minimum of 62 percent alcohol can also be used to disinfect your hands, provided that gross soiling and organic material is removed first. It should also be noted that alcohol-based sanitizers are not effective against all pathogenic bacteria (spores for example), nor against all viruses or protozoa (such as *Cryptosporidium*), so hand washing is still the best means of cleaning your hands and remaining safe.

Following these recommendations, most immunocompromised individuals can have a long, enriching, and loving relationship with their pet for years to come.

Table 7.2
Recommendations for Immunocompromised Individuals around Animals

Avoid owning and coming in contact with:

- Immunosuppressed animals
- Reptiles, amphibians, baby chicks, ducklings
- Exotic/wild animals
- Stray dogs and cats
- Sick animals
- Young farm animals

Hygiene:

- Change litter box and bird cage lining daily. Use of plastic litter box liners encouraged.[†]
- Keep litter boxes out of the kitchen and dining room.
- Pick up dog feces daily.[†]
- Maintain a clean, healthy aquarium.
- Wear gloves when cleaning litter box, picking up dog feces, cleaning bird cage, gardening, handling raw meat, or similar exposures. For aquariums, use heavy rubber gloves.[†]
- Disinfect litter box with hot water and detergent and scrub well.[†]
- For birds, change cage liner daily.
- Spray soiled bird cage liner with 1 percent bleach solution and let sit for 10 minutes before removing paper (do not expose bird to bleach fumes).[†]
- Minimize contact with animal feces, blood, urine.
- Wash pet food bowls regularly, but not in the kitchen sink. Keep the pet feeding area clean.
- Do not bathe infants in the kitchen sink.
- Children under five years should not be allowed to touch or eat pet food, treats, or supplements and should be kept away from pet feeding areas.
- Wash hands for 20 seconds after touching animals, picking up feces, changing litter box, cleaning bird cage or aquarium, gardening, handling meat, handling food or water dishes, feeding pets, and similar exposures—even if using gloves.
- Adults should supervise children around animals and in washing their hands.
- Wash bites and scratches immediately with copious amounts of soap and water.
- Seek immediate medical care for bites and scratches.
- Do not allow pets to lick wounds or face.
- Do not share food or eating utensils with pets.
- Do not kiss pets.

Pets:

- Use flea and tick repellents regularly.
- Have pets examined by veterinarian every six months for preventive care.
- Maintain regular vaccine schedule.
- Do not let pets drink from toilet.
- Keep cats indoors at all times.
- Feed only good quality commercial food, and cook any meat and eggs well before feeding.

- Do not feed raw meat, raw fish, or raw eggs.
- Keep pet nails trimmed.
- Have sick animals seen by veterinarian promptly.
- Have nonimmunocompromised person take any animal with diarrhea to the veterinarian to check for infectious causes. Animals with diarrhea should be separated from immunocompromised owner until healthy.
- Routinely deworm dogs and cats with a broad spectrum dewormer and heartworm preventative.
- Have a fecal exam performed on dogs and cats at least every six months.
- Adopt only adult dogs and cats (at least one year of age).
- Adopt from a private family, where there is less chance of the animal having disease.
- Do not bring a new cat into your home that was an outdoor cat or fed raw meat.
- Have newly adopted pet seen by veterinarian prior to allowing it to live with an immunocompromised person.
- Keep dogs on leash or adequately fenced.
- Do not let animals have access to garbage.
- Do not let pets hunt.
- Do not let pets eat the feces of other animals.

Foods, cooking, and eating:

- Follow USDA-FSIS recommendations for cooking meats. Cook beef, fish, veal, lamb steaks/chops/roasts to 145°F; pork, ground beef, ground veal, and ground lamb, egg dishes, and casseroles to 160°F; leftovers to 165°F; poultry to 165°F.
- Do not eat hot dogs, lunch meat, cold cuts, deli meats, fermented or dry sausage unless heated to 165°F.
- Wash hands well for 20 seconds after handling meats, hot dogs, luncheon/deli meats.
- Do not eat refrigerated paté or meat spreads from refrigerator section of your grocery store. Canned is cooked and safe to eat.
- Do not eat soft cheeses (feta, queso fresco, brie, Camembert, etc.) unless made with pasteurized milk.
- Do not eat smoked seafood unless it is cooked.
- Wash vegetables thoroughly before eating.

Other recommendations:

- To avoid fungal infections from the environment, do not clean out chicken coops or dig where birds roost. Avoid exposure to soil dust, such as at construction sites.
- Do not help during the birthing of animals and avoid being around the birthing area.

---

† Should be performed by someone who is not immunocompromised whenever possible.

FURTHER READING

Centers for Disease Control and Prevention. Bottled water and immunocompromised individuals. Available at: http://www.cdc.gov/healthywater/drinking/bottled/#immuno.

Centers for Disease Control and Prevention. Healthy Pets Healthy People. Available at: http://www.cdc.gov/healthypets/index.htm.

Centers for Disease Control and Prevention. For people at extra risk. Available at: http://www.cdc.gov/healthypets/extra_risk.htm.

Centers for Disease Control and Prevention. Preventing infection from pets. Available at: http://www.cdc.gov/hiv/pubs/brochure/oi_pets.htm.

How to prevent foodborne illness. Foodsafety.gov. Available at: http://www.food safety.gov/.

LeJeune JT, Hancock DD. Public health concerns associated with feeding raw meat diets to dogs. *Journal of the American Veterinary Medical Association* 2001;219:1222–5.

Pets are Wonderful Support. Safe pet guidelines. Available at: http://www.pawssf. org/page.aspx?pid=463.

REFERENCES

1. American Pet Products Manufacturers Association. Industry statistics and trends. Available at: http://www.americanpetproducts.org/press_industry trends.asp. Accessed March 2010.
2. Tizard IR. *Veterinary immunology: An introduction.* 8th ed. St. Louis, MO: Saunders Elsevier; 2009.
3. Davis RG. HIV/AIDS education: Still an important issue for veterinarians. *Public Health Reports* 2008;123:266–75.
4. Turtle-associated salmonellosis in humans—United States, 2006–2007. *MMWR Morbidity and Mortality Weekly Report,* 2007;56:649–52.
5. National Association of State Public Health Veterinarians. Compendium of measures to prevent disease associated with animals in public settings, 2009. Available at: http://nasphv.org/documentsCompendia.html. Accessed March 24, 2011.
6. Stine GJ. *AIDS update 2007.* New York: McGraw-Hill; 2007.
7. Conti L, Lieb S, Liberti T, et al. Pet ownership among persons with AIDS in three Florida counties. *American Journal of Public Health* 1995;85:1559–61.
8. Luppi P. How immune mechanisms are affected by pregnancy. *Vaccine* 2003;21:3352–7.
9. Outbreak of listeriosis—northeastern United States, 2002. *MMWR Morbidity and Mortality Weekly Report* 2002;51:950–1.
10. McClure EM, Goldenberg RL. Infection and stillbirth. *Seminars in Fetal and Neonatal Medicine* 2009;14:182–9.
11. Strohmeyer RA, Morley PS, Hyatt DR, et al. Evaluation of bacterial and protozoal contamination of commercially available raw meat diets for dogs. *Journal of the American Veterinary Medical Association* 2006;228:537–42.
12. Behravesh CB, Ferraro A, Deasy MIII, et al. Human Salmonella infections linked to contaminated dry dog and cat food, 2006–2008. *Pediatrics* 2010; 126:477–83.

Chapter 8

Zoonoses of Concern from Dogs

Carina Blackmore, MS Vet. Med., PhD, DACVPM

INTRODUCTION

The relationship between dogs and people goes back thousands of years. Wolves were taken in by human hunter-gatherers and used for protection, as draft animals, and likely as a source of food and fur. Friendlier and useful animals were kept and bred, and the domesticated dog evolved over time. The dogs quickly spread across cultures around the world, and their roles expanded to herding, hunting and sniffing. Dogs have been kept as companions for many years as well, but the relationship with man's best friend has changed since World War II, when pet dog populations started to increase dramatically. In 2006, 43 million U.S. households owned dogs. Dogs are now more likely to stay inside, are considered part of the family, and provide emotional support to the owners. They also fulfill important roles as guide dogs, service animals, and companions to the sick and elderly.

Dogs provide a great health benefit for the owners. Dog owners have been shown to have better mental and physical health than non–pet

owners; dog owners make fewer visits to the doctor and get more exercise. However, dogs can also cause injury and disease. On average, 76,000
unintentional fall injuries and 387,000 bites are caused by dogs each year
in the United States. Dogs can also transmit infectious disease agents to
people (termed zoonotic diseases or zoonoses). More than 25 different
zoonotic organisms have been documented in dogs, including bacteria,
viruses, nematode worms, mites, cellular protozoans, and fungi. Dog zoonoses can be transmitted to people via several different routes: direct contact between dog and person; contact with the dog's urine, feces, and other
body fluids; and by dog bites or scratches. Disease transmission can also
occur indirectly from the environment (e.g., from soil, clothing, or surfaces contaminated with animal feces) or infected insects, ticks, or mites.
Most zoonotic diseases are rare; however, rabies, hookworms, roundworms, leptospirosis, and a few enteric diseases are more common and
are discussed in detail throughout this chapter.

8.1.   DID YOU KNOW?

- Dogs, unlike cats, seldom develop plague or tularemia illness.
- French microbiologist Louis Pasteur, the father of pasteurization, developed the first rabies vaccine in 1885.
- Approximately 50 percent of all reported salmonellosis
  cases are detected in infants and toddlers. Environmental
  contamination with *Salmonella* is believed to be an important
  transmission source.

RABIES

The rabies virus is spread from animal to person primarily by bites
and infects the nervous system of the host. The brain damage that results
is severe and fatal in almost 100 percent of cases. All warm-blooded animals can get rabies, but certain animal species, including dogs and cats,
are more susceptible than others. There are many varieties (strains) of the
rabies virus, and each strain is maintained in a particular animal host species. The most important rabies reservoir hosts in the United States include raccoons, skunks, foxes, and bats.

Dog rabies used to be a serious public health concern in the United
States, but dog rabies vaccination programs, which started in the 1950s,
have helped control canine rabies in most industrialized countries. The

disease continues to be a serious problem in some parts of Africa, Asia, Latin America, and the Middle East, and dog bites are still the most common cause of human rabies across the world. The last dog infected with the canine strain in the United States was in 2004, and the country has been declared free of this strain since. It is important to note that although the canine rabies virus strain has been eliminated from the United States, dogs and cats can still acquire wildlife strains. On average, 83 rabid dogs were reported in the United States each year between 2004 and 2008.

The rabies virus is neurotropic in all mammals, including humans, which means that it spreads and multiplies inside the nervous system. The virus enters nerves at the site of the bite and travels inside the nerves to the spinal cord and the brain. A few days before the animal or person becomes visibly ill, the rabies virus travels from the brain through the nerves going to the salivary glands and is released into the saliva. One of the areas of the brain the rabies virus infects is the area that controls behavior. Rabid animals can become very aggressive and bite other animals or people they come in contact with. Saliva with rabies virus is injected into the wound of the bite victim and the cycle starts over.

The length of the incubation period (the period between infection and the onset of clinical signs) depends on several factors, including the location of the bite on the body. The further from the brain the bite occurs, the longer the incubation period, because the virus has farther to travel to the brain. A bite breaking the skin is the most important route of rabies transmission; however, the virus can also be transmitted if infected saliva comes in direct contact with open cuts in skin or mucous membranes in the eyes, mouth, or nose. Scratches that break the skin, caused by cats and other animals that frequently lick their paws, may also be a concern. The rabies virus cannot penetrate intact skin and is quickly destroyed by sunlight, drought, the acid present on intact skin, alkaline substances (e.g., soap), and other environmental factors outside the host.

In dogs, the incubation period can vary between 10 days and six months, but most animals become ill between two weeks and three months after the bite. Three phases of rabies disease are recognized in the dog. The first phase (the prodromal phase) usually lasts 2–3 days and is characterized by very small, barely noticeable behavioral changes. The dog may develop a fever and become slightly nervous or restless. Friendly animals may become shy or irritable, and aggressive animals may show unusual affection. The second, excitatory phase is also called the furious rabies phase (Figure 8.1). The dog now is increasingly irritable, restless, or nervous. It may be sensitive to light, touch, or sounds and may be very dangerous, biting at anything nearby. The furious phase can last one to seven days. As more nerve cells become damaged, the disease enters the paralytic phase. During this phase, which also lasts one to seven days, paralysis of the vocal cords may cause a change in the bark, and paralysis of the throat muscles may cause drooling as the dog develops difficulty swallowing. The dog becomes uncoordinated, paralyzed, and, eventually, slips into a coma and often dies of respiratory arrest.[1] Although most dogs show signs of furious rabies, some do not show much aggressiveness and quickly progress into the paralytic phase of the illness (dumb rabies).

Human rabies used to be a much feared disease in the United States. Rabies vaccines for dogs became available in the 1920s, and by the mid-1960s the number of human rabies cases had decreased dramatically, from 100 or more to 2 to 3 cases each year. Most of the human cases that still occur in the United States result from bat bites (the bat strain of rabies) or exposure to dogs in countries where canine rabies (the canine strain) is still common. The last human case due to the canine strain of rabies contracted in the United States was reported in 1994 from Texas. Another reason for the decrease in the number of human rabies cases is because of the availability of highly effective post-exposure rabies prophylaxis (PEP)

Figure 8.1
A dog with furious rabies

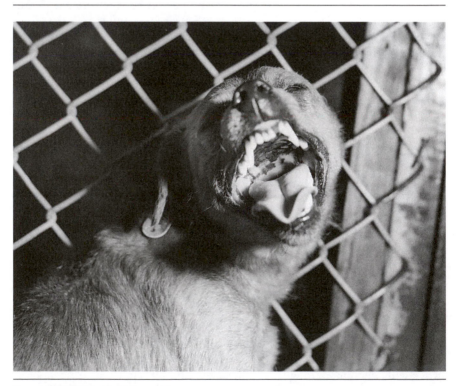

Source: CDC Public Health Image Library.

treatment; none of the patients treated appropriately with PEP in the last 30 years in this country have come down with the disease.

The first symptoms of human rabies are typically flulike, with headache, fever, and lack of energy. The area around the bite wound where the rabies virus entered may also be painful, itchy, more or less sensitive to touch, or have other sensory changes. After a few days, symptoms expand to such abnormal behaviors as anxiety, irritability, paranoia, and confusion. The person may have trouble sleeping, be hypersensitive to light and sound, and experience hallucinations. The patient also develops progressive paralysis. The jaw and throat gradually become paralyzed, and the production of large quantities of saliva and an inability to swallow or speak are typical symptoms during the later stages of the disease. Humans may show panic when presented with liquids to drink, and are unable to satisfy their thirst. The disease was once commonly known as hydrophobia, from this characteristic symptom.

The period between human infection and rabies symptoms is one to three months on average, but can be as long as several years. Death usually occurs within 2–10 days after the first symptoms.[1] Intensive medical care can prolong survival, but people do not generally recover from rabies and most ultimately die from the disease. The few known rabies survivors were almost all left with severe brain damage.

Human rabies can be prevented by avoiding contact with suspect rabid animals. As mentioned above, the most effective way to prevent human rabies exposure is through animal vaccination. There are a number of animal rabies vaccines licensed by the U.S. Department of Agriculture (USDA) for use in dogs, cats, sheep, cattle, horses, and ferrets. Routine rabies vaccinations of dogs, cats, and ferrets are required by many states. Some USDA-approved vaccines for dogs or cats provide a multiyear immunity period. Dogs and cats vaccinated by a one-year rabies vaccine must be revaccinated each year. Both one-year and multiyear vaccines are highly effective. All dogs and cats should be vaccinated at 3 months of age or older and revaccinated 12 months after the first vaccination. Thereafter, the interval between vaccinations will depend on the manufacturer's directions on the vaccine label. People should also avoid contacting, handling, or feeding stray dogs and cats. These animals are at higher risk for rabies infection because they often interact closely with raccoons and other rabies carriers. Wildlife are often attracted to dog and cat food, so leaving food outside for outdoor pets or strays may increase the likelihood of rabies exposure for both pets and people.

Human rabies vaccines are also highly effective. Such high-risk groups as veterinarians or animal control personnel who are in regular contact with suspect rabid animals should consider getting vaccinated against rabies. The vaccination series consists of three shots given over a three-week period. The vaccine is also used to treat individuals who have been exposed (bitten) by a suspect rabid animal. If the exposed person has been previously vaccinated against rabies, two booster doses given three days apart are needed. Unvaccinated rabies exposure victims need four doses of vaccine given over two weeks as well as one shot of human rabies immunoglobulin provided at the time of the first vaccine treatment. Individuals who believe they may have been exposed to a rabid animal should wash the bite wound thoroughly with soap and water then contact their physician regarding the need for PEP.

INTESTINAL PARASITES

Roundworm Infections (*Toxacara Canis*)

Roundworms of the genus *Toxacara* affect both dogs and cats and are probably the most common infections transmitted from these pets to their owners in the United States. Young children who are likely to play in soil contaminated with parasite eggs and then put their fingers in their mouths are at highest risk for infection. In a study from 2007,[2] it was estimated that almost 14 percent of the U.S. population was infected with the *Toxacara canis* parasite. Infections were more common in young individuals and males. People at higher risk included those who owned dogs and those who worked with soil, such as farmers or landscapers.

The worms, which can measure 2.5–4.5 inches in their adult form, live in the intestines of dogs. Puppies usually get infected with *Toxacara* by the mother either during the pregnancy or from her milk. The larvae penetrate the puppy's intestinal wall and are carried in the blood stream to the lungs. Larvae then migrate through the lungs to the throat, where the larvae are swallowed and go on to develop into mature adults in the puppy's intestines. When the puppy is three to four weeks old, the roundworms start to produce large numbers of eggs that spread into the environment through the animal's stool. The larvae inside the eggs need one to two weeks to mature before the eggs are infective (capable of infecting another host). People and older dogs are, for this reason, generally not infected by direct contact with infected puppies but accidentally swallow infective *Toxacara* eggs present in soil or other contaminated surfaces (Figure 8.2).

When older dogs are infected, larvae often travel to muscles and internal organs such as the liver or kidneys where they become dormant. The larvae are often reactivated during pregnancy and may travel from the liver or kidneys to the uterus and mammary glands to infect the newborn puppies.

When people swallow *Toxacara* eggs, the larvae are released from the eggs in the human intestine. Larvae penetrate the intestinal wall and migrate through the organs and tissues of the body. Eventually they settle down and become encapsulated. Most larvae die in the capsule, but some

Figure 8.2
Toxacara canis **parasite life cycle**

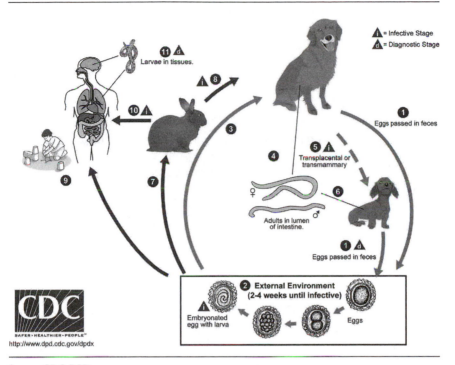

Source: CDC-DPDx.

remain alive for a long time. The symptoms associated with toxacaria-sis depend on the damage the larvae cause during their migration. Most human infections are asymptomatic, but some larvae become encapsulated and cause harm to the eyes or certain internal organs. Ocular larva migrans (OLM) can cause a range of eye diseases affecting many different parts of the eye, including inflammation of the cornea (keratitis), iris (iritis), or the entire vascular layer of the eye (uveitis) and detachment of the retina. Symptoms are generally limited to one eye and the loss of vision can be gradual or sudden. The worms may cause permanent vision loss or blindness from cataracts or scarring of the retina. The damage may take years to develop, so symptoms are most often seen in older children and young adults. The diagnosis is made by microscopic examination of the eye where the worm often is visible. About 700 individuals are diagnosed with OLM in the United States each year.

The immature worms can also travel through other human organs. Symptoms associated with larval movement through internal organs (visceral larva migrans) depend on which organ the larvae have migrated to. Common symptoms include fever, upper abdominal pain, general discomfort, weight loss, and an enlarged liver and spleen. Some patients may also have nausea, vomiting, neurological symptoms, an itchy rash, and coughing, wheezing, or other breathing problems. Symptoms are more common in young preschool children and may persist for months. Visceral larva migrans can be treated with antiparasitic drugs, and both drugs and surgery may be used to limit the damage of OLM. It should be noted that roundworm infections are not spread directly from person to person.

Signs of *Toxocara* infection most often occur in puppies, while adult dogs generally remain symptom free. Typical signs of roundworm infection include poor growth, dull coat, and sometimes a large pot-bellied stomach. More severe signs include coughing, breathing problems, colic, vomiting, diarrhea and even death. Worms may be seen in the stool or vomit of infected pups. Puppies infected with a large worm load can develop pneumonia and die only a couple of days after birth. They might also die if a large number of adult worms develop and cause blockage in the intestinal tract.

Hookworm Infections (*Ancylostoma* Species)

Hookworms belong to a family of nematode worms that live in the small intestine of humans and animals. The parasite has been named after the hooks it uses to attach to the host's intestinal wall to suck blood. Human hookworms (*Necator americanus* and *Ancylostoma duodenale*) are important causes of anemia and stunted growth among children in the tropics and subtropics and can also cause severe symptoms in pregnant women and people who are malnourished.

The dog hookworm (*Ancylostoma caninum*) and the dog and cat hookworm (*Ancylostoma braziliense*) like the warmer climates as well but are found throughout the United States. The worms prefer the warm climate because hookworm larvae spend part of their life cycle outside the animal host (Figure 8.3).

The cycle starts when the parasite eggs, produced by adult worms in the dog's intestine, are released into the environment. The eggs hatch and the larvae mature (molt) in the environment 5–10 days before they are capable of infecting a new host. Dogs are infected when they swallow hookworm larvae or when they eat other animals infected with the immature parasite. The larvae may also burrow directly through the dog's skin. They travel through the host's tissues to the animal's blood vessels and move through the vessels to the heart and lungs, where they are coughed up into the dog's throat and swallowed. The larvae are then transported to the small intestine where they mature to adult worms.

Figure 8.3
Ancylostoma braziliense parasite life cycle

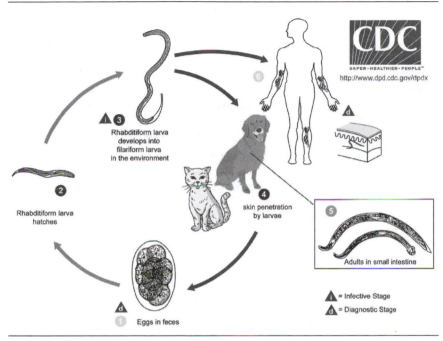

Source: CDC-DPDx.

Rather than migrating to blood vessels, some hookworm larvae travel to muscles and other parts of the body where they become dormant. Similar to *Toxacara canis*, these larvae can be reactivated during pregnancy and infect the unborn pup. The parasites also travel to the mammary gland in large numbers and infect newborn pups through the milk.

Clinical signs of dog hookworm infection include diarrhea, which may be tarry or bloody, poor hair coat, failure to thrive or gain weight, weight loss, pneumonia, and anemia. The illness can be severe and even fatal in young animals, especially in puppies infected with a large number of worms.

People are infected with dog and cat hookworms by swallowing the infective larvae, which then penetrate the intestinal wall and spread throughout the body. Infections can also occur through the skin when worms have prolonged (5–10 minutes or longer) contact with the person's skin surface. However, most animal hookworms have trouble penetrating through the human skin to reach underlying tissues and organs and instead stay and move around in the upper skin layer (cutaneous larva migrans). The traveling worms often cause intense itching and leave visible, red, slightly swollen, snakelike tunnel tracks in the skin generally seen on those parts of the body that are exposed to the contaminated soil, such as legs, hands, and feet.

The incubation period is typically one to two weeks and the infection can last for a few days to weeks until the larvae eventually die. When the hookworm larvae are able to get through the skin or intestinal wall, symptoms depend on which organ or body tissue has been affected. Diarrhea, abdominal pain, muscle pain, and eye problems are a few problems that have been reported.

Hookworm infections are more common in children and in those adult populations with close contact with soil (e.g., gardeners, farmers, and exterminators). The parasites are not spread directly from person to person. The infections can be treated with antiparasitic drugs given orally, or as cream or ointment applied on the skin.

Prevention and Hygiene

Human roundworm and hookworm infections can be prevented by regular deworming of dogs, especially pregnant dogs and puppies. Puppies shed most eggs before they are three months old, so treatment of puppies should begin as soon as two weeks after birth. Infections can also be avoided by removing the waste of dogs or other pets from areas where children play. *Toxacara* eggs can survive for years in the environment and are often found in sandboxes and on playgrounds where dogs and cats have access.[3] Environmental control is very difficult and generally requires the sand or the top soil to be removed or burned; common disinfectants do not kill the eggs. Environmental control of hookworms is easier. Larvae are susceptible to drying and direct sunlight, and surfaces can be disinfected with various chemicals, including bleach solution. Sodium borate can also be used to disinfect soil.

Cat and dog waste should be cleaned up promptly and either bagged and disposed of in the trash or buried. Wearing footwear and gloves when appropriate to avoid prolonged skin contact with contaminated soil can also decrease the risk of infection. In addition, it is important to wash hands thoroughly after playing or working in sand or soil. Children should be taught not to eat dirt and to always wash their hands after playing with pets or after playing outdoors.

LEPTOSPIROSIS

Leptospirosis is one of the most common and important zoonoses worldwide. Human disease was first described by Adolf Weil in 1886, but disease syndromes consistent with leptospirosis have likely occurred for centuries. A leptospirosis-like illness plagued troops in both Napoleon's army at the siege of Cairo and those fighting the American Civil War. The disease is caused by a spiral shaped (spirochete) bacterium (Figure 8.4) of the genus *Leptospira*. There are more than a dozen species and more than 250 subspecies (serovars) of *Leptospira*. Common serovars include *L. canicola*, *L. grippotyphosa*, *L. hardjo*, *L. icetrohaemorrhagiae* and *L. pomona*.

Leptospira can infect a wide range of animal species including mammals, birds, amphibians, and reptiles. Important hosts such as rodents, dogs, cattle, swine, and raccoons can carry the bacteria in their kidneys for months or years without any obvious signs of illness. The organisms are then shed into the environment when the animals urinate. *Leptospira* can be found in almost all parts of the world except the North Pole and South Pole, but they are of greater concern in temperate and tropical climates. The bacteria can survive for weeks or months in soil, survive well in standing water, but do not multiply outside the host.

Human leptospirosis is rare in most of the United States. The bacteria are endemic in fresh water in Hawaii, and about half of the 100–200 cases reported in the United States each year acquire their infections there, but

Figure 8.4
***Leptospirosis* bacteria**

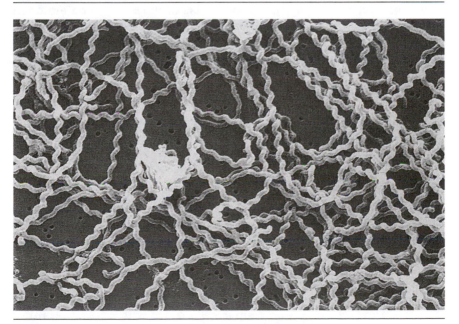

Source: CDC Public Health Image Library. Photo by Janice Haney Carr.

it is likely that a number of human cases of leptospirosis go undiagnosed. The clinical presentation is nonspecific and may easily be confused with influenza or viral meningitis (inflammation of the membranes around the brain).

Humans become infected by direct skin contact with urine or blood from the infected host, indirectly by swallowing bacteria in contaminated water and food, breathing in bacteria in aerosolized water or urine, or by direct skin contact with bacteria in contaminated water and soil. Infections from rodent bites have also been reported. Those who work in fresh water or who are involved in fresh water sports are at particular risk for disease. Residents of urban areas with high rodent populations and children who handle infected puppies are also at higher risk. Person-to-person transmission is uncommon, but transmission via sexual intercourse and breast-feeding has been reported.

Human symptoms can range from subclinical disease to a severe biphasic illness depending on the *Leptospira* species and serovar involved. The acute phase often begins abruptly, typically beginning 7–10 days after exposure, with nonspecific signs including fever, head ache, reddening of the eyes. and severe muscle aches, particularly of the back, thighs, and calves. Nausea, vomiting, abdominal pain, chest pain, and cough may also be present. The symptoms of the initial phase last for about a week and are followed by a one- to three-day period when the fever drops and symptoms improve or disappear. In some individuals, the nonspecific symptoms then come back. In this second phase of illness, bacteria are often found in the patient's urine. The bacteria multiply in the lining of small blood vessels throughout the body and can affect the function of a number of organs. Such signs of meningitis as headache, confusion, and stiff neck are often seen during the second phase of leptospirosis. In addition, about 5–10 percent of all leptospirosis cases develop liver, kidney, or central nervous system disease, sometimes even leading to organ failure. The individual may become jaundiced, with yellow sclerae (the whites of the eyes) and skin color, and develop kidney failure, bleeding disorders, and severe respiratory distress. The symptoms may persist for weeks but generally resolve over time. Infected individuals can also develop eye problems up to a year after recovery from the acute leptospirosis. Luckily, most recover full function of their eyes over time, but recovery may take years. Abortions have also been reported to occur during the first and second phase of the illness. About 1–5 percent of all leptospirosis cases die from the disease. Mortality is higher among immunosuppressed and elderly patients and those with multiorgan failure. Humans, unlike many animals, are accidental hosts and do not become chronic carriers of the bacteria.

Among animals, clinical disease is more often seen in cattle and dogs than sheep and cats. Dogs, like people, get infected with leptospirosis after contact with *Leptospira* bacteria in animal urine, soil, or water. Also similar to people, exposed dogs may remain symptom free or may develop a mild, severe, or potentially fatal disease. Death can occur peracutely without any other evidence of leptospirosis or as a consequence of multiorgan failure. Nonspecific initial signs such as fever, muscle stiffness, shivering, and weakness are usually seen 4–12 days after exposure. The dog may become depressed and lose its appetite. As the disease progresses, the animal may show signs of kidney disease with increased drinking and urinating (polydipsia/polyuria), blood in the urine, and vomiting. Dogs can also develop liver disease (jaundice), cough, diarrhea, weight loss, and abortion. Eye inflammation and bleeding may also be seen in some animals. The infection is generally diagnosed based on clinical signs and blood serum tested for antibodies. The severity of disease depends on the dog's age, route of exposure, infection dose, and vaccination history. Signs also vary depending on the *Leptospira* species or serovar. Dogs are susceptible to infection with many *Leptospira* serovars; however, *L. canicola, L. icterohemorrhagiae, L. bratislava, L. grippotyphosa,* and *L. pomona* are examples of serovars that are important causes of canine illness.

Most dogs recover within two weeks after disease onset, especially if the illness is diagnosed early and the dog is treated with appropriate antibiotics. If the initial signs go undetected or the infection is not treated, some animals can develop chronic kidney problems, and about 10 percent will die.

Younger and larger (more than 15 lb.) dogs living outdoors or with exposure to contaminated surface water, such as hunting, working, or herding dogs, are at higher risk for infection with *Leptospira*. However, dogs living in homes or apartments can also be exposed, either via mice and rats in the home environment or by stepping in contaminated puddles on outdoor walks.

People should keep their home, garage, and animal areas free from rodents. Gloves should be used for cleanup if environmental surfaces such as litter boxes, animal cages, and rodent-infested areas are suspected to be contaminated with animal urine. Prompt hand washing is also important, especially after handling animal feces or body fluids. A number of disinfectants can be used to kill this organism on various surfaces. In addition, people should avoid swimming or wading in water in lakes or rivers likely to be contaminated with *Leptospira*. Dog kennels should be kept clean, and dogs should not be allowed to drink from or swim in water suspected to be contaminated with the bacteria. The risk of infection can be reduced in dogs with routine water exposure by annual, or more frequent, vaccinations against leptospirosis. It is important to note that the vaccine only protects against illness from a handful of the most common serovars, so the common sense precautions discussed here are still very important. If the risk of leptospirosis is high and exposure cannot be avoided, prophylactic antibiotic treatment may be considered.

DIARRHEAL DISEASES

Giardiasis

Giardia intestinalis, sometimes called *Giardia lamblia,* is a protozoan parasite found in the small intestine of many domestic and wild animals worldwide. It is not clear whether animals and humans are infected with the same organism or a group of host-specific, closely related *Giardia* species with a more limited ability to spread among hosts.

The parasite has two stages: cysts and trophozoites. Infections occur when people or animals swallow water and food contaminated with the *Giardia* cysts. The parasite can also spread directly from person to person or animal to animal. After ingestion, trophozoites are released from the *Giardia* cysts in the host's intestine and multiply and form new cysts that are shed in the stool. These cysts can survive for long periods of time in cool, moist environments and can remain alive for several months in cold water. Day-care centers are an important source of *Giardia* outbreaks in young children. Hikers and backpackers who drink untreated water contaminated with *Giardia* in the wild are also at higher risk for disease.

Most people infected with *Giardia* remain healthy, but some individuals do develop a diarrheal illness 1–25 days after exposure, with the majority falling ill within 7–10 days. Symptoms include a sudden onset of foul-smelling diarrhea with pale and greasy, but seldom bloody, stools. The person may experience abdominal cramping, bloating, nausea, and fatigue, but fever and vomiting are uncommon. Weight loss may occur as a result of a disturbed intestinal uptake of fats and fat soluble vitamins. Symptoms generally last one to two weeks and resolve without treatment with antiprotozoal drugs, but chronic infections lasting months to years do occur. HIV infected individuals are at higher risk for prolonged and more severe infections.

Giardia infections are common in puppies and can cause acute, intermittent, or chronic diarrhea. Signs generally appear 5–14 days after exposure and include soft, light-colored foul-smelling, mucous-rich and fatty stools, poor hair coat, bloating, and weight loss. The disease is typically not life threatening, and most dogs recover without antiprotozoal drug treatment. The parasite seldom causes illness in older animals, but it is estimated that 2–10 percent of healthy dogs shed infectious *Giardia* cysts in their stools at any one time. Because asymptomatic carriers of the parasite are so common and the organism is so hardy, animals kept in shelters and kennels are at higher risk for disease.

To prevent giardiasis, people should filter or boil untreated water from lakes, rivers, springs, and shallow wells for at least one minute before drinking or allowing pets to drink. At higher altitudes (more than 2,000 meters), untreated water should be heated to a rolling boil for three minutes or more. Raw fruits and vegetables should be cleaned, and areas contaminated with animal feces should be thoroughly cleaned and dried (the parasite does not survive well in dry environments). Dogs believed to have contaminated their coat with *Giardia* cysts should be washed with a dog shampoo. Protozoan parasites such as *Giardia* are relatively resistant to chlorine disinfectants; however, there are other disinfectants that are effective in killing them.

Campylobacteriosis

Campylobacter are bacteria with more than 20 different strains and are found in birds and mammals, with most human infections caused by *Campylobacter jejuni* or *Campylobacter coli*.

People are infected by consuming the bacteria in food or water or from direct contact with infected infants or animals. Symptoms generally start two to five days after exposure and are seen in people of all age groups. Signs typically include fever, headache, abdominal pain, which sometimes can be mistaken for appendicitis, and watery or bloody diarrhea. The illness typically lasts less than a week. A few individuals can develop such complications as reactive arthritis (formerly known as Reiter's syndrome), and an autoimmune reaction that impacts the joints (arthritis), the urogenital system (urethritis and cervicitis), and the eye (conjunctivitis). Guillain-Barré, an autoimmune neurologic disease resulting in reversible muscle weakness or paralysis, occurs in 1:1,000 cases.

Dogs also tend to get infected by food, water, and direct dog contact. Signs generally develop within three days of exposure and include mild diarrhea, sometimes with mucus or blood, and loss of appetite, vomiting, and fever. Infected adult animals usually remain healthy but can still shed bacteria in their stool. Young, stressed, and weak puppies are more likely to develop severe illness and spread disease to others. Infections with this microbial pathogen can easily be treated with antibiotics.

To avoid infection, it is important that people and pets do not drink water or unpasteurized milk products that could be contaminated by animal feces. It is also important to wash hands after handling raw chicken and not to eat undercooked poultry. People should also wash their hands after handling animals, especially kittens and puppies, and children should not be allowed to handle sick animals.

Salmonellosis

Salmonella bacteria are found worldwide, but are more common in areas with intense farm production. The bacterium was first isolated from sick pigs in 1885 by Daniel Elmer Salmon, an American scientist, and since that time more than 2,500 varieties (serovars and strains) of *Salmonella* have been discovered, some with a greater ability to cause human illness than others. Many animals, including mammals, birds, reptiles, and amphibians are *Salmonella* carriers, they can shed *Salmonella* for months in their stool without showing signs of illness. The bacteria can spread from human to animals, from animals to humans, between animals, and directly from person to person. *Salmonella* bacteria survive well in wet and warm settings, so environmental exposure is also possible.

Dogs can be *Salmonella* carriers, but rarely get sick from the bacteria, but young animals as well as immunocompromised, pregnant, or lactating animals are more likely to become ill. Puppies or adult dogs stressed by boarding or hospitalization can also develop salmonellosis. Signs of disease develop on average three days after exposure and include diarrhea with fever and bloodstream infections (septicemia). Pneumonia, abortion, and chronic recurring infections are also possible, and the more severe infections can be fatal. Animals can be exposed to *Salmonella* through feed, raw meat, raw milk, dog treats made from animal products, water, and from direct animal-to-animal contact.

Salmonellosis is a very common disease in humans with an estimated 1.4 million cases each year in the United States, Most people become infected by eating foods contaminated with animal feces. Humans can also acquire this agent directly from animal or fecal contact. Person-to-person spread of salmonellosis, however, is rare. The time between exposure and disease onset in people is short, ranging from 12 hours to three days. Symptoms can range from no signs to septicemia. Typical symptoms include fever, nausea, abdominal cramping diarrhea that is sometimes bloody, vomiting, headache, chills, and muscle ache. Most people recover spontaneously after four to seven days, but severe dehydration is possible in infant and elderly patients. Blood-borne spread of the bacteria can lead to infections in other organs, such as the lungs (pneumonia), heart valves (endocarditis), kidneys (polynephritis), bones (osteomyelitis), the membranes around the brain (meningitis), and joints (arthritic abscesses). Reiter's syndrome or reactive arthritis occurs in about 2 percent of patients with salmonellosis. The reaction typically appears within one to three weeks of disease onset and lasts three to four months. Relapses are seen in half the patients and some develop chronic arthritis. Deaths from salmonellosis are uncommon except among the very young, very old. and immuocompromised persons. Bacterial shedding usually ends after a few days but may last several weeks, and, unlike some animals, humans rarely become long-term carriers of *Salmonella*.

People with diarrheal disease most often just need supportive care. Antibiotic treatment of these patients is actually contraindicated because antibiotics tend to kill off friendly bacteria normally present in human (and animal) intestines. This die-off may create a more favorable gut environment for the *Salmonella* bacteria and a prolonged shedding. Widespread antibiotic treatment of *Salmonella* infections in other countries have also resulted in the emergence of multidrug-resistant *Salmonella* strains. Such strains have spilled over into dogs as well. In 1999 and 2000, a multidrug-resistant *S. typhimurium* outbreak occurred in three veterinary clinics and one animal shelter causing illness in both dogs and caretakers.[4] Antibiotic use was shown to have facilitated the spread of bacteria in these facilities.

Salmonella infections can be avoided if people make sure to wash their hands after handling animal feces, pets, or pet toys. People with diarrhea should stay away from preparing food or drinks for others, and surfaces contaminated with *Salmonella* should be disinfected with bleach or other effective compounds. Dog owners should not feed their dogs raw meat[5] or raw milk, and they should not allow their dogs to eat trash or the stools of other animals.

Cryptosporidiosis

Cryptosporidium are protozoan parasites that thrive in the intestines of people and many animals. Some are species specific, however, many, including *Cryptosporidium canis,* the dog *Cryptosporidium,* transmit between animals and man. The parasites mate inside the intestinal cell lining and shed eggs (oocysts) into the stool. The oocysts have an outer protective shell allowing them to survive for months in the environment, protecting them from drying and providing some resistance to some disinfectants such as chlorine. People can become infected with *Cryptosporidium* by drinking contaminated water, eating contaminated food, and through direct contact with animals. The parasite is not usually found in municipal drinking water, but it was the source of one of the largest cryptosporidiosis outbreaks detected in the United States. More than 400,000 residents of Milwaukee, Wisconsin, became ill during this 1993 outbreak. As mentioned above, the oocysts survive fairly well in chlorinated water and people can get infected by swallowing contaminated water in swimming pools and recreational fountains.

Human symptoms include a watery diarrhea that is often explosive, abdominal cramping, and weight loss. Some experience nausea, vomiting, and a low-grade fever. Most people recover without treatment after 8–20 days, but disease can be more severe and long lasting in immunocompromised individuals. Patients with HIV may not be able to clear the parasite, and cryptosporidiosis may be a contributing cause of death in these individuals. Infants and their caregivers, travelers, men who have sex with men, and animal handlers are all at higher risk for infection.

In the United States, cattle are the most important animal host of *Cryptosporidium,* while infections in dogs are believed to be less common.

Newborn puppies and immunocompromised animals are most susceptible, whereas older healthy dogs may be asymptomatic carriers, rarely becoming ill. Clinical signs in dogs include diarrhea, poor appetite, weight
loss, and dehydration. Dog-to-human transmission has been documented
from infected puppies in a shelter setting, and dogs are a more important
risk factor of human disease in other parts of the world.

To avoid infection, public areas should be kept free of animal waste.
Any area that becomes contaminated needs to be thoroughly cleaned. A
5 percent ammonia solution can be used to disinfect clean surfaces. Sick
children should not attend child-care centers or schools, swim in pools, or
play in water parks. Sick animals should not be boarded in kennels, and
in animal shelter environments they should be isolated from the other
animals.

OTHER DISEASES

Ringworm

Many owners are aware that dogs can get ringworm. This is true, although *Microsporum canis,* the fungal agent of most concern, is less common in dogs than in cats. In addition, dogs are more likely than cats to
develop a skin rash from the infection. The signs in dogs include focal
hair loss (alopecia), redness (erythema), and scaling and itchiness (pruri-
tus) around the skin lesions. Infections are generally more severe in immunocompromised animals. Animals housed in crowded environments
and young animals are also at higher risk. Human symptoms are similar
regardless of the ringworm species. For more information on ringworm,
see chapter 9.

Methicillin-Resistant *Staphylococcus Aureus* Infection

Another important cause of human skin infection is *Staphylococcus aureus,* a bacteria that can cause blisters, infected hair follicles, and abscesses.
More severe symptoms are seen in a smaller proportion of patients, including pneumonia and septicemia, and the infection can be fatal. Most
such severe infections are a result of surgical wound infections and other
exposures in the hospital setting. Methicillin-resistant *Staphylococcus aureus* (MRSA) bacteria are of particular concern because of their resistance
to certain antibiotics, making infections very difficult to treat. Some people
can carry MRSA bacteria on their skin, in their nasal passages, or in body
fluids without becoming ill. A 2008 study[6] reported that about 1.5 percent
of the U.S. population are MRSA carriers. MRSA is primarily transmitted
from person to person, but the bacteria can be transmitted from people

to dogs, and there is increasing evidence it can also be transmitted from dogs to people. It is also possible for both people and dogs to get infected by having contact with surfaces contaminated with the organism. Risk factors for MRSA infections in dogs include having wounds requiring intense wound care, caretakers with poor hand hygiene, and staying in such crowded conditions as shelters or kennels where sick animals can have direct contact.[7] Dogs living with immunocompromised people, health-care personnel, and small animal veterinarians are also at higher risk. Healthy dogs can carry the MRSA bacteria on their skin or in their nasal passages without becoming ill. However, it does not appear they are an important long-term bacterial source for other animals or people, because, unlike people, dogs appear to clear the bacteria relatively quickly without antibiotic treatment.

Brucellosis

Brucella canis is a bacteria that causes reproductive health problems such as abortions and stillbirth in dogs. Pups of an infected mother can be born normal but develop symptoms later on. Many dogs do not become ill but are asymptomatic carriers of the bacteria and can sexually transmit the infection to other dogs. People who have close contact with infected dogs, in particular direct contact with birthing materials from infected animals, are also at risk. The bacteria can also be shed in urine, saliva, and nasal and eye secretions. Still, human infections are uncommon. Symptoms in people are variable and similar to those associated with other *Brucella* species. Infections begin with a nonspecific, flulike illness and a recurring fever (undulant fever). Symptoms can wax and wane over time and may evolve into such long-term health concerns as joint pain, chronic fatigue, and testicular disease if not successfully treated with antibiotics. Children, pregnant women, and immunocompromised persons are at higher risk of infection. The disease can be prevented if people wash their hands frequently after contact with infected dogs and wear gloves while handling birthing materials or newborn pups from infected dogs. The disease is very difficult to treat in dogs, and many kennel owners elect to euthanize animals infected with *B. canis*. Pet dogs may be neutered and treated with antibiotics. Although the treatment will lower the transmission risk it may not eliminate bacterial carriage in male dogs with chronically infected prostate glands.

Escherichia Coli O157:H7 Infection

Escherichia coli 0157:H7 and other Shiga-toxin producing *Escherichia coli* (STEC) are important human enteric pathogens. The primary symptoms in people include bloody diarrhea and kidney failure. Dogs are not important carriers, but ruminants, particularly cattle, are. STEC infected animals are often asymptomatic but may develop diarrhea. Human infections can be avoided if people wash their hands after handling animals, raw meat, carcasses, and feces.

Scabies

Sarcoptes scabiei mites live in human and animal skin. The mites have evolved into variants that have adapted to a particular host species, but the mites can also jump between hosts. Human symptoms start 20–35 days after exposure, with skin lesions in people often appearing in the webbing between fingers and on genitalia, breasts, and flexor surfaces of the wrists and elbows. Such lesions are very itchy, especially at night. Human scabies is a particular problem among immunocompromised and elderly individuals, and outbreaks are common in long-term care facilities. Scabies is common in dogs as well and can affect all ages and breeds. Scabies in dogs can cause hair loss, which often starts on the abdomen, chest, and ears. Other typical signs include crusting of the skin around the eyes, on the elbows, and hocks (ankles), and like in people can cause intense itching. Puppies from animal shelters or large breeding kennels are at increased risk for infection. Other risk factors for dogs include wildlife contact. Humans are often treated topically with Permethrin 5 percent cream. Dogs can be dipped in lime sulfur or treated topically with Selamectin. Oral treatment with ivermectin is also effective, but this drug is contraindicated in collies and collie crosses. The mites that cause dog scabies can cause scabies symptoms in people but generally do not reproduce in humans, so the infection clears up fairly quickly on its own. The reverse is also true: The mites that cause scabies in humans cause scabies in dogs, but the infection usually clears up without treatment.

Tuberculosis

Human tuberculosis can be caused by several species of the genus *Mycobacterium*, but the most common cause is *Mycobacterium tuberculosis*, a feared disease worldwide. *M. tuberculosis* infections are often difficult to treat, requiring lengthy treatment (sometimes a year or more) and may be fatal if left untreated. The most common symptom in people is pneumonia, but the infection can spread to other organs. The bacteria can be inhaled by other people when infected individuals cough and sneeze. Humans can also on occasion transmit tuberculosis to dogs. Signs in dogs are similar to those seen in humans and include chronic cough and weight loss. Whether dogs can infect people with tuberculosis is not clear. To minimize the risk of transmission between people and pets, people with tuberculosis should cover their coughs around dogs. Humans should also avoid close contact with coughing dogs that have a history of *M. tuberculosis* exposure.

PREVENTION

The most important ways to prevent transmission of diseases from dogs to people are to make sure people wash their hands after handling animals and avoid handling sick or unknown dogs. If other animals can come in contact with pet waste the owner should pick it up, using gloves, and dispose of it in the garbage. They should also keep their dogs healthy by providing them a nutritious diet and not allowing them to eat raw or scrap foods. In addition, the animals should also be brought to a veterinarian for regular checkups (including fecal examination to make sure the dog is free from parasites), for microchipping, vaccinations, and tick prevention medication (Figure 8.5). Core vaccines include vaccines against the canine parvovirus, canine distemper virus, canine adenovirus-2, and rabies. Vaccines against kennel cough (*Bordetella bronchiseptica*) are generally also required for boarding.[8]

Figure 8.5
Routine dog care is important to keep your dog healthy

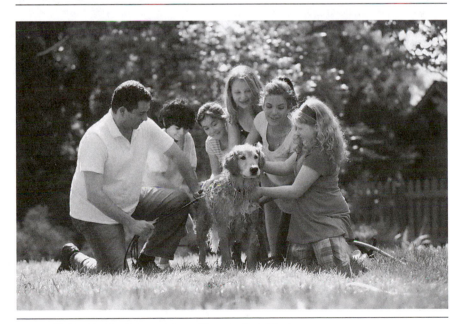

Source: CDC Public Health Image Library. Photo by Cade Martin.

FURTHER READING

American Veterinary Medical Association Website. Methicillin-resistant *Staphylococcus aureus*. Available at: http://www.avma.org/reference/backgrounders/mrsa_bgnd.asp.

Centers for Disease Control and Prevention Website. Healthy Pets Healthy People. Available at: http://www.cdc.gov/healthypets/.

Dvorak G, Rovid-Spickles A, Roth JA. *Handbook for zoonotic diseases of companion animals*. Ames, IA: Center for Food Security and Public Health, Iowa State University; 2008.

Rabinowitz PM, Conti LA, eds. *Human-animal medicine: Clinical approaches to zoonoses, toxicants, and other shared health risks*. Maryland Heights, MO: Saunders Elsevier; 2010.

Rabinowitz PM, Gordon Z, Odofin L. Pet-related infections. *American Family Physician* 2007;76:1314–22.

REFERENCES

1. Baer GM. *The natural history of rabies*. London: Academic Press; 1975.
2. Won KY, Kruszon-Moran D, Schantz PM, Jones JL. National seroprevalence and risk factors for zoonotic *Toxocara* spp. infection. *American Journal of Tropical Medicine and Hygiene* 2008;79:552–7.
3. O'Connell E, Suarez J, Leguen F, et al. Outbreak of cutaneous larva migrans at a children's camp—Miami, Florida, 2006. *MMWR Morbidity and Mortality Weekly Report* 2007;56(49):1285–7.
4. Wright JG, Tengelsen LA, Smith KE, Bender JB, et al. Multidrug-resistant *Salmonella Typhimurium* in four animal facilities. *Emerging Infectious Diseases* 2005;11(8):1235–41.
5. Lefebvre SL, Reid_Smith R, Boerlin P, Weese JS. Evaluation of the risks of shedding *Salmonellae* and other potential pathogens by therapy dogs fed raw diets in Ontario and Alberta. *Zoonoses and Public Health* 2008;55:470–80.
6. Gorwitz RJ, Kruszon-Moran D, McAllister SK, et al. Changes in the prevalence of nasal colonization with Staphylococcus aureus in the United States, 2001–2004. *Journal of Infectious Diseases* 2008;197:1226–34.
7. Soares Magalhaes RJ, Loeffler A, et al. Risk factors for methicillin-resistant *Staphylococcus aureus* (MRSA) infection in dogs and cats: A case-control study. *Veterinary Research* 2010;41:55.
8. American Animal Hospital Association (AAHA) Canine Vaccine Task Force. 2006 AAHA Canine Vaccine Guidelines, Revised. 2007. Available at: http://www.aahanet.org/PublicDocuments/VaccineGuidelines06Revised.pdf.

Chapter 9

Zoonoses of Concern from Cats

Ken Thorley, BVSc, MVS, MACVSc

Please note: A glossary is provided at the end of this chapter to describe several words that may be unfamiliar to the reader. Words bolded within the text, except for headings, are included in the glossary.

Cats have been domesticated for around 10 millenia. Originally, they were prized for their ability to keep rodent numbers down. These days, there are around 100 million pet cats in America, and the merits of cat ownership are more related to the joys of companionship that they provide and the positive psychological health benefits that accrue from that relationship. However, although owning a cat can be very rewarding, there are a few trade-offs, one in particular being zoonoses—those diseases than can be transmitted from animals to people. Some of these zoonoses are of particular importance in cats, which is the focus of this chapter. Cat owners and health-care workers should be aware of the various zoonoses of cat and how to avoid them.

Like zoonoses associated with other species, the conditions described in this chapter may occur as a result of direct contact with cats, from contact with a contaminated environment shared by cats, or contact with disease-transmitting insect **vectors** (particularly fleas and ticks) brought into the environment by cats. The zoonoses discussed here may affect anyone, but are more likely to be clinically significant and more severe in those with deficient immune systems. This includes infants, elderly individuals, those receiving immunosuppressive drugs, AIDS patients, and many others.

BARTONELLOSIS

Bartonella infection is the most common direct zoonosis acquired from cats. The bacterium *Bartonella henselae* is the main causative agent of cat scratch disease (CSD) in humans, and cats are the main **reservoir** hosts for this organism. Cats are healthy, inapparent carriers of *Bartonella*, and generally more than 20 percent of cats are infected,[1] but this rate varies markedly between geographical areas and the subset of cats studied. Based on the presence of **antibodies** to the organism, twice the percentage (40%) of currently infected cats show evidence that they have been infected at some time in their lives. The prevalence is higher in areas with warmer temperatures and more rainfall, which are the areas that have the highest prevalence of fleas. The prevalence of *Bartonella* infection is highest in kittens, outdoor cats, and in multicat environments (households or shelters).

Bartonella species are usually transferred to cats by fleas. Fleas ingest the *Bartonella* when feeding on infected cat blood and the organism is then excreted by the flea, which can survive for nine days in flea feces. Cats become infected when they ingest the flea feces while grooming themselves. Flea feces can also contaminate cats' nails, from where the infection is transmitted to humans via a scratch.

Cats can remain infected with the bacteria for many months before eliminating the infection on their own, and are typically healthy during this time. Some cats may become ill from *Bartonella* infection, but with such a high percentage of the cat population testing positive for this organism, it is often difficult to prove that *Bartonella* is the cause of the cat's illness. In an ill cat that has tested positive for *Bartonella* by serological antibody testing or polymerase chain reaction (PCR), has responded to treatment with antibiotics to which *Bartonella* are known to be susceptible, and has no other likely causes of the illness, bartonellosis must be suspected as the cause. While it is still not clear what illnesses this organism causes in cats, thus far bartonellosis has been documented as the cause of ocular disease, **endocarditis**, osteomyelitis, and a few other clinical diseases in cats.

Cat scratch disease, with an **incubation period** in humans of 3–14 days, is more common in children and adolescents. Most infected humans develop no symptoms or very mild symptoms approximately one week after becoming infected. Symptoms that may occur include a small raised **papule** at the site of the bite or scratch and/or an enlarged, painful **lymph**

node near the site of inoculation, which presents as a large painful lump under the skin usually in the region of the neck, groin, or armpit. A mild fever occasionally accompanies this. Antibiotics are of questionable efficacy in the treatment of CSD so are not prescribed for mild to moderate cases. In most cases, the infection usually resolves itself without treatment, but occasionally severe disease may occur. In such severe cases, the symptoms the person may experience are a persistent fever lasting more than two weeks, lethargy, muscle and joint pain, weight loss, enlarged spleen, conjunctivitis, and **uveitis**. Rarely, infections of the heart, brain, and retina may occur. Immunocompromised people are more likely to develop serious illness. In these individuals *Bartonella henselae* may cause bacillary angiomatosis, a condition in which blood vessel proliferation results in tumorlike masses appearing in the skin and organs. Also in immunocompromised individuals, *B. henselae* has been associated with peliosis hepatis, in which blood-filled cavities develop in the liver.

The available methods (blood **culture**, **serology**, and PCR) used to detect *Bartonella* infection in cats can all return false positive and false negative results. A positive PCR test does not indicate that the organism is alive, and false positives can occur. A positive serology test can tell us that the cat was once infected, but does not tell us whether the organism is still present. Blood cultures are often falsely negative as the appearance of the organism in the blood is cyclical. If cultures are positive, the question arises of what to do about it, especially with the organism being present in such a high percentage of the feline population. Antibiotics to which *Bartonella* are susceptible cannot reliably eliminate the organism from the cat, have not been found to lower the incidence of CSD in their owners, and may allow the *Bartonella* organism to develop resistance to the antibiotic. Accordingly, testing and treatment of healthy cats for *Bartonella* is not currently recommended.

To prevent the zoonotic acquisition of *Bartonella* infection from cats the following steps should be undertaken: prevent cats from becoming infected with *Bartonella* by rigorous year-round flea control; keep cats indoors to minimize exposure to fleas and other potential arthropod vectors such as ticks; trim cats' nails regularly and avoid bites and scratches; and do not encourage rough play with a cat. Wounds resulting from bites or scratches should be thoroughly washed as soon as possible with soap and water. Do not allow cats to lick open wounds. Immunocompromised individuals should avoid contact with cats of unknown health status and should only adopt healthy adult cats over one year of age that have no known history of fleas.

TOXOPLASMOSIS

Toxoplasmosis is one of the most important feline-associated zoonoses, but it is also one of the most misunderstood. Approximately one-third of the human and cat populations are infected with this organism, yet it is rare for people to acquire it directly from a cat. Indeed, studies have shown no correlation between cat ownership and increased risk of toxoplasmosis.

An appreciation of the life cycle of the causative organism, *Toxoplasma gondii,* is essential to an understanding of toxoplasmosis and the way in which it infects humans. Cats are the definitive host for *T. gondii,* meaning that the organism must infect a cat to complete its life cycle. Cats are usually infected by eating infected prey such as rodents or birds. In a cat that has not previously been infected by the organism, *T. gondii* undergoes sexual reproduction in the cat's intestine. This results in millions or billions of oocysts (eggs) being excreted in the cat's feces for a single brief period of one to three weeks, typically 7–10 days. Once a cat has been infected, it will not excrete the oocysts again, so usually those that excrete *T. gondii* are young cats. The excreted oocysts are not able to infect other animals or humans until these oocysts have undergone further internal division, a process that takes a minimum of 24 hours and sometimes up to five days. In damp conditions, the survival of infective oocysts in the environment is inversely proportional to the ambient temperature: At 39 degrees Fahrenheit they may remain viable for up to 2.5 years, while at 95 degrees Fahrenheit they can only survive one to two months. The oocysts contaminate soil or water where the cat has defecated, including gardens and children's sandboxes.

9.1. DID YOU KNOW?

- Before 1990 there were only two *Bartonella* species that had been recognized and named. Now there are more than 20!
- The isolation of *Bartonella* DNA from the teeth of an 800-year-old cat in France showed that the infection of cats with this organism is not just a recent phenomenon.
- *Coxiella burnetii* is so contagious that a single inhaled organism is enough to cause infection.

When a human or other animal eats food that has been contaminated by *Toxoplasma* oocysts they may become infected by the organism, which replicates and invades their bodies. This process is accompanied by either no symptoms at all or a very mild, transient fever and malaise. Most people never know that they have been infected. If the host animal or human has a competent immune system, the organism will be walled off in tissues as cysts, where it usually lies dormant causing no illness for the rest of the host's life. However, when an uninfected animal or human ingests meat that contains these cysts, they may become infected with the organism. The tissue cysts can be destroyed, and hence meat rendered safe to eat, by cooking the meat to at least 160 degrees Fahrenheit.

There are two categories of people who are at risk from toxoplasmosis: those without a competent immune system and unborn fetuses. If a person is immunosuppressed (e.g., receiving immune-suppressive drugs, is elderly, or has some other type of immunosuppressive condition), the organism may escape from the patient's tissue cysts and cause severe illness, including inflammation of the brain, nervous system, heart, liver, and eyes. If a woman that is already infected with *Toxoplasma* falls pregnant there is no risk to the unborn fetus. However, if a woman who has not previously been infected by *Toxoplasma* becomes infected with the organism during pregnancy there is a risk that *T. gondii* may cross the placenta and infect the fetus, with the potential to cause stillbirth or neurological or ocular disease in the child.

So what can we do about *Toxoplamsa gondii?* First, it is important to remember that this is a ubiquitous organism and can be found in soil and animals worldwide. Based on the average infection rates in humans, there is a one in three chance that you are already infected by *Toxoplasma gondii*, and likely you will not suffer any adverse health consequences from it. However, there are some simple precautions that can be taken to prevent infection with *Toxoplasma*, and these guidelines should be strictly followed by pregnant women and immunocompromised individuals. Make sure all meat is cooked thoroughly to 160 degrees Fahrenheit, or medium-well done, or greater. This will kill any *T. gondii* cysts that it might contain. Wash hands after handling raw meat. Thoroughly wash and/or peel all vegetables to remove any sporulated oocysts that may have come from the soil in which they were grown. Wear gloves when gardening for the same reason, and wash your hands afterward. Cover children's sandboxes when not attended to prevent cats from defecating in them. As cats are usually infected with *Toxoplasma* by eating infected prey or undercooked meat, prevent them from hunting or eating raw meat. It is very rare for an indoor cat fed only commercial cat food to become infected with *Toxoplasma*. Feral or stray cats are a more significant source of oocysts than pet cats. As oocysts are not able to infect humans for at least 24 hours after excretion by the cat, ensure that all feces are removed daily from the litter box. Consider using a disposable litter box liner to prevent the tray becoming contaminated with oocysts that have been present for more than one day, and scald the litter tray with boiling water when you clean it and let it sit for five minutes, but be careful not to burn yourself in the process!

Remember, most cats become infected when they are kittens and excrete the infective oocysts only for one very brief period lasting not more than three weeks, after which they are no longer a potential source of this zoonosis. Pregnant women and immunocompromised individuals should not acquire new kittens, but if they already own a cat, they do not need to get rid of it. Someone other than a pregnant woman should be in charge of litter box cleanup. If that is not possible, gloves should be worn by the woman when cleaning the litter box, and she should wash her hands well afterward.

It is not advisable to test your cat for *Toxoplasma* because it is not common for humans to be infected with *Toxoplasma* directly from cats, and serological testing cannot predict whether a cat is **shedding** oocysts or not. People usually acquire the infection from eating raw meat, ingesting oocyst-contaminated soil or vegetables, but not from cats. The oocyst excretion period is so brief that by the time serological tests reveal that a cat has been recently infected this period would have already finished. Also, because of the brevity of the excretion period, testing for the presence of oocysts in cats' feces is not recommended because the chances of discovering this brief excretion period are remote.

As previously mentioned, *Toxoplasma* can only cross the placenta (potentially resulting in disease of the fetus) if a woman is infected with *T. gondii* for the first time while she is pregnant. Hence, if a *Toxoplasma* test were to be performed, it would be more useful to test the mother prior to becoming pregnant, rather than to test the cat. If the mother tests positive, it means that she has already been infected, *T. gondii* will not cross the placenta, and the fetus is not at risk. If the test turns out to be negative, she needs to be careful, but the advice is the same: Follow the guidelines outlined previously.

Studies have also found that, because they are such fastidious groomers, cats' coats are not contaminated by *Toxoplasma* oocysts even when excreting the organism, so there is no risk of acquiring this particular infection from touching or petting cats. It has also been shown that HIV-positive individuals with a cat in the household are not at any greater risk of acquiring toxoplasmosis than those without a cat.[2] If an AIDS sufferer does develop clinical or symptomatic toxoplasmosis, it usually results from previously acquired tissue cysts becoming reactivated. There is thus no need for an HIV-positive person to relinquish ownership of a cat.

Although clinical toxoplasmosis may respond to appropriate antimicrobial medications, there is no benefit to treating a healthy cat for *Toxoplasma*, as this will not clear the organism from the cat.

DERMATOPHYTOSIS

Dermatophytosis is one of the most common and most contagious zoonoses. Colloquially, it is often called ringworm, because the classical lesion has a ring or circular shape, but this name is a confusing misnomer because the infection is caused by a fungus, not a worm. Most dermatophyte infections in dogs and cats are due to one of three species: *Microsporum gypseum, Microsporum canis,* and *Trichophyton mentagrophytes.* Cats are three times more likely to develop dermatophyte infections than dogs and so are the most common source of this zoonosis. Most dermatophyte infections in cats are due to the species *M. canis,* and cats are considered the natural reservoir of this organism. Infection with the less common dermatophyte species (*T. mentagrophytes* and *M. gypseum*) is more likely in outdoor cats, which tend to acquire them from hunted rodents or from the soil.

Generally, dermatophytosis is spread directly from cat to cat, but the infective fungal spores can survive in the environment for long periods of time and infection can be transferred indirectly when cats inhabit areas contaminated with hair or dandruff from an infected cat. *M. canis* can survive in the environment for 18 months, although this is dependent on ambient conditions. Dermatophytosis is more common in tropical and subtropical climates, and is more common in countries with significant numbers of feral or outdoor cats with poor health. Also, the condition is much more common in kittens, in longhaired and pedigree cats, and in such multicat environments as catteries or shelters.

Cats and dogs infected by dermatophytosis display classical lesions that are circular, hairless, but not itchy. However, the lesions in cats can vary widely in appearance such that there may be only subtle hair loss, with varying degrees of redness, itchiness, crusting, and inflammation. The nail beds may also become infected. Lesions are initially localized, usually on the head or front legs, but can spread and become more generalized. In people the appearance tends to be more characteristic with red, circular, slightly raised and itchy lesions.

In both animals and humans, immunity to dermatophytosis develops with time. As a result, it tends to be a self-limiting condition. Chronic infection in the cat may occur due to a defect in the cat's immunity, either inherited or acquired. Likewise, the infection has the potential to be more severe in immunocompromised people, in whom it may invade through the skin to deeper structures and spread to other parts of the body. Some cats may carry the organism on their coats yet not show any signs of infection. These cats may be a source of spread of dermatophytosis, although the chances of animals or humans acquiring an infection from such a cat is lower since the dose of the organism that they carry may not be sufficient to cause infection. The most common source of infection is typically kittens, especially those that have come from a multicat environment where there has been a history of dermatophytosis.

The appearance of typical lesions on a cat may be enough to allow a veterinarian to make a presumptive diagnosis. The veterinarian may also highlight the infected hairs with a special ultraviolet lamp, or recommend laboratory culture of the organism in a medium that favors fungal growth. Although the condition is often self-limiting and may resolve without the need for medication in kittens or puppies, treatment is usually warranted to minimize environmental contamination and its spread to other animals or humans. Treatment of affected cats and dogs involves application of antifungal creams and the use of medicated shampoos and rinses. Oral drugs are generally administered unless the lesions are small and focal, or the animal is not a suitable candidate for these drugs. Treatment may be necessary for a long period, such as one to two months or more, and resolution can be determined by negative fungal cultures of hair brushings or pluckings. Where possible, the infective spores must be removed from the environment by detailed and repeated cleaning and disinfection. This involves vacuuming of carpets and furnishings and washing of surfaces with dilute bleach. Vacuum bags need to be tied closed and disposed of or burnt. Although a commercial vaccine is available to prevent and treat dermatophytosis in cats, trials have found it to be ineffective, and when given to clinically affected cats, it may result in them becoming asymptomatic carriers of the organism; hence, it is not recommended.

The eradication of dermatophytosis from a cattery, shelter, or multicat premises can be especially difficult. Ideally, all cats in the facility should be treated, but this is often not possible or practical. Alternatively, a system of quarantine and treatment of affected or suspect cats in separate rooms is necessary, with return to an infection-free room when proven to be no longer carrying the organism.

As kittens are the most likely source of infection, they should be acquired from sources that do not have a history of dermatophyte infection. Such sources may include private breeders with a small numbers of cats or well-managed catteries and shelters. Studies have shown that 50 percent of people exposed to a dermatophyte-infected cat will become infected.[3] In approximately 70 percent of households with an infected cat, at least one family member will acquire the zoonosis.[4] Accordingly, children and immunocompromised people should avoid handling a new cat until it has been examined by a veterinarian. This applies especially to cats acquired from multicat facilities and to kittens. People who develop any suspicious skin lesions should be checked by a physician. Treatment in people may involve local creams or medications and, in more severe cases, oral antifungal medications.

PASTEURELLA MULTOCIDA

Four to five million people are reported to be bitten by animals in the United States every year, but the actual number is much higher because many more are not reported. Cats are responsible for only 5–25 percent of these occurrences, but a bite from a cat is much more likely to become

infected than a bite from a dog. In fact, the infection rate in people bitten by cats is estimated to be 20–80 percent, while the range from dogs is
approximately 3–18 percent.[5] Dog bites tend to cause more open wounds
resulting from crushing or tearing of tissues, but cat bites usually involve
deep needlelike punctures inflicted by their thin canine teeth, wound
tracts that provide ideal environments for the growth of bacteria normally inhabiting their mouths. Although many disease-causing bacteria
have been isolated from infected animal bites, the most common of these
is *Pasteurella multocida,* which is the infectious agent in around three-
quarters of infected wounds resulting from cat bites.

Bacteria normally inhabit the mouths of animals and people, and *P.
multocida* is no exception. This organism has been found in the nasal cavity, pharynx, and mouth of most cats, where it forms part of the normal
bacterial **flora**, and it can be found in kittens less than seven days of age,
where it is presumed to be spread by the mother to the kittens when she
licks their faces. Alternatively, it might be picked up by the kittens from
the mother's skin when suckling. The presence or absence of the organism
in a cat's mouth is not related to such other factors as environment, age,
gender, or breed. *Pasteurella* are also present in dogs' mouths, but with a
lower frequency, so a person is less likely to acquire infection from this
organism from a dog bite. Many cats and dogs have *Pasteurella* in their
saliva, but this is unlikely to cause infection in humans unless inoculated
in a wound.

In humans, when a wound from a bite develops a *Pasteurella* infection,
it usually appears as a localized tissue inflammation or abscess, with redness, heat, swelling, pain, and/or pus. The draining lymph node may be
enlarged. Fever, malaise, and weakness may occur. Symptoms can start
as soon as 2 to 12 hours after the bite, and if not attended to may worsen
over the following days. There is the potential for infection to migrate
into deeper structures such as bones, joints, and tendons, particularly if
not treated promptly. Rarely, it may disseminate via the bloodstream or
lymphatics and cause serious complications at more distant sites in the
body, such as the heart (endocarditis) or brain (meningitis). Immunocompromised or **splenectomized** patients are particularly at risk of these more
serious complications.

To avoid *Pasteurella* infection when bitten by a cat, a person should immediately wash the wound thoroughly with soap and water and visit a
physician promptly. In many cases antibiotics will be prescribed, and their
early administration is crucial to preventing an established infection.

PLAGUE

Plague is caused by *Yersinia pestis,* a bacterial species that is highly
infectious to humans. This organism has caused the death of hundreds

of millions of people throughout history as it struck in the form of several catastrophic pandemics, including Justinian's Plague in Rome from 540 to 590 C.E., the Black Death of 1347 to around 1400 C.E., and the Great Plague of London in 1665 C.E. Except for Australia and Antarctica, the disease is present on all continents, with endemic areas in some parts of Africa, Southeast Asia, South America, the Middle East, and the western third of the United States, where it is endemic in the states between the Rocky Mountains and the Pacific Ocean, especially northern New Mexico, southern Colorado, California, and northern Arizona. It can also be found is some of the Plains states. It is a disease that is more common in semi-arid locations, with many cases reported in children in southwestern Native American reservations. The U.S. incidence of reported cases has increased since 1970, and this may be related to increasing semiurban development encroaching on areas where the disease is endemic.

Wildlife reservoirs of *Yersinia pestis* primarily include wild rodents, such as rock and ground squirrels, chipmunks, prairie dogs, wood rats, deer mice, and voles, among which a low level of disease is maintained with occasional deadly outbreaks. The disease is spread by the fleas that infest these animals. Cat and dog fleas are not efficient or significant spreaders of the disease, but in the states where plague is endemic, dog and cat fleas are not common, so fleas found on companion animals in these areas could be rodent fleas and carriers of plague. The organism may infect domestic rats, which historically have been the source of urban plague epidemics. Farm animals and dogs, however, are largely resistant to developing illness. This is evidenced by the finding of antibodies to plague in dogs that did not develop any signs of illness, although in some rare cases dogs have shown fever and inflammation of lymph nodes. Most dogs recover spontaneously and have not been associated with transfer of the disease to humans. Cats, however, show a similar spectrum of disease to that seen in people and have been implicated in transmission to people.

Cats are infected either by ingestion of infected rodents or rabbits or, after being bitten by, or ingesting, rodent fleas. Humans are usually infected after being bitten by infected fleas but can also acquire the infection from contact with an infected animal, including rodents, lagomorphs, or the carnivores that eat them. Of those carnivores, most have been cats. Cats that have the pneumonic form of plague (infection of the lungs) can infect people who are in close contact through coughing, breathing, and sneezing. Between 1977 and 1988, contact with infected cats resulted in 23 cases of human plague, which was 7.7 percent of the total number of cases of human plague.[6] These cases resulted from bites or scratches from infected cats, nursing of sick cats, and contact with dead carcasses. Other carnivores that may infect humans include bobcats, coyotes, skunks, raccoons, and badgers; trappers and hunters need to be very cautious in endemic areas. Infection can also be transferred to humans by contamination of mucous membranes or abraded skin with secretions (saliva, blood) or exudates (pus from a wound). Person-to-person spread is possible (pneumonic form), but this has not occurred in the United States since 1925.

Clinical signs can appear within one to two days in experimentally infected cats, whereas the incubation period in humans is one to eight days. Both cats and humans may develop the three classical forms of plague: bubonic, **septicemic** (infection of the bloodstream), and pneumonic. In both species, bubonic is the most common, consisting of markedly enlarged swellings under the skin. These are infected lymph nodes (known as buboes) that are painful and contain pus, the discharges from which are highly infectious. In cats, the swollen nodes are most commonly located around the head because this species is usually infected by ingestion of a rodent and the organism enters the cat's body through the oral mucosa. In humans, the buboes are commonest in the armpit, but may be found in the neck, thigh, or groin, depending on where the organism entered the body. Infection via flea bites is more likely to cause enlarged nodes in the groin or femoral area, whereas infection from a cat bite or scratch generally causes enlarged nodes in the neck or armpit. In both humans and cats, the buboes may be accompanied by fever, lethargy, malaise, and inappetence. Death may follow, especially if the administration of appropriate antibiotics is delayed.

In cats and humans, the septicemic form may occur directly or indirectly following the bubonic form. In septicemic cases, infection spreads via the bloodstream to cause multiorgan failure, shock, and death. The pneumonic form may occur due to spread from the other two forms or may occur due to primary infection via aerosolized droplets from an animal or human with the pneumonic form. This most alarming mode of transmission means that even being in close proximity (within two meters) to a cat that has the pneumonic form is dangerous. Close contact with a human infected with the pneumonic form is also potentially dangerous.

A presumed diagnosis, based on clinical signs shown by the cat and the finding of the typical safety pin-shaped bacteria in buboes, may be made by a veterinarian and treatment started. This is followed by laboratory confirmation. Extreme caution should be exercised. The condition is a reportable disease: State health authorities must be informed and those exposed to the cat should urgently see a physician. Infected animals should be isolated and veterinary personnel must wear a protective gown, mask, gloves, and eye protection. After 72 hours of appropriate antibiotics, cats will no longer be infectious to humans. Surfaces contaminated by secretions and fluids from infected cats should be cleaned with routine disinfectants. The cat and its home environment should be treated for fleas, and other animals in contact with this cat at home should be treated.

Mortality in untreated human and feline cases is high, but when antibiotics are administered early enough most will recover. Surgical drainage of buboes may be required.

In endemic areas, cats and dogs should be kept indoors and not allowed to roam or hunt, and strict flea control should be implemented. Potential sites of rodent infestation should be removed by cleaning up piles of wood, rocks, and junk around houses, and animal food should not be left outside. Health authorities may advise fumigation of likely rodent and flea-infested areas.

Q FEVER

Q fever was first recognized in 1937 in Australian abattoir workers and is caused by the bacterium *Coxiella burnetii*. Initially, it was thought that this zoonosis mainly affected farm and abattoir workers, but in the 1980s in the maritime states of Canada, outbreaks of Q fever were documented after exposure to cats giving birth, indicating that other animals also served as sources of infection for humans. The prevalence of infection in cats is still uncertain, but 20 percent of shelter cats in one study conducted in southern California had antibodies to *C. burnetii*, indicating past or present infection.[7] Another study found the organism's DNA in the uterus of 8.5 percent of client-owned cats in north-central Colorado.[8]

In 1991, an article was published in a medical journal highlighting the risk from parturient cats.[9] This article described a family reunion that occurred over a three-day period at the home of the grandparents in Gouldsboro, Maine, a small coastal fishing village. All family members reported direct or close contact with a cat that was giving birth and her kittens shortly after birth. Within two to three weeks, all 11 adults and the older children attending the reunion had developed acute Q fever, which included headaches, high fever, cold sweats, muscle pain, nausea, vomiting, or cough.

C. burnetii is found worldwide and is potentially highly infectious. Natural reservoirs for the organism are ticks and many animal species, both domestic and wild, including birds and amphibians. The most important of these with regard to human zoonoses are cattle, sheep, goats, and cats. There is no evidence that ticks transfer the disease to humans, although ticks do spread the disease between animals, particularly from wild animals to domestic species. Domestic animals do not require ticks to transfer infection, as the placenta and birth fluids of these species may contain high numbers of *C. burnetii*, which contaminate pasture and soil when birth occurs. The organism is resistant to extremes of temperature and desiccation, so it can readily spread by wind-blown dust once it dries. Hence, living on a road traversed by farm animals as they move between paddocks has been found to be a risk factor for people acquiring Q Fever.

However, the route of infection in humans is usually by direct aerosol spread from placental membranes and amniotic fluids of animals giving birth or aborting. The organism has also been found in the urine and feces of infected animals. Rarely, consumption of infected, raw (unpasteurized) milk or dairy products can lead to human infection, and human-to-human spread has also been reported.

Cats may become infected by ingesting a contaminated carcass or prey, from a tick bite, or via aerosol from a contaminated environment. Although infection has been associated with abortion in animals, at which time large numbers of the organism are excreted with the placenta, most animals, including cats, are usually asymptomatic. Exposure to stillborn kittens presents a particularly high risk for human infection with Q fever.

The disease in humans can be inapparent, acute, or chronic. Most human infections are asymptomatic or consist of nonspecific flulike symptoms, hence, it may go undiagnosed. Symptoms of acute human infection begin within two to four weeks of exposure and include fever, chills, muscle and joint pain, headache, and malaise. Pneumonia and hepatitis are common manifestations of disease, and occasionally it can infect the brain, heart, and other organs. Chronic Q fever can present as a chronic fatigue syndrome, with lethargy, muscle and joint pain, sleep disturbances, headaches, and fever. In some cases, relapses have occurred decades after recovered acute infections. Early treatment with antibiotics and other drugs is important, and mortality occurs in less than 1 percent of cases.

The organism has been cultured from the uterus of cats 10 weeks after parturition and in urine for 8 weeks after experimental infection. Subsequently, cats that appear to be apparently healthy may be infectious when giving birth. Indeed, it is not yet known whether the organism causes fetal deaths, abortions, or stillbirths in cats. Accordingly, humans should take care when a cat is giving birth. Direct contact with the birth fluids and placenta of cats should be avoided, and early spaying of female cats should be considered, especially if the cat's owner is immunocompromised.

RABIES IN CATS

As cycling of rabies infection does not occur amongst cats, infection in cats is regarded as a spillover from other species. In skunks, raccoons, foxes, and bats, spread of rabies may occur between members of the same species, maintaining a presence of the virus in the environment. In the United States, cats (and dogs) need to be infected by another species, a rabies reservoir species (skunk, raccoon, fox, bat); there is no feline or canine strain of the virus in this country.

The species and strain of rabies that infects cats depends on the geographical area. In the U.S. Midwest, it is the strain spread by skunks, while on the Atlantic coast it is usually the raccoon strain. In developing countries, it is usually the dog strain, and, as a result, dog rabies is still the most important cause of human rabies worldwide. However, in the United States since 1980, more cases of rabies have been reported in cats than in dogs. In 2009, there were 300 cases of rabies in cats compared to 81 cases of dogs.[10] Despite these figures, fewer people seek rabies protection after cat bites than after dog bites.

It usually takes two months after exposure to a rabid animal before cats show clinical signs, although this can vary from two weeks to several months. Rabid cats are usually unvaccinated, over one month of age, and with a history of outdoor access in an endemic area. Behavior changes are typically present and may be noticed first, such as unusual friendliness, shyness, irritability, vocalization, or voice change. Unexplained paralysis or weakness is often present, sometimes presenting as lameness of a hind leg. Clinical signs can be subtle and variable for one to two days, including vomiting, inappetence, fever, diarrhea, lethargy, or depression, sometimes with neurological signs. The furious and dumb forms may occur in cats. The furious form is seen in 90 percent of rabid cats, with trembling, pacing aimlessly, rage, fearfulness, viciousness, and attacking inanimate objects. Clinical signs in cats worsen over three to five days. Death occurs within 10 days, often within 3–4 days.

A classic situation regarding rabies was described of a family on vacation that stopped at a fast food outlet in Texas.[11] There the two daughters found a very friendly kitten and talked their parents into letting them take it home, unaware that they were in grave danger. Despite being checked after the family returned home the next day by their local veterinarian, the kitten was judged to be healthy and routine vaccines, including a rabies vaccine, were administered. The cat seemed very quiet for the rest of the day, but the following day was found hiding apprehensively in a closet. On the third day it was taken back to the veterinarian. At this time it appeared extremely nervous, with slight hind limb lameness, but otherwise normal. However, as the examination was concluding, the kitten unexpectedly attacked violently, repeatedly biting the veterinarian and the veterinary assistant. Although the family lived in a rabies-free area, the cat was euthanized, and subsequently confirmed to be rabid. The family was advised of the diagnosis and referred to their physician, while the veterinarian and veterinary assistant, who had previously been vaccinated against rabies, were given two further doses of rabies vaccine.

The above story highlights the risks to humans posed by stray cats or cats of unknown vaccination status. Stray cats should be approached with caution. Even if they appear healthy, handling of rescued cats should be considered with caution. Infected cats start shedding the virus in saliva about three days before they show illness, and continue to do so until death. Theoretically, they can transfer the virus to humans by licking as well as biting, so a cat that bites a human should be confined and observed for 10 days, during which time the cat should not receive a rabies vaccination. If the cat shows signs that are suspicious of rabies during the quarantine period, it should be euthanized, local health authorities informed, and the cat submitted to an approved laboratory for rabies testing.

In countries where rabies is endemic (such as the United States), all cats should be vaccinated against rabies. If a fully vaccinated cat is bitten by a suspected or proven rabid animal, it should receive an immediate rabies booster vaccine and be placed into quarantine for 45 days. If a cat that is not currently and fully vaccinated against rabies is bitten by a potentially rabid animal, it should be euthanized and tested for rabies. Alternatively, if euthanasia is not performed, the cat should be placed in quarantine for six months and vaccinated against rabies during this time. Consultation with a veterinarian and local animal control officials should be performed in these circumstances, and public health authorities should be informed immediately about any suspected human rabies exposures. Individuals exposed to a potentially rabid cat (or other animal) should visit a physician as a matter of urgency.

OTHER ZOONOSES OF CATS

This chapter has highlighted several important zoonoses associated with cats, but there are numerous others. These include a number of infectious agents of the gastrointestinal tract that have the potential to infect humans. *Dipylidium caninum* is a tapeworm that can infect both cats and humans through the ingestion of infected fleas. Human infection is uncommon, but when it occurs it is usually in children, in whom it may cause abdominal pain, diarrhea, or anal itchiness. Roundworms, which may colonize the gut of dogs or cats, can infect humans when they ingest eggs passed in the feces of these animals. The conditions known as visceral larva migrans and ocular larva migrans may result, which refer to the migration of these worms into the organs or eyes of humans with subsequent inflammation and damage. Hookworm is another worm that may infect cats and is zoonotic. When hookworm eggs contact the skin of a person (typically when a person has contact with soil that is contaminated by excreta from infected dogs and cats), the person may develop cutaneous larva migrans, which refers to very itchy worm-shaped tracts visible in the skin. Accordingly, all cats should be regularly dewormed under the supervision of a veterinarian.

Cats may also be infected with zoonotic protozoa, such as *Giardia* or *Cryptosporidium,* or by zoonotic bacteria such as *Campylobacter* and *Salmonella,* which can cause diarrhea in humans. However, it is much more likely that humans will become infected by these agents from environmental sources such as contaminated food or water rather than by direct contact with cats. Higher numbers of potentially zoonotic organisms are excreted in the feces of cats with diarrhea, so to minimize the risk to humans, cats with diarrhea should be examined by a veterinarian.

Human tularemia, caused by the bacterium *Francisella tularensis,* is usually transmitted by infected ticks, but can sometimes come from contact with infected animals, including cats. Cats in turn may be infected by ticks or through the ingestion of infected rabbits and rodents. Infection of humans via cat bites or scratches is uncommon, and various forms of the disease can occur in people depending on the route of infection. Infected cats usually exhibit inflamed lymph nodes and abscessed organs. To reduce the risk of spread from cats to humans, owners should use tick preventative products on their cats and prevent them from hunting.

Sporotrichosis is a fungal infection caused by contamination of skin wounds with the organism *Sporothrix schenckii,* which is found in soil, but can be associated with plants and plant material. Cats probably become infected during fights through scratches from cats with contaminated nails, and humans may be infected when the organism contacts broken skin. Infected cats and humans develop ulcerative, purulent skin lesions, which may spread via the lymphatic system. The fungus multiplies in infected cats and is then passed in large numbers in their feces and wound discharges, with the potential to infect humans. Gloves should be worn when working with infected cats, and hands should be thoroughly washed when done.

Chlamydophila felis is a bacterium that causes conjunctivitis and mild sneezing in cats. It can also cause conjunctivitis in people who touch ocular discharges from infected cats, and occasionally has caused infections of the lungs, kidneys, and heart of humans. People, especially immunocompromised individuals, should avoid contact with ocular or respiratory discharges of cats.

Fleas and mites, including *Cheyletiella, Sarcoptes,* and *Notoedres* can spread from cats to humans, causing skin disease. There are numerous rinses, sprays, and spot-on products available to prevent infestation of cats with these parasites.

GENERAL RECOMMENDATIONS

When adopting a new cat, the safest choice with regards to protecting human health and preventing zoonotic disease transmission will be a healthy indoor adult cat with no ectoparasites (fleas, ticks, or mites) from a private family. Such a cat is of very little risk to humans because it comes from an environment that is least likely to be contaminated by many different cats and many different organisms. The new cat should be quarantined from immunocompromised individuals until it has been checked by a veterinarian; thereafter, it should be checked by a veterinarian at least yearly, and whenever it is sick. It should be vaccinated against rabies, dewormed regularly, and commercially available flea and tick control products should be used year-round to prevent infestation with these parasites.

Litter box liners should be used and litter boxes cleaned at regular intervals with detergent and scalding water. Feces should be removed daily, preferably not by an immunocompromised person. If an immunocompromised person must clean the litter box, gloves should be worn and hands washed thoroughly afterwards Hands should be washed after handling cats and other animals, and the handling of animals that are unfamiliar should be avoided. Cats and dogs should be prevented from drinking from toilets. Children's sandboxes should be covered to prevent cats defecating in them. Gloves should be worn when gardening and handling meat, and hands washed thoroughly with soap and water afterward. All meat should be cooked to at least 160 degrees Fahrenheit (medium-well). Keeping cats indoors is encouraged as it reduces their exposure to many potentially zoonotic agents. Cats should not be allowed to lick your face, and food utensils should not be shared with them. Cats' nails should be kept trimmed to avoid skin penetration when scratched, and cats should not be provoked into biting or scratching. If a person is scratched or bitten, he or she should apply first aid and be checked by a physician.

GLOSSARY

Antibodies: proteins produced by the body to combat infectious organisms.

Culture: to grow an organism in a prepared medium in a laboratory.

Endemic: an organism or disease is present in a locality or region.

Endocarditis: inflammation of the lining of the heart

Flora: a population of microorganisms living in or on the body.

Immunosuppress: to suppress a person's natural immunity to illness.

Incubation period: the time between infection with an organism and the onset of illness.

Lymph nodes: glands that form part of the immune system and drain and filter lymph from tissues.

Papule: a small red elevation of the skin.

PCR: polymerase chain reaction; a method of detecting an organism's DNA.

Reservoir: an organism in which a pathogen maintains a presence in the environment.

Septicemic: infection of circulating blood with infectious organisms accompanied by illness

Serology: analysis of blood for antibodies.

Shedding: releasing an infectious organism into the environment.

Splenectomize: to remove the spleen.

Uveitis: inflammation of the uvea; a part of the eye.

Vector: an animal, such as an insect or arthropod, that can transmit an infectious organism between animals or to humans.

FURTHER READING

American Association of Feline Practitioners. 2006 Panel report on diagnosis, treatment, and prevention of Bartonella spp. infections. Available at: http://www.catvets.com/professionals/guidelines/publications/index. aspx?ID=175.

Breitschwerdt EB, Maggi RG, Chomel BB, et al. Bartonellosis: An emerging infectious disease of zoonotic importance to animals and human beings. *Journal of Veterinary Emergency and Critical Care* 2010;20(1):8–30.

Center for Food Security and Public Health Plague information page. Available at: http://www.cfsph.iastate.edu/DiseaseInfo/disease.php?name=plague& lang=enGreene.

Centers for Disease Control and Prevention (CDC) information pages. Available at: http://www.cdc.gov/rabies/

http://www.cdc.gov/ncidod/diseases/submenus/sub_q_fever.htm

http://www.cdc.gov/nczved/divisions/dfbmd/diseases/dermatophytes/

REFERENCES

1. Lappin MR, Griffin B, Brunt J, et al. Prevalence of Bartonella spp., Mycoplasma spp., Ehrlichia spp., and Anaplasma phagocytophilum DNA in the blood of cats and their fleas in the United States. *Journal of Feline Medicine and Surgery* 2006;8:85–90.
2. Wallace MR, Rossetti RJ, and Olson PE. Cats and toxoplasmosis risk in HIV-infected adults. *Journal of the American Medical Association* 1993;269:76–7.
3. Pepin, GA, Oxenham M. Feline dermatophytosis. The diagnosis of subclinical infection and its relevance to control. *Veterinary Dermatology Newsletter* 1997;11:21.
4. Pepin, GA, Oxenham, M. Zoonotic dermatophytosis (ringworm). *Veterinary Record* 1986;118:110–11.
5. Griego R, Rosen T, Orengo I, et al. Dog, cat, and human bites: A review. *Journal of the American Academy of Dermatology* 1995;33:1019–29.
6. Gage KL, Dennis DT, Orloski KA, et al. Cases of cat-associated human plague in the western US, 1977–1998. *Clinical Infectious Diseases* 2000;30:893–900.
7. Randhawa AS, Dieterich WH, Jolley WB, et al. Coxiellosis in pound cats. *Feline Practice* 1974;4:37–8.
8. Cairns K, Brewer M, Lappin M. Prevalence of Coxiella burnetii DNA in vaginal and uterine samples from healthy cats of north-central Colorado. *Journal of Feline Medicine & Surgery* 2007;9:196–201.

9. Pinsky RL, Fishbein DB, Greene CR, et al. An outbreak of cat-associated Q fever in the United States. *Journal of Infectious Diseases* 1991;164:202–4.
10. Blanton JD, Palmer D, Rupprecht CE. Rabies surveillance in the United States during 2009. *Journal of the American Veterinary Medical Association* 2010; 237:646–57.
11. Clark, KA. Rabies. *Journal of the American Veterinary Medical Association* 1988;192:1404–6.

Chapter 10

Zoonoses of Concern from Small Mammals

Jeffrey L. Rhody, DVM

INTRODUCTION

A few decades ago veterinary medical professionals divided the world of animals into companion small animals (dogs and cats), food animals (cows, sheep, pigs, chickens, etc.), equine (horses), and zoo animals. Today things have changed. While the divisions of food animals and equine remain unchanged, we look at companion animals differently. People no longer consider dogs and cats as the only house pets. Birds and reptiles are also commonplace in homes and are considered valued family members. Parrots and tortoises are even placed in owner's wills to allow for their continued care in the likely event they outlive their owners.

This chapter addresses a rapidly growing segment of the pet population—small mammals. Small mammals kept as pets include rabbits, rodents, ferrets, sugar gliders, African pygmy hedgehogs, Virginia opossums, and fennec foxes. Pet rodents include mice, rats, hamsters, gerbils, guinea pigs, chinchillas, degus (de/-gyu with a short e sound), squirrels, chipmunks, and prairie dogs. These pets deserve high quality medical care as much as any other species. In fact, in 2009, the American Board of Veterinary Practitioners offered the first board specialty exam for veterinarians to become an "exotic" small mammal specialist.

When we share our lives and our homes with animals, we accept certain responsibilities—not the least of which is to provide the best possible care for them. Many of the exotic small mammals discussed in this chapter have specialized requirements. For example, guinea pigs require vitamin C in their diet, and chinchillas and degus need regular dust baths. Nutritional requirements differ with each species. How we house, feed, and interact with our pets plays a large role in their ability to stay vibrant and healthy. Proper care of a specific species translates into less likelihood of infectious disease. Less infection in our pets translates into less potential for people to be exposed to zoonotic infections. Consequently, keeping our pets healthy helps keep us healthy. This chapter also addresses common small mammalian wildlife species that can transmit diseases to humans, including wild rodents, wild rabbits and hares, raccoons, foxes, wild hedgehogs, and squirrels.

REALITY AND THIS CHAPTER

This book is designed to educate readers about animal diseases and their impact on human health. In the following pages you will learn about diseases that small mammals can carry and consequently transmit to people. This chapter will address zoonoses from pet, laboratory, and wild small mammals. Do not let the material presented color your view of the world. Microbes are ubiquitous in nature. They are spread via contact, air, food, and water, and by insects, especially mosquitoes and fleas, because they suck blood from their hosts. If we were able to see microscopically with our naked eyes, the world would look like one large bug-infested planet. Bacteria and fungi would be everywhere. If we could see through an electron microscope as we walked around, we would see viruses everywhere. Whether we like it or not, what looks "clean" to us is really not— well it is, it is just not free of microorganisms. The world we live in is not sterile.

If you dwell on the prevalence of microorganisms in the world, you might obsess about getting sick. You would not garden, you would not touch anything barehanded, and you might not even eat. The microscopic world can be dangerous; however, we could not survive without bacteria. In your body now, millions of millions of bacteria live and thrive. Most, if not all, of these bacteria are harmless to you. Many are beneficial. If our bodies were sterile, our immune system would be compromised, and our digestion would be impaired. All bacteria, fungi, and viruses are not pathogens (microbes that cause disease), nor do all parasites cause disease.

As you read this chapter, do not lose sight of the fact that while there are many microbes around you, most are harmless. The information provided is informative and educational. You should be aware of zoonotic diseases and how to prevent them, but should not be scared into living life through plastic wrap. This chapter is intended to promote disease awareness and not intended to create disease paranoia.

10.1. DID YOU KNOW?

- Hunters can acquire tularemia from sick rabbits, which is likely responsible for the adage, "Never shoot the slow rabbit."
- Rat bite fever is most common in Japan, where it is called Sodoku.
- Leptospirosis, once a disease of rural areas and associated with livestock, is commonly carried by rodents in urban areas.
- Mice commonly get pinworms, but these are not the same as human pinworms and will not cause disease in people.

WHAT IS NOT IN THIS CHAPTER

There are many zoonotic illnesses that can be transmitted by small mammals that are not discussed in detail in this chapter. Rabies is perhaps the most important zoonotic illness carried by warm-blooded animals. Because pet small mammals carry rabies very rarely, it will not be discussed. *Salmonella* is a bacterium that causes gastrointestinal illness in people. We will discuss it briefly in this chapter, but a wider discussion of salmonellosis can be found in other chapters in this book. Finally, the list of potential zoonoses from small mammals is long. I will list all known potential diseases, but will discuss in detail only a relative few.

BACTERIAL ZOONOSES

Tularemia

Caused by *Francisella tularensis*, tularemia is one of the most common bacterial zoonoses from small mammals in the United States, Europe, and Asia. Tularemia, however, is uncommonly associated with captive or pet animals. Wild rodents and lagomorphs (hares and rabbits) are the primary reservoir hosts. *Francisella* is usually transmitted to people via insect bites (ticks and deer flies), via drinking water contaminated by dead hosts, or contact at slaughter or ingestion of dead animals. Tularemia is sometimes called rabbit fever or deer fly fever.

In the United States, tularemia was first described in 1911 and has since been reported in all states except Hawaii. According to reports from the Centers for Disease Control and Prevention (CDC) over 70 percent of human cases are associated with a tick bite. Hunters and landscapers are at an increased risk of exposure. Insect bite-related exposure is increased in spring and summer, but hunters more often get infected during the fall and winter hunting seasons.

Infected people develop skin lesions, respiratory disease, and/or meningitis (inflammation of the membranes around the central nervous system tissues). Symptoms show up 1–10 days after infection and can show up in one of six syndromes (a constellation of symptoms comprise a syndrome). The most common clinical syndrome is ulceroglandular. Ulceroglandular tularemia causes a skin ulcer at the site of infection (e.g., tick bite), swollen or painful lymph nodes, fever, chills, headache, and exhaustion.

It is recommended that all forms of tularemia be treated with antibiotics. Treated tularemia has a very low mortality rate. Untreated tularemia (especially in the lung and other internal organs) can be fatal in 40–60 percent of the cases.

Prevention and control of tularemia is straightforward and easy. People at risk should use insect repellents and check themselves daily to remove ticks. Chlorination of the water supply reduces contamination. All meat (especially wild rabbit) should be cooked well, and hunters should wear gloves and a mask when slaughtering their kill.

Rat Bite Fever

Rat bite fever (RBF) is a rare but serious zoonosis spread by laboratory or pet rodents worldwide. The bacteria involved are *Streptobacillus moniliformes* and *Spirillum minus*. In rats, the bacteria can cause infection of the lymph nodes in the neck, arthritis, gangrene, and infections in the throat. In the guinea pig, *Streptobacillus* (not *Spirillum*) causes infection of cervical (neck) lymph nodes (causing what is known as caseous lymphadenitis— the medical term for cottage cheese-like pus in a lymph node).

Streptobacillus and *Spirillum* can be found normally in the rat pharynx (the very front part of the throat) and can be passed on to other animals and people via bites of normal rats. People can also be infected via the bite of an infected animal or the contamination of wounds with infected fluids. *Streptobacillus* can also be inhaled or ingested by way of milk or water contaminated with rat feces. In the United States, RBF is most common in animal caretakers in research laboratories.

The incubation period (time from infection until symptoms develop) in people is 2–14 days for streptobacillary infection, and can be up to 60 days for spirillary infection. Symptoms include relapsing fever, chills, vomiting, muscle soreness, and enlarged lymph nodes in the region of the bite. Streptobacillary infections can also cause a rash.

Treatment with antibiotics is recommended, and untreated cases have a 7–10 percent fatality rate. Preventive measures to reduce prevalence of RBF include pasteurization of milk and elimination of access for rodents to contaminate food. Proper handling of laboratory and pet rats is important to avoid being bitten and to avoid acquiring this agent. All rat bite wounds should be thoroughly cleaned as soon as possible, and a physician should be consulted.

Plague

Plague, caused by *Yersinia pestis*, is covered in detail in chapter 9, "Zoonoses of Cats"; however, since rodents play a key role in this disease, the basics will be covered here as well. Plague is not a zoonosis of concern from pet rodents but is from wild rodents, which outdoor cats hunt. Cats then acquire the infection and can potentially pass the infection to their owners or anyone else who comes in close contact with them, such as veterinary staff.

Known mostly as the cause of the Black Death in the 1300s, plague is still seen in scattered rural areas of the United States. While only 5–15 cases per year are seen in this country, the World Health Organization reports a global incidence of 1,000 to 3,000 cases per year.

Yersinia pestis is spread primarily via the bite of the rodent fleas and causes three clinical forms of plague in people: bubonic, septicemic, and pneumonic. A flea takes a blood meal from an infected rodent (e.g., chipmunk, prairie dog, squirrel, mouse, and rat) or wild lagomorph (e.g., hare or rabbit). When that flea bites a human, *Yersinia* is released into the bloodstream and can cause bubonic plague. Typically, a person notes a painful swelling of a lymph gland. This swollen gland is called a bubo and is the reason for the name bubonic plague. Other symptoms include fever, chills, headache, and extreme exhaustion. *Yersinia* can then spread to the rest of the body via the bloodstream (septicemic plague) and to the lungs (secondary pneumonic plague). Primary pneumonic plague can occur when a person has close contact with another host (person or cat) that has secondary pneumonic plague. The person inhales *Yersinia pestis* when a host with secondary pneumonic plague talks, coughs, or breathes, aerosolizing the bacteria.

Bubonic plague in humans is most often associated with wild animals and their fleas, not usually pet animals, and has an incubation period of one to six days. Outbreaks of plague have been associated with guinea pigs farmed for food in the Andean regions of South America.[1]

Pneumonic plague patients show fever, weakness, and rapidly develop pneumonia and shortness of breath. Chest pain, cough and sputum that may be bloody or watery are also typical. Sometimes patients are nauseous, painful in their abdomen, and may vomit.

Prevention of zoonotic plague is associated with measures to reduce wild rodent populations and implementing flea control. According to the CDC, a vaccination is not available in the United States. People with pneumonic plague should be isolated while in the hospital setting, and people who have had contact with them should be treated with antibiotics preventively.

Leptospirosis

Leptospira is a special bacterial type called a spirochete, and these particular spirochetes tend to infect the liver and kidneys. Rats frequently get infected via contact with an infected rat's urine, which contaminates the environment with leptospira bacteria.

A reported case of leptospirosis in a veterinarian sends rat owners and veterinarians a cautionary message. In this case, a veterinarian had minor wounds on his hands from gardening when he examined a seemingly healthy pet rat. As rats are prone to do upon handling, it urinated on his hand. The veterinarian later developed fever, chills, and malaise and was later diagnosed with leptospirosis[3]

While leptospirosis (or lepto) is treatable with antibiotics, people with chronic kidney disease have a 20 percent mortality rate. When a person is urinated on by a rat or contacts rat urine, the area contacted should be washed as soon as possible, and gloves should be worn when handling rats if the handler has wounds on her hands. For more about leptospirosis, please see chapter 8, "Dog Zoonoses."

Typhus

Typhus is an illness caused by rickettsial bacteria, and there are three types of typhus: murine, epidemic, and scrub. In most cases, typhus in people causes high fever, rash and flulike symptoms. Murine typhus (also called endemic typhus) occurs when feces from a rodent flea that contains *Rickettsia typhi* contaminates wounds on people, thus infecting the person. Rats and opossum are the primary sources of these fleas. Worldwide in distribution, murine typhus in the United States occurs mostly on the Gulf Coast. Epidemic typhus is related to infected lice and their bites, and the animal reservoir is typically the flying squirrel. Consequently, hunters are at an increased risk of contracting this disease. Scrub typhus is due to chigger bites (chiggers are the larval form of trombulid mites) and is more common in Asia. Murine and scrub typhus are rarely fatal. Epidemic typhus has a high mortality rate without treatment.

Salmonellosis

Salmonellosis is a bacterial infection that can affect humans and animals. Many healthy animals carry this bacterium, and feces from these

Table 10.1

Bacterial Zoonoses from Small Mammals

Organism	Disease name (if any)	Potential carriers of disease
Bordetalla bronchiseptica	—	Rodents, lagamorphs
Campylobacter (multiple species)	Campylobacteriosis	Ferrets, hamsters, hedgehogs, rats
Corynebacterium kutscheri	—	Mice, rats, rabbits, hamsters
Francisella tularensis[1]	**Tularemia**	Rabbits
Leptospira[1]	**Leptospirosis**	Rats, mice, raccoons, skunks, hedgehogs
Listeria monocytogenes	Listeriosis	Ferrets
Mycobacterium (multiple species)	Mycobacteriosis	Ferrets, possums, raccoons
Pasteurella multocida	—	Rodents, rabbits
Streptobacillus moniliformes[1] **Spiriullum minus**	**Rat bite fever**	Rats
Salmonella[1] (multiple species)	**Salmonellosis**	Rodents, lagamorphs, sugar gliders, hedgehogs, prairie dogs, ferrets
Streptococcus pneumoniae	—	Guinea pigs, rats
Yersinia pestis[1]	**Plague**	Rats, prairie dogs, ground squirrels, guinea pigs
Yersinia pseudotuberculosis	—	Rodents, Lagamorphs
Yersinia enterocolitica	—	Chinchillas, Rabbits, Prairie Dogs, Other Rodents
Clostridium piliforme	Tyzzer's disease	Prairie Dogs, Guinea Pigs, Lagamorphs
Borrelia burgdorferi	Lyme disease	Squirrels, Hedgehogs, Hares, Rabbits
Rickettsia[1] (multiple species)	**Typhus**	Fleas from Rats, Opossums and Mites from Rodents
Helicobacter (multiple species)	—	Ferrets (potentially)[2]

[1] Discussed in chapter text.

[2] *Helicobacter* spp. may not be zoonotic.

animals can be infectious to other animals and people. Small mammal pets that can carry salmonella include rodents (including guinea pigs and chinchillas), ferrets, rabbits, prairie dogs, sugar gliders, and African pygmy hedgehogs. Salmonella is most commonly a foodborne pathogen (e.g., from undercooked chicken). It is estimated that only 3–5 percent of all human salmonellosis is associated with exposure to exotic pets.[4] With regard to small mammal-associated human salmonellosis, the incidence is very low. Most of the pet-associated salmonellosis is related to improper handling of reptiles. Prevention of salmonella involves basic hygiene. Hands should be washed after contact with any potential carrier species, after touching or cleaning the cage or food bowls, before eating, and before handling or preparing foods.

VIRAL ZOONOSES

Influenza

Local outbreaks of seasonal flu in people can be associated with epizootics (animal outbreaks) in ferrets. Influenza viruses A and B are responsible for the typical seasonal flu affecting humans, and it is of interest to note that ferrets can be infected with either of these. Influenza A causes an upper respiratory infection in ferrets, and just as with humans, immunocompromised ferrets with influenza infection can develop pneumonia and die. Influenza B is less common in people and causes milder clinical disease. Transmission of influenza virus is via respiratory aerosol containing the virus or contact with nasal discharge.

During the H1N1 outbreak in 2010, a few pet ferrets were infected, but all survived. During the outbreak, veterinarians were often contacted regarding the risk of infection posed to children by classroom rodents and ferrets. While rodents can be infected, they do not get ill or spread influenza. The classroom pet ferret has no risk of acquiring the flu virus unless a human transmits it to them. Therefore, humans pose more of a risk to the ferret than the ferret does to humans. If a classroom ferret develops the new H1N1 or seasonal flu, this provides indirect evidence that someone who had been in contact with the ferret was infected. This reasoning holds true unless a) the ferret is removed from the school (e.g., on the weekend) and gets infected by a human being or another ferret and returns to school and becomes ill, or, b) the ferret has been present in the classroom for less than one week and could have contracted influenza before it arrived.

Prevention of influenza virus infection is very important during the flu season. It is recommended that people, especially those with a high risk of serious complications from infection, receive annual flu vaccines. Anyone with flulike symptoms is encouraged to stay home from work, school, camp, mass gatherings, and shopping malls for at least 24 hours after fever disappears (without the use of fever-reducing medication). In the health-care setting (e.g., doctor's office, hospital, long-term care facility), more stringent control measures are recommended. Health-care workers and hospital visitors should stay away from hospitals for seven days from onset of symptoms or until symptoms resolve—whichever is longer. Other measures that may help reduce the spread of the virus include frequent washing of hands, avoiding sharing of eating utensils, and covering noses and mouths when sneezing or coughing. People who are coughing should sit at least 3–6 feet away from other people.

It is interesting that influenza A viruses infect a wide variety of species. While ferrets can be infected with avian flu virus (H5N1), seal flu virus (H3N2 and some H6 subtypes), and equine influenza H1N1), only the type A H1N1 and type B strains of flu will cause a ferret to become ill.

Lymphocytic Choriomeningitis Virus (LCMV)

LCMV was first isolated in 1933 and is a virus that is carried by rodents. Symptoms in people can range from no symptoms, a mild flulike illness

Table 10.2

Viral Zoonoses from Small Mammals

Organism	Disease name (if any)	Potential carriers of disease
Orthomyxovirus[1]	**Influenza A and B**	Ferrets
Influenza virus (H7N3/O2)	Avian flu	Ferrets,[2] mice[2]
Hantavirus[1]	**Hantavirus pulmonary syndrome**	Wild deer mice
Lyssavirus	Rabies	Any warm-blooded animal[3]
Arenavirus[1]	**Lymphocytic choriomeningitis**	Mouse, Guinea Pig, Hamster
Mouse Reovirus-3	—	Mice
Orthopoxvirus[1]	**Monkeypox**	Prairie dogs, Gambian rat
Herpes Simplex 1[4]	Herpes	Rabbits

[1] Discussed in chapter text.

[2] Ferrets and mice can be infected with the virus isolated from Pakistani chickens but no cases have been reported.

[3] Mostly associated with wildlife, especially raccoons and foxes, but has been isolated from ferrets, lagomorphs, and many rodents. Clinical rabies infection has been reported in rabbits.

[4] Herpes Simplex 1 has been shown to cause disease in rabbits but to date has never been associated with a human infection.

that is self-limiting, to severe neurologic problems. For those people who do become ill, signs usually begin 8–13 days after exposure to the virus. Classically, LCMV has two phases in humans consisting of a biphasic febrile illness. Biphasic fever occurs when fever goes away only to recur soon. The first phase, which can last up to one week, is typical of the flu, with symptoms that include fever, malaise, lack of appetite, muscle soreness, headache, nausea, and vomiting. Occasionally, sore throat, cough, joint aches, chest pain, painful testicles, and pain in the face and neck may be seen in phase one. Phase two begins a few days after recovery from phase one and includes symptoms such as meningitis (fever, headache, and a stiff neck), encephalitis (drowsiness, confusion, weird sensations, and maybe abnormal movements or severe weakness or paralysis), or both (meningoencephalitis). Rarely, acute hydrocephalus (increased fluid pressure in the brain) occurs and may require surgical intervention. There may also be an association with LCMV infection and inflammation of the heart muscles. All manifestations of the viral infection include inflammation of tissues without bacterial infection.

In most cases, recovery from LCMV infection is complete. No chronic infections have been reported. Sometimes scarring of the nervous system tissue from prior inflammation can cause temporary or permanent symptoms. Nerve deafness and arthritis have been reported as sequelae of infection. One of the major concerns about LCMV involves infection of a fetus. If a woman in the first trimester of pregnancy becomes infected and passes the infection (through the placenta) to the developing fetus, the virus can cause severe and permanent developmental defects. These defects include congenital hydrocephalus, chorioretinitis (inflammation in the eye resulting in blindness), and mental retardation. Although the disease lymphocytic choriomeningitis (LCM) has a mortality rate of less than 1 percent, fetal death has been reported. Treatment is supportive and not specific. Sometimes corticosteroids (cortisonelike medications) are used to reduce inflammation of tissues; however, there are no effective antiviral medications for LCMV.

LCM and milder LCMV infections are considered worldwide in distribution, but there have been no reported cases from Africa or Australia. Wild mice are the most common reservoir of infection, and it is estimated that about 5 percent of these mice in the United States carry LCMV. Prevalence of human LCMV infection is likely more widespread than reported. Serologic studies in urban areas report that 2–5 percent of people test positive for exposure to LCMV.

The primary source of human infection is the wild house mouse (*Mus musculus*), although LCMV can be carried by pet mice, guinea pigs, and hamsters as well. Infected mice shed the virus in their saliva, urine, and feces for the duration of their lives and usually do not show any signs of illness. Hamsters with LCMV can shed the virus for at least eight months.

Breeding rodents will transmit the virus to their offspring. Occasionally, infected animals will show symptoms of malaise, lack of appetite, and a rough hair coat. Severely affected rodents can show weight loss, a hunched posture, photophobia (fear of light), inflamed eyelids, tremors, and convulsions. Rarely, an infected rodent will die.

Human LCMV infections are almost always due to exposure to wild mice via contact with feces or urine or via a bite. Infected people are not contagious to one another, with the notable exception of vertical transmission (mother to fetus). It has been noted recently that transplantation of infected organs may cause LCMV infection in the recipient. Arthropod parasites (e.g., bedbugs, cockroaches, fleas, flies, lice, midges, mites, mosquitoes, and ticks) can act as vectors if they obtain virus from an infected rodent and bite a person or contaminate food items.

While domesticated mice, rats, guinea pigs, and hamsters can carry the virus, they represent a minor but potential risk for infection. Pets are usually infected at the breeder, in the pet store, or at home by exposure to wild mice feces and urine. In 1973–1974, a LCM epidemic occurred in the United States involving 181 cases in 12 different states.[5] Epidemiologists and public health officials found the source of the infection—a single location in Alabama that housed and sold hamsters for distribution to other sites.

Prevention of LCMV infection is important for at-risk individuals. Laboratory workers who work with either the virus or handle infected animals are at significant risk of infection. However, this risk can be minimized by taking proper protective measures to reduce contact with the virus or rodent feces and urine. Proper handling and protective gear can prevent rodent bites. Laboratories should also use only those animals that come from sources that regularly screen their animals for LCMV.

For people who live in environments with a large population of house mice, it is recommended to avoid handling mice and their excrement. Be sure to check all food materials in the area for penetration by wild mice, which are very good at eating through cardboard boxes and paper bags. When cleaning up a rodent infested area, the CDC advises a three phase approach. Phase one (Seal it up) is designed to seal the area from future mice incursions. Phase two (Trap up) is designed to catch mice currently living in the area. Finally, Phase three (Clean up) is designed to clean up the dead rodents and their droppings. If you note mouse feces in your home or garage, it is best to wear gloves and a mask, spray the feces with 1:10 bleach to water solution and allow it to sit for five minutes. Sweep up the droppings and discard all open food or drink containers from the area. Details of these phases can be found on the CDC websites listed under Further Reading at the end of this chapter.

Owners of pet mice, hamsters, and guinea pigs are at relatively low risk for LCMV infection. Prevention of infection starts with preventing exposure of pets to LCMV. Pet rodents should not be exposed to or in contact with wild rodents. Other measures to reduce pet-to-human transmission include washing hands after handling pets or their excrements, keeping cages clean and unsoiled, cleaning cages in a well-ventilated area, and not kissing pet rodents.

While the risk of LCMV infection is minimal, preventive measures should be taken by all pregnant women. Strict avoidance of contact with wild rodents is imperative. If there is a wild rodent infestation, the woman should not be involved with the Seal it up, Trap up, and Clean up protocol. Pet rodents should be kept separate from the woman's living quarters. Pregnant women should not be involved in cage cleaning or direct handling of the pet. Ideally, they should avoid staying in the same room as the hamster, mouse, or guinea pig for long periods.

Monkeypox Virus

Monkeypox is an illness limited mostly to Africa, where the natural viral reservoir are rodents, primates, and rabbits. Clinical disease in people resembles influenza (fever, headache, chills, muscle soreness, and sweats) but is followed within 10 days by a skin rash with some vesicular and pustular lesions.

Monkeypox virus is genetically related to the smallpox virus, probably the most devastating disease in history. For centuries, repeated smallpox epidemics swept across continents and decimated populations. Smallpox reportedly killed Queen Mary II of England, Emperor Joseph I of Austria, King Luis I of Spain, Tsar Peter II of Russia, Queen Ulrika Elenora of Sweden, and King Louis XV of France. Survivors of the disease were often left with deep pockmarks in their face and body, and many were left blind. Smallpox is now eradicated, and vaccination for this disease is no longer necessary.

In 2003, there was a human monkeypox outbreak in the United States. Before this time, monkeys were presumed to be the primary reservoir host. More than 70 human cases of monkeypox were identified in Wisconsin and central states, and all infected people reported close contact with prairie dogs. Epidemiologic investigation revealed that most of these prairie dogs were imported and sold from a single Illinois pet store, and most of these prairie dogs were also clinically ill. Sick prairie dogs had inflammation of the eyelids and conjunctivitis (inflammation of the membranes under the lids and over the white of the eyes). Some animals died; no human fatalities were reported. The mortality rate for monkeypox outbreaks in humans in Africa is typically low (1–10%).

Coming on the heels of the September 2001 terrorist attacks and at a time when concern regarding bioterrorism was very high, this monkeypox outbreak created genuine concern and received a lot of publicity. It is now thought the imported prairie dogs were exposed to infected Gambian giant pouched rats, which were, at the time, allowed to be imported legally. Thanks to epidemiologists, veterinarians, and public health workers, widespread panic about monkeypox or smallpox bioterrorism was averted, the outbreak controlled, and the virus eliminated from the United States. It is no longer legal to import Gambian giant pouched rats, as well as several other animals that were being imported from Africa at the time.

Hantavirus

Hantavirus causes two different human disease syndromes: hemorrhagic fever with renal syndrome (HFRS) and hantavirus pulmonary syndrome (HPS). HFRS occurs mostly in eastern Asia, Russia, and Korea and carries a case-fatality rate of around 5–15 percent.

Exposure to hantavirus occurs via contact with rodent urine and feces that have contaminated the local environment. This virus is almost always associated with wild rodent populations, but in Europe and Japan, captive rodents have been implicated.[6] In the United States, HPS is a wild rodent-associated infection, which when suspected should be reported to the CDC. Each year, 20–40 cases of HPS are reported in the United States. People over the age of 17 are most commonly infected, and children under the age of 10 are rarely infected.

HPS patients experience a 7–10 day period of nonspecific viral symptoms, after which an abrupt and severe respiratory compromise ensues. Patients are often placed on a ventilator to support their breathing while in respiratory distress. The case fatality rate is high, at approximately 36 percent.

In 2009, HPS was reported in five young children in four different states. All cases were evaluated for environmental contamination, and rodent droppings were found in the house walls, bedroom, food, buildings in the yard, backyard play areas, and the garage. The most common reservoir in the United States is the deer mouse (*Peromyscus maniculatus*). The deer mouse has a range that encompasses all of the United States and parts of Canada and Mexico. Recommendations for environmental rodent control and decontamination can be found on the CDC website listed at the end of this chapter.

PARASITIC ZOONOSES

Cryptosporidiosis

Cryptosporidiosis is a disease caused by the protozoal coccidian organism cryptosporidium. Human illness is typically caused by *Cryptosporidium parvum*, and the illness is usually self-limiting. Severe illness is seen only in people with compromised immune systems (e.g., AIDS patients). Exposure to cryptosporidial organisms is via ingestion of spores, which are found in the feces of infected humans and animals. Exposure to cryptosporidium most often occurs via such fecal-contaminated water sources as swimming pools.

Cryptosporidia has many different species. Gene mapping of the organisms allows comparison of organisms within the genus or the species more accurately. Not all species of cryptosporidia are capable of causing infection in humans. By far the most common animal hosts for human cryptosporidial infections are cattle.[7,8] Whether species of animal hosts or species of cryptosporidia other than *C. parvum* are a risk for human infection is a matter of ongoing scientific investigation.

Rabbits rarely carry cryptosporidia, but experimentally they can be infected with *C. parvum*. In the summer of 2008 in the United Kingdom, there was a waterborne outbreak of human cryptosporidiosis that was traced to a wild rabbit that entered a treated water tank. A study from China found that *C. parvum* from hamsters and pet Siberian chipmunks had the same gene markers as *C. parvum* isolated from a human being in the Netherlands.[9] While research into animal vectors of *Cryptosporidia* continues, pet rodents and perhaps pet rabbits should be considered rare but potential sources of infection.

Hymenolepiasis

Hymenolepis nana, also known as the dwarf tapeworm, is the most common tapeworm infection in humans in the world today. Infection is not generally a major health concern, and most infected people show no symptoms. Symptoms, if they occur, include nausea, loss of appetite, diarrhea, abdominal pain, and weakness. Young children can develop a headache, an itchy anus, and may have difficulty sleeping. Diagnosis is via identification of microscopic worm eggs in the stool, and treatment is very effective.

Infections are commonly diagnosed in children, in people living in institutions, and in people who live in areas with poor sanitation or who do not practice adequate personal hygiene. People become infected by ingesting tapeworm eggs, and once infected a person can re-infect themselves or infect others in the house if sanitation or hygiene is poor, so naturally contact with an infected person's feces poses a risk for infection.

Wild rodents are the primary source of environmental contamination with eggs. Some insects (e.g., beetles) that have ingested infective eggs can transmit the infection if the insect is eaten. Contaminated water, food, and soil present an increased risk for people to inadvertently ingest the eggs. Infected pet hamster feces can sometimes contain these eggs, which is a good reason why children should be encouraged not to eat while handling their hamster (or other pets) and to wash their hands after handling the hamster or its droppings.

Prevention of dwarf tapeworm infection is relatively easy. Hands should be washed with soap and water after using the toilet, after handling pet hamsters, and before handling food. Pet cages should be cleaned regularly. Childcare providers should wash hands thoroughly after changing diapers or contacting feces—even if gloves are worn. When travelling to countries where food may be contaminated, all raw vegetables and fruits should be washed, peeled or cooked with safe, potable water before they are ingested.

Trixacarus Mites

These mites are microscopic arthropod parasites that infect guinea pigs and can be transmitted to people[6]. Most guinea pigs with these mites do not show any signs of illness, but some guinea pigs get a rash, become intensely itchy, and can have itch-induced seizures. *Trixacarus caviae* mites are in the sarcoptid family of mites and are similar to the parasite that

Table 10.3

Parasitic Zoonoses from Small Mammals

Organism	Disease name (if any)	Potential carriers of disease
Cryptosporidium[1]	**Cryptosporidiosis**	Ferrets, hedgehogs, rabbits, rodents, possums, foxes
Encephalitozoon cuniculi[1]	Encephalitozoonosis	Rabbits
Giardia (multiple species)[2]	Giardiasis	Rodents, ferrets
Hymenolepsis nana[1]	**Tapeworm infection (Hymenolepiasis, Cestodiasis)**	Rodents
Taenia (multiple species)	Tapeworm infection	Rats, mice, rabbits
Trixacarus caviae[1]	—	Guinea pigs
Sarcoptes scabiei	Scabies	Ferrets
Liponyssus bacoti[3]	Typhus, Q fever, Plague	Rats
Cheyetiella parasitovorax[1]	Cheyetiellosis	Rabbits
Baylisascaris procyonis[1]	—	Raccoons

[1] Discussed in chapter text.

[2] *Giardia* spp. from small mammals may not be zoonotic.

[3] This organism is actually a parasite of the rat called the tropical rat mite. Its importance lies in the ability to transmit severe disease to people.

causes scabies in dogs and people. Symptoms in people with these mites include itchy small red bumps on the hands, arms, or neck. Infection may be self-limiting, but treatments with prescription dermatologic medications help resolve the infection and itch rapidly.

Cheyletiella Mites

Cheyletiella parasitovorax is a common sarcoptid mite that infects rabbits. Infected rabbits can appear normal or show hair loss and significant scaly dandruff. In fact, this mite causes enough dandruff that it occasionally carries the flakes with it as it moves. For this reason, it is also known as the walking dandruff mite. Humans can get a red papular rash associated with mite bites that can be very itchy. Infections in humans are self-limiting since the mite cannot reproduce off the rabbit host.[6] Cheyletiella infection in humans is uncommon, and it is not listed on the Centers for Disease Control and Prevention website as a zoonotic illness.

Baylisascaris

Baylisascaris is the intestinal roundworm parasite of raccoons. In urban and suburban areas in the United States, raccoons are often found around or near people's homes. Human infections occur when infected raccoon feces contaminate food, soil, or water and the eggs then ingested. People at the highest risk of infection are children and developmentally disabled persons that spend a lot of time outdoors. At-risk populations also include hunters, trappers, taxidermists, and wildlife handlers.

This roundworm infection is very common in raccoons, but human infections are rarely diagnosed. While only 25 cases have been reported in the United States as of 2003, *Baylisascaris* infection is likely either misdiagnosed as other infections, underdiagnosed, or underreported. Symptoms of infection depend on how many eggs are ingested and where the worm migrates in the body. Ingestion of a small number of eggs may not result in symptoms or illness. Ingestion of large numbers of eggs can be associated with severe illness. Symptoms can include nausea, fatigue, liver enlargement, loss of coordination, lack of attention to surroundings and people, loss of muscle control, blindness, or coma. *Baylisascaris* infections in humans is frequently fatal.[10]

Prevention of infection involves avoiding direct contact with raccoons and their feces. Prevention guidelines found on the CDC *Bayliscaris* website (listed at the end of this chapter) include:

1. Do not feed raccoons or keep them as pets.
2. Neighborhood cooperation to discourage raccoons from living in and around your home by preventing access to food, and sealing

trash containers. The CDC also recommends closing off access to attics and basements, keeping sandboxes covered, removing all fishponds and other sources of water, removing bird feeders, and clearing all brush from terrestrial surroundings.
3. Removal of feces and all contaminated materials should be done carefully, and all material should be burned, buried, or sent to a landfill.
4. Humane trapping and relocation of raccoons may be recommended in certain situations.

Encephalitozoon

Encephalitozoon cuniculi (EC) is part of a family of microsporidia. For years microsporidia were classified as spore-forming parasites. They have recently been reclassified as fungal organisms. Microsporidia are ubiquitous in nature.

EC is a common rabbit pathogen causing kidney, eye, and central nervous system disease. The spores are shed from rabbits in the urine and feces.

Microsporidiosis is a serious intestinal opportunistic infection of severely immunocompromised patients. AIDS patients are most commonly affected when the T cell count falls very low. With the advent of good immunotherapy for HIV/AIDS, microsporidiosis is no longer considered to be a significant risk for most patients. Even if microsporidial infection is diagnosed, it is very rare for EC to be the offending organism.

FUNGAL ZOONOSES

Ringworm

Ringworm is the only zoonotic fungal infection from small mammals (for more information on this disease, see chapter 9, "Zoonoses of Cats"). Ringworm is a dermatophyte infection of the skin like that of athlete's foot (tinea pedis), jock itch (tinea cruris), and nail bed infections. There are multiple species of dermatophytes that cause ringworm, only a few of which are zoonotic. *Microsporum canis* is a common cause of ringworm in dogs and cats and is the most common zoonotic dermatophyte.

Trichophyton is another zoonotic dermatophyte genus; however, the incidence of zoonotic transmission is much lower than with *Microsporum canis*. Typically, *Trichophyton* causes scalp and beard infections in people. Rodents can carry these dermatophytes, and while many rodents show no rash or signs of infection, some rodents with *Trichophyton* will demonstrate skin infection and rash.

Prescription medications are available to treat skin fungal infections effectively, and prevention of infection involves washing skin and clothes after handling pet rodents.

NONZOONOTIC ILLNESSES ASSOCIATED WITH SMALL MAMMALS

No discussion of human disease associated with small mammals would be complete without mentioning allergies. Allergies to animals are caused by an adverse reaction to fur, dander, or saliva. Most allergies manifest as itchy skin with or without a rash. Nasal congestion and watery eyes are also common, but severe respiratory effects such as bronchitis and asthma have occurred. Anaphylactic reactions (a rapid-onset, potentially fatal reaction that is sometimes associated with severe bee stings) have been reported from exposure to rabbits.

Rodents and rabbits can cause allergic reactions in people, and many veterinarians report allergies to rabbits. There is a 1999 report of three people who developed an urticarial (skin hive) reaction upon contact with pet hedgehog spines.[11] The hives developed soon after contact with the spines, and in two cases resolved quickly. The authors called this condition hedgehog hives.

While allergies are not infections and therefore cannot be considered zoonotic, they nonetheless represent a human ailment that can be directly linked to close contact with animals. Some pet owners will eliminate the offending pet from their homes or lives. A Dutch study reported that 2 percent of the population studied reported never owning pets because of health reasons. In the same study, more than 12 percent reported having removed pets from their home for health reasons in the past.[12] Some people will choose to undergo medical and immunotherapy to reduce the allergic symptoms. It is the latter group of people who illustrate the strength of the human-animal bond and demonstrate that this bond extends to many species of animals including nontraditional pets.

CONCLUSION

Small mammals are a part of everyone's life, and if you keep small mammal pets, you share your home and hearts with them. Even if you do not keep pets, wild small mammals still live in and around your environment.

All animals are capable of transmitting disease agents to other animals as well as to humans, and vice versa (e.g., infecting ferrets with influenza). This chapter was dedicated to the presentation of the scope of known zoonotic diseases related to small mammals and a discussion of some of these diseases in depth. In this discussion of zoonoses, a common theme is apparent. Prevention of zoonosis is usually possible with proper sanitation, good personal hygiene, and clean food storage and food preparation areas. Despite the numbers of potential zoonotic diseases, the incidence of human disease associated with animals is low.

It is the author's hope that after reading this chapter, the reader is better educated, informed, and aware. The author is a strong advocate for pet ownership and has a deep respect for the bond that develops between people and their pets—whether that pet is a dog, a rabbit, a lizard, or a fish. Scientific studies have proven many beneficial health effects that come from contact with domesticated animals. It is the author's unabashed belief that for most people, the benefits of pet ownership greatly outweigh any health risk incurred.

The author would like to thank Danielle Yaakov, DVM, for her assistance and technical review of this manuscript.

FURTHER READING

From the Centers for Disease Control and Prevention website:

Bacterial Zoonoses

Tularemia: http://www.cdc.gov/Tularemia/
Rat bite fever: http://www.cdc.gov/nczved/divisions/dfbmd/diseases/ratbite_fever/
Plague: http://www.cdc.gov/ncidod/dvbid/plague/qa.htm
Leptospirosis: http://www.cdc.gov/nczved/divisions/dfbmd/diseases/leptospirosis/

Viral Zoonoses

Influenza: http://www.cdc.gov/flu/
Lymphocytic choriomeningitis: http://www.cdc.gov/ncidod/dvrd/spb/mnpages/dispages/lcmv.htm
Monkeypox: http://www.cdc.gov/ncidod/monkeypox/
Hantavirus (rodent control): http://www.cdc.gov/rodents/

Parasitic Zoonoses

Hymenolepiasis: http://www.cdc.gov/ncidod/dpd/parasites/hymenolepis/2004_PDF_Hymenolepis.pdf
Baylisascaris: http://www.cdc.gov/ncidod/dpd/parasites/baylisascaris/default.htm

REFERENCES

1. Ruiz A. Plague in the Americas. *Emerging Infectious Diseases* 2001;7:539–40.
2. Veterinary Information Network website: Available (to members) at: http://www.vin.com/Members/Associate/Associate.plx?from=GetDzInfo&DiseaseId=1374.

3. Baer R, Turnberg W, Yu D, et al. Leptospirosis in a small animal veterinarian: Reminder to follow standardized infection control procedures. *Zoonoses Public Health* 2010;57:281–4.

4. Woodward DL, Khakhria R, Johnson WM. Human salmonellosis associated with exotic pets. *Clinical Microbiology* 1997;35:2786–90.

5. Deibel R, Woodall JP, Decher WJ, et al. Lymphocytic choriomeningitis virus in man: Serologic evidence of association with pet hamsters. *Journal of the American Medical Association* 1975;232:501–4.

6. Mitchell MA, Tully TN. Zoonotic diseases. In: Quesenberry KE, Carpenter, JW, eds. *Ferrets, rabbits, and rodents: Clinical medicine and surgery.* 2nd ed. St. Louis: Saunders, 2004.

7. Xiao L, Feng Y. Zoonotic cryptosporidiosis. Federation European Microbiologica Societies, *Immunology and Medical Microbiology* 2008;52:309–23.

8. Snel SJ, Baker MG, Venugopal K. The epidemiology of cryptosporidiosis in New Zealand, 1997–2006. *New Zealand Medical Journal* 2009;122:47–61.

9. Lv C, Zhang L, Wang R, et al. *Cryptosporidium* spp. in wild, laboratory, and pet rodents in China: Prevalence and molecular characterization. *Applied and Environmental Microbiology* 2009;75:7692–9.

10. Okulewicz A, Bunkowska K. Baylisascaris—A new dangerous zoonosis. *Wiad Parazytol* 2009;55:329–34. Abstract available at: www.ncbi.nlm.nih.gov/pubmed/20209804.

11. Fairley JA, Suchniak J, Paller AS. Hedgehog hives. *Archives of Dermatology* 1999;135:561–3.

12. Brunekreef B, Groot B, Hoek G. Pets, allergy and respiratory symptoms in children. *International Journal of Epidemiology* 1992;21:338–42.

Chapter 11

Zoonoses of Concern from Pet Birds

Niklos Weber, DVM, DABVP (Avian, Canine, Feline)

Pet birds are becoming more and more popular in these days of improved breeding practices and the availability of better veterinary care. According to a national 2009–2010 pet owner survey conducted by American Pet Products Association, there are approximately 15 million pet birds in the United States among 6 million households,[1] making birds the fourth most popular household pet after dogs, cats, and fish. Bird fanciers and pet bird owners cherish their pets for their plumage, song or speech, and companionship. While pet birds can be a delight for their human companions, there are a few health risks of which owners and those contemplating owning a pet bird should be aware of, especially if they are elderly, have a compromised immune system, or have young children in the household. In rare incidences, birds can transmit certain bacteria, fungi, viruses, or parasitic diseases to people. Owners should be aware of these diseases and the measures they can take to prevent them.

Much more is known today about proper husbandry and dietary requirements of different species and disease processes than 20 years ago, so it is much easier to prevent and treat disease, and birds live much longer than they used to. Problems still exist in determining when a bird is sick, but it is quite difficult for most owners to ascertain subtle signs of the beginning of an avian illness.

This chapter mostly deals with zoonotic diseases (diseases transmissible from animals to humans) in pet parrots, but includes some information on passerines (finches, canaries, mynahs, etc.), columbines (doves and pigeons), poultry (chickens, turkeys, etc.) and waterfowl (ducks and geese). It is not meant to be a definitive and comprehensive resource on all zoonotic diseases of birds, but to highlight the major zoonotic risks that birds may pose to their owners and their families. Owners with questions or concerns should consult an avian veterinarian for more information. This chapter will discuss and highlight zoonotic risks to people, measures that should be taken by caretakers, clinical signs in sick birds, symptoms of disease in humans, and general treatment and prognosis of diseases in birds. Diseases that are covered include Psittacosis (*Chlamydophila*), salmonellosis, *Campylobacter, Mycobacterium* (avian tuberculosis), histoplasmosis, cryptococcosis, avian influenza, viral encephalomyelotides (including equine encephalomyelitis and West Nile virus), giardiasis, and *Dermonyssus* (fowl mite) ectoparasitism. Most of these diseases, however, only have poultry or wildlife as their reservoirs. Of the diseases discussed, the only zoonoses that are common in pet birds are psittacosis and giardiasis; others are rare or do not transmit directly from pet birds to humans.

Additional zoonotic diseases that can occur in pet birds but are not discussed in this chapter include: colibacillosis caused by *Escherichia coli,* Newcastle disease, pasteurellosis, and erysipeloid. These diseases are only rarely transmitted to humans from birds or cause mild disease in humans. Questions or concerns about these rare diseases should be directed to your veterinarian, your physician, or even your state public health department, where you will hopefully find a veterinarian to help answer these questions.

THE BASICS OF BIRD HEALTH AND ILLNESS

The determination of illness in birds is more difficult than in dogs and cats for three reasons. First, they have not been domesticated for as long as dogs and cats, and, as such, they are not generally as comfortable around humans, so they do not show weakness as readily. Second, for the most part, they are prey species; in the wild obviously weak individuals will be culled from the flock by predators, so an instinct for hiding illness for as long as possible is advantageous. Third, most avian species have evolved to live in flocks with distinct dominance hierarchies, and any member that shows weakness is immediately relegated to a lower dominance status. Because a lower dominance state corresponds to fewer breeding opportunities and an inferior food selection, birds strive to avoid this state at all costs.

When birds are sick for long periods of time, they are subject to a great deal of stress, both in fighting the disease and striving to hide it. Chronic stress of this type causes certain hormones to increase, which suppresses the immune system, usually exacerbating health problems and predisposing them to infections. The stress hormones cause changes in metabolism and the way the bird absorbs and deposits fat, sugar, and protein. They also cause overusage of certain vitamins and minerals, which results in deficiencies and further illness. Immune suppression and exacerbation of an illness will cause higher numbers of pathogenic organisms and higher rates of shedding. However, many times a bird that transmits zoonotic disease can be asymptomatic and shed the organism that causes disease without showing any signs. For this reason, birds should be tested for certain diseases before exposing immunocompromised people to them (e.g., before placing the bird in a elderly care facility).

Fortunately, avian medicine has advanced by leaps and bounds over the past decade. In recent years, avian veterinarians have developed many new diagnostic and therapeutic techniques and have researched new drug dosages and nutritional requirements. For example, the use of endoscopes, intraosseous fluids (intravenous fluids given into the bone), complete blood workups on very small samples, safe anesthesia, and other techniques are now commonplace in avian medicine. There is even a specialty board (the American Board of Veterinary Practitioners) that certifies specialists in avian practice. Currently, birds receive veterinary care on par with that of dogs and cats. Occasionally, even ducks and chickens receive CAT (computer-assisted tomography) scans and MRIs (magnetic resonance imaging). Similarly, public health medicine has advanced greatly in recent years, resulting today in a greater ability to detect early and contain an outbreak of a zoonosis, treat human cases more effectively, and prevent further cases through such rapid control and preventive measures as the use of vaccination campaigns.

PREVENTING TRANSMISSION OF DISEASE

Transmission of disease-causing organisms from birds to humans is actually fairly difficult. The organisms that cause diseases in birds have evolved to live and reproduce at higher than human body temperatures, so they only survive with difficulty in the human environment. A normal human immune system can also fight off most of these organisms easily, and in addition, most organisms have evolved to infect one particular species, so many diseases are not transmissible even to other species of birds. Some viruses (such as avian influenza) need to mutate in order to become pathogenic to humans.

People who are immunocompromised have immune systems that do not work as well as they should, so they are at increased risk for complications or severe outcomes if they become infected with a contagious disease. Examples of immunocompromised people, of which there are many, include very young children, the elderly, people with diseases such as AIDS or other conditions that suppress the immune system, and people receiving chemotherapy treatment. These groups of people should be especially vigilant with biosecurity protocols. They should wash their hands after animal contact and after cleaning up after animals, and they should avoid contact with bird feces and discharges. If an immunocompromised person is unable to be vigilant on their own (such as a small child), then that person should be supervised and assisted by a capable adult.

Biosecurity is a term referring to the preventative measures taken to reduce transmission of infectious disease between people, animals, or geographic areas. Important aspects of biosecurity include quarantine, isolation, vaccination, disease treatment, and biocontainment. Quarantine refers to isolating an animal that has been potentially exposed to a disease to confirm that it does in fact develop the disease, and isolation is the segregation of an infected and contagious animal to prevent spread of diseases to others. Vaccination and treatment help prevent or cure diseases and aid in reducing spread of the disease. Biocontainment is the process whereby people avoid carrying contaminated material between groups of animals, by washing hands between handling two birds, cleaning and disinfecting shoes before walking between aviaries, or showering and changing clothes before traveling between chicken farms, for example.

It is important to keep pet birds healthy and minimize stress because sick and stressed birds tend to shed higher numbers of infectious organisms. Breeding aviaries and lofts should be built with adequate air circulation to minimize inhalation of potentially infectious aerosolized fecal particles and dander, as well as to control levels of toxic gases in the environment. High levels of ammonia in particular (normally released by volatilization from the uric acid component of avian fecal material) can damage the cells (epithelium) of the avian respiratory tract, which can easily lead to secondary infections. There are no published recommendations for air exchanges per hour for aviaries, but there should be enough airflow so that no odor can be detected and dust should not be visible floating in the air. Adequate space in the aviary is important to minimize the physical and mental stresses associated with territorial and dominance infighting, which can be constant depending on the level of crowding and the species involved. Aviary protocols should be in place to minimize stress and provide hide boxes and escape areas for certain species that need to escape from aggressive mates. New birds should always be tested for infectious disease before adding them to the household or flock because moving to a new place is always stressful on birds and will result in increased pathogen shedding. Pet birds should be examined and blood work performed by an avian veterinarian yearly to make sure they remain healthy.

Most infectious zoonotic diseases from birds are transmitted via the fecal-oral route. This means that the virus or bacteria is shed in the feces of the bird, dries out, and becomes airborne when attached to dust particles. These dust particles can be inhaled or inadvertently ingested by humans and enter the body through the gastrointestinal or respiratory tract, where they are either killed by the immune system and other body defenses (such as stomach acid), or they cause disease. Some diseases are similarly transmitted by dried aerosolized respiratory secretions from affected birds. Some viruses, such as West Nile virus, are spread via arthropod (insect) hosts like mosquitoes or fleas, so pet birds do not have a high potential to be a source of infection—insect borne diseases are much more of a concern with wildlife.

Common mistakes made by bird owners that can lead to zoonotic infection include cleaning cages and accessories without adequate personal protection, lack of hand washing, and inappropriate contact with the bird. Cage and accessory (perches, toys, dishes, etc.) cleaning should be done using appropriate personal protection equipment (PPE) such as gloves, safety goggles or face mask, a N95 dust mask or respirator for dusty aviaries, and coveralls if needed for large aviaries. The usage of PPE minimizes the risk of dust inhalation and the chances of contaminated material splashing into the eyes and mucous membranes of the face.

Hand washing is the most important procedure that can be performed to prevent disease transmission. Almost all birds defecate indiscriminately and then walk in the feces, so many birds have contaminated feet. They also preen themselves frequently and can easily contaminate their beaks or oral cavities. When owners play with their birds, it is very important to wash this miniscule amount of fecal material off of their hands before eating or touching their faces. Simple hand washing can reduce disease by 25 percent or more, according to the Centers for Disease Control and Prevention (CDC).[2]

Many owners like to kiss their birds or feed them food directly from their mouths. These behaviors, in addition to potentially causing behavioral problems (inappropriate mate bonding, for example) creates a high risk for zoonotic disease transmission. Other owner behaviors that can lead to direct fecal-oral transmission of disease include letting the bird climb on the face, sleeping with the bird, feeding the bird during (human) meals, or situating the bird's cage close to food preparation and dining areas. These behaviors should be avoided as much as possible. In large aviaries or lofts, owners should take care to keep the mouth closed when capturing birds as well as while cleaning or feeding.

Wild bird feeders should be cleaned and disinfected frequently with diluted bleach, and the areas around them should be kept clean as well. The ground around feeders or areas where birds congregate should have the feces removed so there is no buildup of bacterial or fungal organisms.

Children should not play in these areas nor should food be prepared, such as on a barbecue grill. If dead birds are encountered they should not be handled, and if West Nile virus is a concern in the area or is suspected, the appropriate public health authorities should be contacted. Most at-risk states have West Nile websites through which these authorities can be contacted.

BACTERIAL ZOONOSES

Psittacosis

Psittacosis is a common infectious disease in parrots and pigeons, caused by the primitive intracellular bacteria *Chlamydophila psittaci*. Psittacosis is spread to humans and other birds in dry aerosolized nasal discharge, dust, and feces. It can cause pneumonia in humans and a wide range of clinical features in birds. Around very dusty birds such as cockatoos, cockatiels, or pigeons, humans are at high risk of breathing the bacteria into their lungs, especially while cleaning the aviaries or otherwise stirring up the dust and dander. Some people have breeding aviaries inside their homes; these setups tend to have inadequate air circulation. People living in these conditions have the highest risk of contracting psittacosis because not only is their whole house full of potentially infectious dust (and they spend more time breathing it), but the birds also can be sicker than usual because of the air flow inadequacy. As was stated earlier, sick birds shed a greater number of infectious organisms.

In birds, *Chlamydophila* can cause a range of disorders. In pigeons and some parrots it causes eye and upper respiratory infections, while in other parrots such as cockatiels it can cause fatal liver failure. Clinical signs can range from eye discharge, conjunctivitis, and sneezing to green urates (the normally white part of the stool), lethargy and severe illness. Some birds, especially cockatiels, may not show any clinical signs at all, yet still shed large numbers of *Chlamydophila* organisms into the environment. The incubation period is usually between three days and three weeks, depending on the species of the bird, the immune status of the bird, and the strain of the *Chlamydophila* involved.

Diagnosis is usually fairly straightforward via PCR (polymerase chain reaction, a method of amplifying DNA to aid in organism identification) testing on blood and choanal, cloacal, or environmental swabs, but can sometimes require multiple tests, biopsies, and/or special stains. Other tests that are used include microimmunofluorescence (MIF) and cell culture. MIF can distinguish between acute and chronic infections. If an aviary infection is suspected, PCR testing can also be done on environmental swabs. Treatment of avian psittacosis is also usually fairly straightforward and includes doxycycline or other tetracyclines, but these antibiotics need to be given for months because the intracellular nature of the bacteria protects it from the effects of the drugs. There are even commercially available diets that incorporate tetracycline so as to allow easier treatment of entire flocks.

Human signs of psittacosis begin after a 5–14 day incubation period. Psittacosis presents as an atypical pneumonia, with high fever, diarrhea, joint pain, splenomegaly, and conjunctivitis. Occasionally, the infection will become systemic and signs of endocarditis, hepatitis, or encephalitis can occur. Diagnosis in humans is based on cell culture and antibody titers. Treatment is with doxycycline or other tetracyclines or macrolides (such as azithromycin), and most infected people are expected to recover.[3]

Since psittacosis is an important zoonotic disease, most states require animal and human cases to be reported to the department of public health (DPH). When the DPH gets a report of a positive case, they will closely monitor the treatment and outcome of the case and work closely with animal authorities in the state in investigations to quickly identify the source of infection and prevent further human cases.

There are a number of steps that can be taken to help prevent the transmission of *Chlamydophila*.[4] Education of people at risk is very important—people working with birds should be trained on protective equipment, hand washing and disinfecting procedures, as well as accurate record keeping for large collections. Birds should be tested and quarantined for at least 30 days after they are purchased, and purchase or adoption of birds that appear sick should be avoided. In multiple bird households or collections, cages or enclosures should be positioned so there can be no aerial transfer of dust or particulates between the cages, and biosecurity should be practiced when moving between enclosures (hands should be washed and nothing should come into contact with different birds without cleaning in between). Birds with frequent public contact should be tested frequently to make sure they do not become infected, and birds that have ever tested positive for *Chlamydophila* should not have contact with the public.

Salmonellosis (Also Called Paratyphoid or Fowl Typhoid)

Salmonella is a bacteria that may infect both birds and people. There are many serotypes of *Salmonella* bacteria, but the serotype that commonly causes foodborne illness in humans (*S. enteritidis*) normally lives in the intestinal tracts of people and many other animals. This serotype is usually of avian origin but is not usually associated with exposure to pet birds. Infection in people is almost always a result of improper food handling or preparation. Occasionally, infection with this agent is associated with exposure to pet reptiles or wild birds, but these cases are also rare. It typically causes illnesses in humans when it is transmitted through uncooked or unwashed foods contaminated with animal or human feces. Transmission of *Salmonella* can also occur by handling contaminated food or water and subsequently touching the mouth before the hands are washed.

Salmonella usually causes a self-limiting but still very unpleasant diarrhea with fever in people, but in some cases it can cause much more serious disease, especially in the very young, the very old, and people who are immunocompromised. Human infection is more likely when the person is taking antacid or antibiotic medications because these drugs impair the stomach's immune defenses by reducing acid and commensal bacteria, respectively. There are around 2–3 million cases of human salmonellosis reported every year in the United States, and around 45,000 different isolates (bacteria types). A nationwide outbreak of salmonellosis in shell eggs in 2010 in the United States caused disease in almost 2,000 people and resulted in a recall of 380 million eggs originating from one group of farms in Iowa, after the CDC traced the serotype to the chicken feed used at the farms.

There are two *Salmonella* species that infect only birds (*S. pullorum* and *S. gallinarum*) but are not public health threats. *S. enteriditis* infection in chickens can rarely cause an oviduct infection leading to infection of the eggs, but this is very rare and has been estimated to occur at a rate of 1:300,000 eggs. Even the infected eggs are not a concern if they are cooked properly before eating. More commonly, eggs and meat from poultry are infected with *Salmonella* by exposure to feces during processing via surface contamination and water baths, and live chickens, turkeys, and pigeons are exposed through rodent feces in the feed and water.

Clinical signs of salmonellosis in birds include lethargy and diarrhea with associated dehydration. Lories can get severe acute disease, which is sometimes fatal. Pigeons and some other birds can get arthritis from joint infections; affected birds become lame and have hot swollen joints and may become septic and die. *Salmonella typhimurium* is the species usually isolated from birds, which is quite different from the *S. enteriditis* associated with human food poisoning.[5] Diagnosis is usually arrived at with a bacterial culture of the feces on special growth media. In some cases and outbreak, the lab or the department of public health will run tests to discover the exact genetic identity of the serotype so that its origin can be traced. A fecal gram stain can be a quick in-house test on pet birds—it will not tell if the offending bacteria is *Salmonella* specifically, but it can find gram-negative bacteria (of which *Salmonella* is one type) in the feces and appropriate antibiotic therapy may be instituted while the bacterial culture is pending. Treatment in pet birds is fairly straightforward as well; appropriate antibiotics are administered.

Campylobacter jejuni is another bacteria that causes diarrhea in humans. *Campylobacter* is transmitted the same way *Salmonella* is, through consumption of contaminated poultry meat and eggs. Most birds that have

Campylobacter infections show no clinical signs, but large flocks might have a higher amount of young bird mortality. Diagnosis is via fecal culture and treatment is with an appropriate antibiotic. *Campylobacter* is considered a low risk for transmission to people from pet birds.

Mycobacterium avium (or **Avian Tuberculosis**)

Avian tuberculosis caused by *Mycobacterium avium* is a rare disease in pet birds but may cause disease in immunocompromised humans. Most of the cases of human *M. avium* infection have been found to be of environmental origin rather than from birds, but sometimes both the bird and the human can be infected from the same environmental source. There have been reports of birds infected with *M. tuberculosis* (human tuberculosis) and *M. bovis* (bovine tuberculosis), but there have been no reports of birds passing these diseases to people.

Mycobacterium organisms normally live in soil and occur everywhere in the world. Infection is by ingestion or inhalation of the infected soil by the bird, and some avian species (e.g., pheasants, sparrows, budgerigars, and cranes) are more sensitive to avian tuberculosis than others. Turtle doves, turkeys, and guinea fowl are relatively resistant to the disease. Mycobacteria cause granulomatous masses (tubercles) in many different organs, so the clinical signs can be variable, but most birds become rapidly emaciated in spite of an increased appetite. Diarrhea, lameness, respiratory disease, and abdominal fluid may also be seen.[6]

Humans can get infected with *M. avium* via the respiratory and/or the gastrointestinal tracts. Immunocompetent people tend to get respiratory disease, which presents as a chronic cough with congestion and weight loss. People with compromised immune systems such as AIDS patients can contract the gastrointestinal form, which presents as a fever with weight loss and abdominal pain and infection in the gastrointestinal tract. Young children can get enlarged lymph nodes, which tend to resolve spontaneously. Diagnosis is through acid-fast staining of sputum or culturing the blood in people with systemic disease. Biopsies and serology can also be performed. Treatment is through long-term multiple antibiotic therapy, and in certain cases surgery may have to be done to remove pulmonary nodules.[7]

Diagnosis is difficult in the live bird, but abnormalities such as very high white blood cell counts and the presence of acid-fast staining positive bacteria in the feces increase the index of suspicion. Specific tests (such as serology to detect immune proteins and PCR testing) are available. Intradermal testing similar to the TB tests performed in people and poultry have been shown to be unreliable in parrots and other avian species.

Treatment of avian tuberculosis in birds is difficult and requires at least four months of therapy due to the intracellular nature of the infection and the slow growth of the *Mycobacterium*. Multiple antibiotics are usually used in combination, but these antibiotics are not generally used for many other diseases so they can be difficult to find and/or expensive. Infected birds should be considered to be infected for life, due to the difficulty in diagnosing and treating the disease and so should be permanently quarantined from other birds. It is very difficult to remove the organism from the environment as well, so other birds should never be kept in the same areas as the affected bird. It is not unreasonable to euthanize affected birds because of the public health risk, but some owners would rather keep the bird under isolation for life since human disease is unlikely to be contracted from a bird that is not showing clinical signs of disease. These birds must be monitored closely, however, and blood work and cultures must be done frequently in case the disease recurs.

FUNGAL ZOONOSES

Cryptococcosis and Histoplasmosis

Cryptococcus neoformans var. *neoformans* and *Histoplasma capsulatum* are fungal organisms found ubiquitously in soil, especially soil contaminated by wild pigeon feces. Birds occasionally become infected by these fungi, and the feces or nasal discharge from affected birds may be infectious to humans, dogs, and other animals. *Histoplasma* is found throughout the world and is endemic in the Ohio River and lower Mississippi River valleys, East Africa, and northern Argentina, while *Cryptococcus* is found worldwide, especially in cities with large pigeon populations.

Clinical disease in birds is usually characterized by upper respiratory infection and copious mucoid nasal discharge, progressing to pneumonia. Fungal infections cause granulomas (masses or nodules of infection and inflammation), and these fungi can lead to deformation of the beak and sinuses. Infection of the gastrointestinal tract can lead to diarrhea, anorexia, or regurgitation; and infection of the nervous system can lead to seizures and other neurologic signs. Many birds do not show clinical signs at all, yet continue to shed the organisms.

Disease in humans can occur after inhalation of the fungal spores from the contaminated soil or dried feces or discharge from infected birds. The disease usually causes pneumonia, but in immunocompromised people it can progress to fungal meningitis, at which point it is difficult to treat. Another species of *Cryptococcus*, *Cryptococcus gatti*, has been known to infect healthy, immunocompetent people. *C. gatti* has not been associated with soil contaminated with pigeon feces and only occurs in tropical and subtropical zones.

Diagnosis of *Cryptococcus* and *Histoplasma* in humans and animals is fairly straightforward most of the time: the organisms are easily seen on stained slides of exudate or biopsy specimens. There are also antibody (serologic) tests for both diseases. Treatment can be difficult as the fungi are resistant to antifungals because of their thick capsules. Additionally, many of the available antifungal drugs are fungistatic, which means they prevent reproduction of the organism rather than killing it outright and they rely on the animal's immune system to kill the organism. Fungistatic drugs require a long treatment period and leave an opening for the fungus to sporulate and protect itself and stay in the body until a time where it can reproduce again. Amphotericin B and some of the newer drugs kill the organism directly and are better choices for treatment of these systemic fungal infections in humans and animals, but still require long-term treatment. The drugs also can be quite expensive.

11.1. DID YOU KNOW?

- The oldest parrot on record lived to 104 years old.
- There are more than 350 species of parrots, ranging from 3¼ inches (pygmy parrot) to 40 inches (hyacinth macaw) in length.
- Chickens outnumber humans on earth four to one.
- The fastest recorded homing pigeon in the United States flew a 102-mile race in 1 hour and 1 minute, averaging over 100 mph!
- Crows and ravens commonly use tools and can solve logic puzzles.

VIRAL ZOONOSES

Avian Influenza

Avian influenza, or as the media have labeled it, bird flu, is caused by an influenza A virus. Influenza viruses tend to mutate frequently, and occasionally a mutation of a species-specific virus type will cause it to become infectious to another species (for example, a duck-specific virus can mutate so that it becomes infectious to humans). In general, since the mutated virus is new, there is little immunity to the novel form in the new target species, and depending on the infectivity of the new virus, an epidemic can be the result. The wild reservoir of avian influenza A virus is waterfowl (ducks and geese), and in areas of the world where biosecurity is lax, it is common for poultry to contract influenza. When a flock or an area is found to have a zoonotic strain of avian influenza virus, the poultry in the flock or area is depopulated to prevent spread of the virus to humans.

Strains of influenza A virus are designated by the primary antibody types associated with two virus proteins (hemagglutinin and neuramidase), called H and N. There are multiple antibodies differentiated by number in each group, so typical strains might be named H1N1, H5N1, or H9N2, for example. Most of the strains are not very infectious or virulent, but in particular the H5N1 strain has a high potential to cause disease and even death in humans. Another reason the H5N1 strain is important is because its particular mutation can cause the virus to become transmissible from human to human (which has happened very rarely to date), while the other strains are only zoonotic from birds. Other avian strains that have been reported to cause human disease are H7N3 and H9N2, but these are rare and not as virulent. Seasonal influenza in humans is caused by types H3N2 and H1N1 (the first one in which the virus proteins were discovered, hence H1 and N1); these strains do not come from birds. The H1N1 virus is of the same type, although genetically different, as those H1N1 flu viruses that caused the 1918 and 2009 human pandemics.

The high pathogenic (HP) H5N1 strain was first seen to transfer to humans in Asia in 1997. There were a number of outbreaks in China, Thailand, and Vietnam between 1999 and 2004. Low -pathogenic H5N1 strains have only been found in wildlife and have not been reported to infect humans. HP H5N1 spread over the first decade of the 2000s to the point where it is enzootic in many parts of the world. In 2010, there was concern that a minor mutation could result in the ability of the virus to transmit directly from human to human in an airborne form, at which point it could result in a worldwide pandemic and the death of millions of people. However, between 2006 and 2008 the number of outbreaks decreased almost sixfold worldwide due to increased biosecurity, education of workers, and flock vaccination programs.[8]

Most of the human cases of H5N1 originate in people who work with poultry and acquire infection through inhalation of aerosolized dried feces or respiratory secretions. Symptoms in humans are different from seasonal flu because the H5 part of the avian virus attacks the lungs and causes viral pneumonia rather than the upper respiratory disease caused by the H1 of seasonal flu virus. Obviously, pneumonia is more dangerous than the common cold so human mortality is higher, reported to be up to 60 percent of hospitalized patients. The World Health Organization (WHO) is currently working on vaccination programs and vaccine manufacturing plans in the event of a pandemic. As of January 2011, WHO reported that there had been 516 confirmed human cases of avian influenza in humans between 2003 and 2010, of which 306 (59 percent) were fatal.[8]

The H5N1 strain of avian influenza can cause high mortality in flocks of poultry. Most other strains are asymptomatic or only cause respiratory or intestinal disease, or may only cause a drop in growth rate or egg production. Testing involves typing the virus to determine which of each antibody the particular isolate reacts with, and there is no treatment in poultry except depopulating the flock to prevent further spread. There have been few reported cases of avian influenza in pet parrots or pigeons and no reports of spread from parrots to humans, so it is not a concern for most cage bird owners.

Arthropod-Borne Viral Encephalomyelitides

The common viral encephalomyelitides (viruses that cause encephalomyelitis, inflammation, and/or infection in the brain) present in the United States include the togaviruses of Western, Eastern and Venezuelan equine encephalitis viruses (WEE, EEE, and VEE) and the flaviviruses of West Nile virus, St. Louis encephalitis virus, and a few other rare viruses. All of these viruses are transmitted by arthropod vectors, usually mosquitoes, and all can infect humans as well as other animals, including mammals, amphibians, and reptiles. Wild birds are the reservoir for these viruses and cage birds can uncommonly contract the viruses as well. Most infections are from arthropod bites, but there have been reported cases of human-to-human virus transmission via contaminated blood transfusions and infections in cats and alligators fed infected meat. For this reason, all donated blood since 2003 has been screened for West Nile virus.

Humans and horses can get severe disease from togavirus infection, commonly WEE and EEE in the United States. Eastern equine encephalitis is the more severe disease and results in about 33 percent human mortality and over 90 percent permanent brain damage in the survivors, while WEE is more common (500 cases in the United States since 1964, compared to 150 for EEE) but results in about 3 percent mortality and 25 percent permanent brain damage.[9] The flavivirus that causes St. Louis encephalitis is much more common, averaging about 200 confirmed cases per year with a mortality rate of 10 percent, but it is estimated that only about 1 percent of the infections are clinically apparent so most infections are not reported. Venezuelan equine encephalitis occurs in sporadic outbreaks mostly in Central America and South America and is rare in the United States.

West Nile virus was discovered in 62 human cases in New York State in 1999 and spread rapidly until 2003, when there were 9,389 cases reported in the United States. Between 2004 and 2007, the number of cases was steady around 4,000, and then in 2008 the number began to drop, so that fewer than 1,000 cases were documented in 2010. The fatality rate for

West Nile virus in humans has varied between 2 and 5 percent in recent years; in the beginning it was 6–15 percent because it was such a new virus and immunity was rare.[10] To further reduce the numbers of infections in recent years, there have been more mosquito abatement protocols used throughout the United States, which has reduced transmission of this and other diseases.

Togaviruses are transmitted by mosquitoes, and as the mosquito bites, it injects the virus into the body. The virus enters the white blood cells and is carried to various organs where it reproduces and causes severe inflammation. In humans, inflammation in the brain causes the headache, fever, and neurologic signs characteristic of these diseases, and eventually can cause scarring, which can result in permanent brain damage.

Clinical signs of viral encephalomyelitides in birds are usually acute, severe, and result in death. Some bird species are more resistant and show mild gastrointestinal disease, from which they recover. West Nile virus causes high mortality in corvids (crows, ravens, and jays), but can infect parrots or any other species as well. Diagnosis is through serology (testing for antibodies) in live birds and humans, and by histopathology (looking at tissue sections under a microscope to visualize changes or virus inclusions) and immunofluorescence antibody tests (staining the virus itself with a fluorescent immunoglobulin dye and looking at it with a special microscope) in dead birds.

There is no treatment for any of the togaviruses or flaviviruses in humans or pets except supportive care to allow the body's immune system to cure the disease. There are vaccines available for horses against EEE, WEE, VEE and West Nile virus, but none is yet available for humans or pet birds. There have been a number of research studies using the equine West Nile vaccine for birds, but the results showed that the vaccine was not efficient.

PARASITIC ZOONOSES

Dermanyssus Gallinae (Fowl Red Mite)

Dermanyssus gallinae, the fowl red mite, is an ectoparasite of poultry and other birds. It is quite common and can infest other mammals and humans as well, but it needs an avian blood meal in order to reproduce. Occasionally these mites are seen in caged birds, especially at night—if a white sheet of paper is laid out the 0.5–1mm long mites are easily seen. They are photophobic, so during the day they hide in cracks, and for this reason birds will rarely be seen carrying the mites during the day. It is common to see these mites in multiple birds from the same pet store or breeding aviary, because they spread rapidly, even between cages.

Clinical signs in birds include feather loss, pruritis (itching), and erythema of the skin. Sometimes in severe infections self- trauma will be seen, and there can be skin infections secondary to inflammation or the self trauma. In humans, the mites cause papules and urticaria, which are extremely pruritic. Diagnosis is straightforward if the mites are seen, and treatment can be achieved with a number of different miticides. Ivermectin or selamectin are usually used in chickens or pet birds, but the environment must also be cleaned well because the mites can live for months off of the host. If a house is infested, local pest-control companies are able to treat the premises.

Giardiasis

Giardiasis is caused by a protozoal intestinal parasite, *Giardia lamblia*. Most of the time, giardiasis is contracted by humans and animals by drinking water contaminated by feces of infected wild birds and animals or livestock. However, there is potential for spread directly to humans from pet birds and mammals via the fecal-oral route. The *Giardia* organism and cyst are not killed by freezing (i.e., ice made from contaminated water is still infectious) but are killed by boiling and cooking. In addition, most water filters easily remove the organisms and cysts from the water. Cysts can survive in the environment for months and are very resistant to many disinfection methods.

The Giardia parasite is ingested in cyst form, and turns into a trophozoite in the small intestine, where it attaches to the intestinal lining and begins reproduction. The attachment of the parasite to the intestinal lining causes malabsorptive diarrhea, severe gas, abdominal cramping, and steatorrhea (greasy stools) in humans. In birds, it causes diarrhea (which may be extremely odiferous), anorexia, and occasionally feather picking. Some humans and birds can become infected without any clinical signs. Among cage birds, cockatiels are the most commonly affected species, and it is common for them to be asymptomatic. The most common source of infection for pet birds is ingestion of the feces from an infected bird, and occasionally the water in a flock or loft environment.

Diagnosis of giardiasis is made with fecal examination. The cysts can be seen on a direct fecal smear, but multiple fecal examinations may be needed. There are also antigen tests available for use on the feces. Due to the likelihood of false negative tests, many patients are treated presumptively on the basis of the clinical signs. Treatment in birds and humans usually involves metronidazole (Flagyl™), which is usually very efficacious.

CONCLUSION

The concern of zoonoses in pet birds is not very excessive given the low frequency of infection in birds and the ability to test and treat them for the most common zoonoses (psittacosis and giardiasis). Care should always be taken, however, to prevent all kinds of transfer of bacteria and other infectious organisms when handling a pet bird, and birds should be frequently tested for these diseases to ensure they are not contagious. The recommended testing frequency is variable depending on each individual case; an avian veterinarian should be consulted for each bird and potential exposure to new birds and humans should be evaluated. For example, a singly owned bird that never leaves the house would require less frequent testing than a bird that lives in a classroom, retirement home, or breeding aviary. Poultry workers and pigeon fanciers should exercise more extreme caution and utilize more personal protective equipment when working with their flocks because of the increased risk and greater number of potential zoonoses.

FURTHER READING

Avian nutritional information is available at: http://www.harrisonsbirdfoods.com/learningcenter/handbook.html.
   To find an avian veterinary specialist, go to: http://www.abvp.com/FindDiplomate.aspx
Doane BM. *The parrot in health and illness.* New York, NY: Macmillan General Reference; 1991.
Gallerstein, GA. *The complete bird owner's handbook.* New York, NY: Simon & Schuster Macmillan; 1994.
Psittacosis medical information is available at: http://emedicine.medscape.com/article/227025-overview and www.nasphv.org/Documents/Psittacosis.pdf.

REFERENCES

1. American Pet Products Association, Industry Statistics & Trends: Pet Ownership. Available at: http://www.americanpetproducts.org/press_industry trends.asp.
2. Centers for Disease Control and Prevention, Hand hygiene in healthcare settings. Available at: http://www.cdc.gov/handhygiene/.
3. Beeckman DS, Vanrompay DC. Zoonotic Chlamydophila psittaci infections from a clinical perspective. *Clinical Microbiology and Infection* 2009;15:11–7.
4. National Association of State Public Health Veterinarians (NASPHV). Compendium of Measures to Control Chlamydophila psittaci Infection Among Humans (Psittacosis) and Pet Birds (Avian Chlamydiosis), 2010. Available at: www.nasphv.org/Documents/Psittacosis.pdf.
5. Harrison GJ, Lightfoot TL, eds. *Clinical avian medicine.* Spix Publishing, Palm Beach, FL; 2006.
6. Manarolla G, Liandris E, Pisoni G, et al. Avian mycobacteriosis in companion birds: 20-year survey. *Veterinary Microbiology* 2009;133:323–7.
7. eMedicine: Mycobacterium Avium-Intracellulare: Treatment and Medication. Available at: http://emedicine.medscape.com/article/222664-treatment.

8. World Health Organization. Cumulative number of confirmed cases of avian influenza A/H5N1. Available at: http://www.who.int/csr/disease/avian_influenza/country/cases_table_2011_01_05/en/index.html.
9. Centers for Disease Control and Prevention. Eastern Equine Encephalitis. Available at: http://www.cdc.gov/easternequineencephalitis/.
10. Centers for Disease Control and Prevention. West Nile Virus. Available at: http://www.cdc.gov/ncidod/dvbid/westnile/index.htm.

Chapter 12

One Health

Radford G. Davis, DVM, MPH, DACVPM

GLOBAL HEALTH TODAY

Based on what we face in the media on a daily basis, it would seem that the human population is losing the battle for health, well-being, and personal safety. With each passing day, safeguarding our health appears almost futile in the face of emerging diseases that perplex scientists and confound the best-laid public health plans, frightening citizens as well as those experts we have come to rely on to protect us. Natural catastrophes, wars, and civil unrest can easily override the balance of well-being and good health and the seemingly adequate public health infrastructure that we have established, a balance that is tenuous at best in some areas of the world. So many factors, known and unknown, seem to impact and influence our health. With each passing month there are reports of newly identified causes of cancer, new evidence for or against the health benefits of a given food or vitamin or supplement, new drug discoveries, drug and food recalls, nostrums that promise younger skins and longer life. So, we ask ourselves, is it possible to win the war on public health when so much of our health is dependent upon external factors? A natural extension of this question is another: Is it possible to also improve the health of animals and our environment, and would doing so improve our health?

Public health has been defined as the "science and art of protecting and improving the health of communities through education, promotion of healthy lifestyles, and research for diseases and injury prevention."[1] Taking this a step further, we can speak of global public health. "Global public health is the collective action we take worldwide for improving health and health equity, aiming to bring the best available cost-effective and feasible interventions to all populations and selected high-risk groups."[2]

Our image of health today is far different from what it was at the turn of the 20th century. In 1900, infectious diseases topped the list of causes of death (see Table 12.1).

By 2030, things will look radically different, with only two infectious causes among a list of chronic, mostly preventable, diseases.[3] Smoking, in fact, is the leading cause of death in the world, killing an estimated 5 million people annually.

Our world is slowing moving away from communicable diseases as a major cause of death; indeed, by 2030 noncommunicable conditions will cause more than 75 percent of all deaths.[3] AIDS, tuberculosis, and malaria will all cause fewer deaths than they do today, but we still remain at risk for the emergence of new deadly diseases and always will. Though predicting the next pandemic is the focus of many researchers and organizations, such prognostication is not within our grasp in the foreseeable future.

In the last three decades, the world has made great progress in many areas of public health: the eradication of smallpox, the eradication of

Table 12.1

Top 10 Causes of Death in Humans—1900

1. Pneumonia
2. Tuberculosis
3. Diarrhea/enteritis
4. Heart disease
5. Stroke
6. Liver disease
7. Injuries
8. Cancer
9. Senility
10. Diphtheria

Table 12.2

Top 10 Causes of Death in Humans—2030[3]

1. Ischemic heart disease
2. Cerebrovascular disease
3. Chronic obstructive pulmonary disease
4. Lower respiratory infections
5. Road traffic accidents
6. Trachea, bronchus, lung cancers
7. Diabetes mellitus
8. Hypertensive heart disease
9. Stomach cancer
10. HIV/AIDS

rinderpest, the near eradication of polio and guinea worm, an increase in life expectancy in most areas of the world, and a global decline in childhood mortality.[2] Yet vast inequalities in health, health care, and life expectancy remain throughout the world.

The health field, and in particular public health, has the human as its focus, which seems logical. After all, we have a certain amount of selfishness when it comes to our own preservation, so people are naturally the basis for these disciplines. However, for understanding the full scope and meaning of health, for ideal prevention and utilization of health resources, for efficient education and even for providing the best treatment, there is good reason to expand our focus to animals and our environment in our full examination of health. People have substantial interactions with animals as companions, as food, for farming, hunting, as co-inhabitants—for better or worse—as we expand our cities, managing to coexist with them as intruders, and we do this in an environment that is in constant flux and at the mercy of human restraint, demands, divisions, and business evolution.

Within the last generation we have discovered approximately 40 new diseases, and most new diseases emerging (75% of them) are zoonotic diseases—diseases that are transmissible from animals to people. In fact, it is believed that of the 1,425 known human pathogens, 61 percent of these are zoonotic by nature. Bovine spongiform encephalopathy (mad-cow disease), severe acute respiratory syndrome (SARS), West Nile virus, H5N1 avian influenza, Ebola virus—these are all notorious disease agents that have caused illness, death, fear, and panic in humans, and they all have animals as their reservoirs. We cannot simply look at the humans to find the solutions to these diseases, so it makes sense when we speak of health to speak of health in a big picture, all-encompassing way—a One Health way. Indeed, the only way we will be able to meet the health needs (both human and animal) of our world in the future is to think in a One Health way.

WHAT IS ONE HEALTH?

One Health takes our previous definitions of health into account and builds upon them by taking into consideration the animal (both wild and domestic) and environmental aspects of health, building and advocating a holistic approach to improving health for all species (human and animal) and for the environment—the triad. Collectively, health professionals, conservationists, veterinarians, wildlife experts, public health workers, environmental experts, policymakers, researchers, and others have finally come to embrace the notion that disease, prosperity, and morbidity among one of the triad has direct and indirect impact upon the others.

One Health has been defined by the American Veterinary Medical Association as "the collaborative efforts of multiple disciplines working locally, nationally, and globally to attain optimal health for people, animals, and our environment."[4] Laura H. Kahn, MD; Bruce Kaplan, DVM; and Thomas P. Monath, MD, contemporary pioneers in the area of promoting One Health, state the following on their One Health website: "Recognizing that human and animal health and mental health (via the human-animal bond phenomenon) are inextricably linked, One Health seeks to promote, improve, and defend the health and well-being of all species by enhancing cooperation and collaboration between physicians, veterinarians, and other scientific health professionals and by promoting strengths in leadership and management to achieve these goals."[5]

The concept of One Health is not new. From ancient times it has been recognized that food, and meat in particular, can cause illness and death unless it is clean and safe to eat. The Greek historians Herodotus and Plutarch both document that during the times of ancient Egyptian rule, animals that were served as offerings to the gods and as food for the priests had to be carefully inspected, and only meat of clean animals could be used. During the early times in Athens there were market police who ensured the proper conduct of the meat traffic, and in ancient Rome, meat inspection was implemented to protect public health. One of the first responsibilities of early veterinarians was that of protecting the food supply through meat inspection and ensuring good animal health, thereby protecting human health.

The concept of One Health and the connectedness of human and veterinary medicine was recognized by Rudolf Virchow, a German physician in the 19th and early 20th centuries, an advocate of public health, and the first person to coin the term zoonosis. Virchow said, "between animal

Figure 12.1
**One Health: Humans, domestic animals, and wildlife share the same
environment, often with overlapping territories, and have influence over
one another. Where they overlap (center black) is where diseases are most
likely to emerge and where the application of One Health strategies will be
needed the most, though not exclusively. Climate change influences all life
and impacts health, human and animal movement, disease transmission,
crops, and livelihoods, among other things. Health, humans, animals, and the
environment cannot be separated from each other; therefore, the answer to
much of today's intertwined health problems cannot be found by focusing on
just one aspect of this complex picture.**

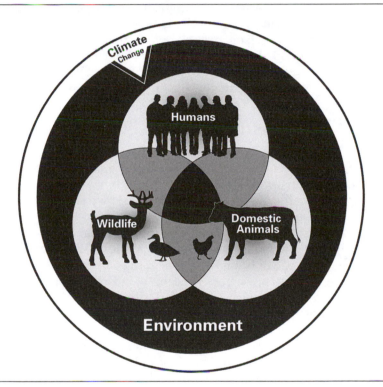

and human medicine there are no dividing lines—nor should there be."[6]
James Law, the first professor of veterinary medicine in the United States,
was a believer that veterinarians should receive public health training and
physicians should be taught about zoonoses. Calvin Schwabe, a veterinary epidemiologist and parasitologist, was a champion for many years
for more unification between human and veterinary medicine to tackle
zoonoses and coined the term One Medicine, which many have renamed
One Health.

From the early days and with the growing realization that the health of people is inextricably tied to the health of animals and to the health of our planet, we are now seeing many national and international organizations beating the One Health drum and advocating the adoption of this fresh, though not new, viewpoint on health. Across the world numerous national and international health and scientific organizations, including the American Medical Association (AMA) and the American Veterinary Medical Association (AVMA), as well as hundreds of experts in the fields of public health and human and veterinary medicine, have pledged their commitment to support One Health.[5] The World Health Organization (WHO), the Food and Agriculture Organization (FAO), the World Organization for Animal Health (OIE), the United Nations Children's Fund (UNICEF), and the World Bank have all demonstrated an interest in seeing One Health succeed. They all recognize that One Health is an avenue to correcting global deficiencies in human health care, alleviating poverty, and preventing illness and hunger—improve the health of animals and the environment, improve the health of the people. Simple.

ONE HEALTH AT THE GRASSROOTS

Although the concept of One Health appears at first blush to be a global-sized, idealistic, almost unwieldy view on health, we can find many examples of One Health and its benefits within our own communities, even within our own homes.

It has long been recognized that animals play an important role in our lives and that the human-animal bond has significant salutary value; that is to say, owning a pet, or being in the presence of a pet, has a positive impact on the mental and physiological health of individuals. In fact, in 1860 Florence Nightingale commented on the positive health effects small animals had in those with chronic illness.[7] Pets serve as topics for conversation—social lubricants, if you will—and become our companions, our friends, helping to decrease feelings of loneliness, anxiety, and depression, helping also in relieving the burden of social isolation. It has been shown that pet owners experience fewer minor health problems such as hay fever, headaches, and painful joints, and having a pet appears to protect owners against heart disease, or at least slows its progression. While exercising pets, we also exercise, keeping us fit and healthy. Pets need a sound, healthy diet, exercise, routine veterinary exams, vaccinations, baths, and a clean, comfortable, safe place to rest. So, as we provide for the health and well being of our pets and extend their lives, we in turn provide for the health and well being of ourselves and extend our own lives.

The use of pets to aid healing in carefully planned and monitored situations, also known as animal-assisted therapy (AAT), has been demonstrated to be useful in many settings, including mental health facilities, nursing homes, and hospitals and is usually conducted with a goal in mind. AAT is meant to enhance human physical, social, emotional, and/ or cognitive function. A good example of the direct benefits of animals can be seen in a study that was conducted in 2009, which demonstrated that a visit by a dog reduced pain perception significantly among children in a pediatric hospital.[7]

Animal-assisted activities (AAA) tend to be more casual meet-and-greet venues of animals and people, such as visitation programs in nursing homes, with no specific treatment goals in mind. The injured child undergoing intense rehabilitation or the elderly woman in a nursing home may look forward to the weekly visits of the animal, anticipating the touch and warmth of the pet and the joy the animal shows at recognizing the person, which in turn lifts the spirits of the person. In the presence of pets, residents of nursing homes tend to be more alert, responsive, and happier, hold longer conversations, and interact more socially.[8] Pets have been used in the treatment and recovery of wounded veterans, children with autism, and others who suffered physical, emotional, cognitive, or social challenges.[8] Remarkably, animals have been trained to aid those with various physical or mental disabilities or those with such illnesses as diabetes, to alert people to impending seizures in those with epilepsy, and have even been trained to sniff out things such as bedbugs and breast cancer. People with psychiatric conditions have benefited from therapeutic horseback riding or working with farm animals, and dolphin interactions have been shown to alleviate depression.[8] In programs where children with severe conduct disorders take responsibility for caring for animals, those children lower their aggressive tendencies and improve their ability to take responsibility, to nurture, show affection, play, teach others, and to respond more appropriately to adult authority. Such animal-based programs have also been successful in helping children with attention-deficit disorders and other learning disabilities in public schools.[8] Pets are even used to help rehabilitate criminals. In the Puppies Behind Bars program (www.puppiesbehindbars.com), prisoners take responsibility for caring for puppies and leading them through training that will produce a dog capable of sniffing out explosives or a dog that will help the disabled, a wounded veteran, or an elderly person, all the while helping prisoners simultaneously develop compassion, a sense of purpose and responsibility, and feelings of success.

The animals in all of these situations just listed must be kept healthy, physically and mentally. If they are in poor health they cannot do their job, which means human health will also suffer, for we humans have come to link our health and well-being with that of the animal's.

Another example of One Health at the grassroots level can be seen by looking closely at your local animal shelter. Animal shelters have a mission, among many missions, to help reunite stray animals with their owners, thereby reestablishing that human-animal bond and the inherent health benefits that go with it. Most animal shelters are also involved in spaying and neutering pets, thus helping control the stray animal population while at the same time reducing the likelihood of the transmission of infectious diseases between domestic animals (dogs, cats, horses, and livestock), to and from wildlife, and to people. Spaying and neutering also has direct beneficial health effects for the animal. Our local shelters and animal control agencies also work to keep dangerous animals out of our communities, simultaneously protecting human and animal health. Vicious dogs incite fear, particularly in children, and can inflict significant harm, even death, in people and animals. Keeping such dogs under control and off the streets is imperative. Dangerous animals, however, are not just limited to dogs. Many exotic or wild animals are also kept as pets and can be very dangerous. Monkeys, apes, tigers, bears, and other wild animals are unpredictable, threaten human life, and should not be kept as pets. Shelters may also find themselves caretakers of abused animals when law officials intervene in domestic violence situations, which oftentimes have both human and animal victims.

ONE HEALTH ON THE NATIONAL LEVEL

Just as there are many examples of One Health initiatives at the local level, there are also many at the national level, such as the surveillance among migratory waterfowl in Alaska or in poultry across the nation for H5N1 avian flu, which has caused hundreds of human deaths around the world and had enormous public health implications since its discovery in 1997 in Hong Kong. We keep watch on the migratory waterfowl, the carrier of all strains of influenza, in the hopes of detecting any incursion of H5N1 avian flu into the United States so that we can quickly eradicate it before it causes significant illness or morality in our flocks, in us, or even in other animals, which might be possible if this highly mutable virus were to change and become infective for other species.

Nationally, we conduct surveillance among animals and report positive cases (animal and human) on many zoonotic diseases: anthrax, plague, brucellosis, tuberculosis, and a good many others. Animals can be used as sentinels for disease agents that can infect humans, and from these animals, and from the epidemiological picture of the disease in the animal populations, we get an idea of the degree of risk we humans face, and we may also uncover clues that will help us predict the human impact. Once we have a snapshot of the disease or the disease agent in animals (or in mosquitoes or fleas or even kissing bugs), we can make recommendations to people on how best to avoid infection.

Knowing how common tuberculosis (*Mycobacterium bovis*) is in deer in Michigan, for example, and what counties of the state are affected, lets us make recommendations to hunters on whether they should consume their kill or if they should submit the carcass for testing. *M. bovis* is a well-known zoonotic disease of significant public health and socioeconomic importance that afflicts livestock worldwide, causing production losses in dairy and beef herds and creating financial hardship for farmers and their families where it occurs. Before pasteurization came into widespread use in the 1930s in the United States, *M. bovis* was passed to people in raw milk, causing tuberculosis. This agent has health implications for the deer, for other wildlife (such as coyotes that consume deer), livestock, and people. Tuberculosis in dairy cattle means economic losses in international trade, because no country wants to import this disease, and restrictions on moving cattle interstate, because no other state wants it either. Over the last 100 years, the United States has expended much money and effort in an attempt to control and eradicate this zoonotic disease, and we are very nearly there. One of the primary objectives of meat inspection is to keep animals with this disease, and other diseases, out of the food chain. Unfortunately, domestic livestock and wildlife can share pastureland and infectious agents. In 1994, a hunter-killed deer in Michigan was found to have *M. bovis,* demonstrating that this agent now had a wildlife reservoir. Eradicating a disease from livestock, which are often confined and identifiable, is much easier than eradicating a disease from wildlife, which are highly mobile, live in the wilderness, and are hard to track.

Rabies is probably one disease that virtually all Americans have heard of and is an excellent example of One Health. Rabies, a disease of mammals (including people), is a concern for U.S. communities as well as many countries and continents across the globe. Known since antiquity, the disease kills an estimated 55,000 people annually and continues to be a significant problem in the United States among wildlife (particularly raccoons, skunks, bats, and foxes), but also remains a concern among our domestic animals. In 2008, 294 cats, 75 dogs, and 59 cattle were reported to have rabies in the United States, but this was a small number compared to the nearly 7,000 wild animals found rabid that year. Nowhere does the issue of controlling stray animal populations become more vital than in the efforts to control and prevent rabies. By removing and reducing stray pets from our communities we reduce the odds a pet will contract rabies from a wild animal and pass that infection on to other animals or to humans, where infection is 100 percent fatal if proper treatment is not received before signs develop.

Rabies among U.S. domestic animals has dropped considerably since the early part of the 20th century when the canine strain was still circulating and dog-to-dog transmission was quite common. Through rabies vaccination campaigns in dogs we eliminated the canine strain of rabies in the United States (though we have several other strains of rabies and pets should still be vaccinated), simultaneously reducing the number of human cases. The rabies vaccine has the benefit of protecting the dog or cat against rabies if it is bitten by another rabid animal, but that wasn't why it was developed. The vaccine was developed to break the cycle of dog-to-dog transmission and the dog-to-human transmission. Every time a dog or cat is taken to the veterinarian for a rabies vaccination, that is a public health preventive measure, a One Health measure—that protects animal and human health simultaneously. Today, we extend this line of thinking to our use of oral rabies vaccination baits that are used in at least 15 states. These fishmeal-based baits contain a pouch of vaccine and are dropped in areas experiencing high levels of rabies in raccoons, gray foxes, or coyotes. When the wild animal eats the bait they become vaccinated, protecting them against rabies, preventing the spread to other wild animals, to our pets, and ultimately to us.

ONE HEALTH INTERNATIONALLY

In many countries, wealth is measured by the number of livestock a person owns. Social events and transactions of property and services around the globe are occasions that often involve the exchange of livestock.[9] Livestock are the principle users of land throughout the world and serve as a source of livelihood for 1 billion people, 800 million of which are poor. The ability to afford such staples of everyday life as clothing, education, health care, and food, therefore, are tied directly to the health and prosperity of the livestock of the indigenous people. Any disease that impacts the health of animals used for food (cattle, sheep, chickens, pigs, etc.) subsequently impacts human health and prosperity. A notorious example is rinderpest.

Rinderpest is consider by many to be the world's most devastating cattle disease, killing up to 90 percent or more of infected cattle in 10 days. Brought to Europe from Asia in the herds of invading tribes, it caused outbreaks in the fourth century of the Roman Empire and has since killed millions of cattle and wildlife in Europe, Africa, the Middle East, and India. An outbreak of rinderpest in an economy based on cattle, where the communities are dependent on draft power, meat, milk, skins, and manure could be devastating, triggering famine and economic depression. Fortunately, in 1962, Walter Plowright, a British veterinary pathologist, developed a simple, affordable vaccine that has brought this disease to its end. Dr. Plowright's efforts not only contributed to veterinary science, but helped alleviate hunger, bolstered economies large and small, helped agrarian families survive and herds thrive, and ultimately contributed to global One Health.

With its eradication, rinderpest becomes only the second disease to ever be eradicated from the globe through humankind's efforts, the first being smallpox. The Food and Agriculture Organization estimates that the cost of eradicating the virus was less than $3 million,[10] but, because of these efforts, Africa was able to produce an additional $47 billion in food and India an estimated $289 billion.[10] This is truly One Health in action.

The tracking of zoonotic diseases, which can adversely impact the health of animals and people alike, is accomplished in many regions of the world using various methodologies, including the testing of animals, animal products (hides, meat, milk), people, and the environment. Study of the organism is done at the molecular level to learn more so that we are better able to control the microbe, or even eradicate it; however, detailed knowledge of any disease is worthless unless it helps in preventing new cases, improves health, and enhances the quality of life. Influenza, with its diversity of strains and substrains that arise from animals, affects numerous animal species and humans, impacts global commerce, and is a very good example of how One Health efforts in the fields of molecular science complement the fields of human and veterinary medicine and public health. What we learn from the genetic makeup of the virus can tell us a good deal about how the virus came to be, where it came from (geographically and its likely animal reservoir), its zoonotic potential, the likelihood for future outbreaks and control, and what is required to make an effective vaccine.

Today our global influenza surveillance network is better than ever in picking up novel influenza strains. The World Health Organization Global Influenza Surveillance Network, established in 1952, has 131 institutions in 102 countries that submit patient samples to its collaborating centers, which in turn test the sample to determine the exact strain of influenza. Surveillance within the United States is comprised of five components: virus testing in WHO collaborating laboratories, reporting of patients who visit their physician with influenza-like illness, reporting of influenza-associated deaths, hospital surveillance, and reports from state health departments on influenza activity and level of spread within their state.

We are constantly on the lookout for new influenza viruses so that we may quickly discern their potential to harm public health and animal health. As with any disease, the earlier we find new microbes, the better. Economies and industries can also suffer in the face of an influenza (or any other zoonosis) epidemic—people may think influenza is transmitted through food (it is not), so they avoid chicken or pork, and tourism suffers when no one wants to visit a country experiencing an outbreak. Highly pathogenic avian influenza (H5N1) has already caused more than $20 billion in economic losses globally. The new 2009 H1N1 influenza strains stirred fears of a coming pandemic and propelled us to get vaccine to market in a hurry.

Worldwide, numerous governments and organizations are looking at wildlife, poultry, and other species in hopes of detecting that newest flu virus at the earliest possible moment, but they are also keeping tabs on what the viruses we already know about are doing. Are they changing? Are they becoming more easily transmissible between animals? Between people? Are they becoming deadlier? But while we have a great many genome sequences from human influenza cases stored in our genetic warehouses, we have far fewer sequences from dogs, cats, horses, seals, mink, and other animals. Enhanced efforts to look more closely at these species and the influenza viruses that circulate within them can lead to a greater understanding of the dynamics of influenza, its evolution and its epidemiology, and ultimately how to prevent its spread and its subsequent morbidity and mortality.

ECOLOGY, OUR ENVIRONMENT, AND ONE HEALTH

Humans have a tremendous impact upon the Earth, and that impact, good or bad, has direct or indirect consequences upon our future, the way we live, where we live, our jobs, our recreation, what plants we can grow for food, and, ultimately, consequences upon our health and the health of animals. Many examples can be given of how humans have sullied the environment, causing ourselves harm, from air pollution to mercury contamination of our lakes and fish, water contamination with human and animal sewage or industrial runoff, and so on. Such topics already fill volumes.

Invasive species is a One Health problem that has grown with the dispersal of humankind. Invasive species are "plants, animals or microorganisms whose introduction and/or spread into a new ecosystem threatens biodiversity, food security, human health, trade, transport and/or economic development"[11] and pose the biggest threat to biodiversity and constraint to economic development. Invasive species also pose the biggest single threat to food security and human health.[11] As we move around the globe, we transport, either intentionally or unintentionally, species of bacteria, viruses, fungus, plants, and animals. The mixture of plant and animal species in a given region before human interference was reached through long periods of evolution and adaptation, creating a balanced ecosystem, thriving until such time as events alter that balance, forcing change, adaption, and evolution once again. The introduction of nonnative plants, animals, or microbes can be beneficial or harmful to those established species, including humans. Such alteration ultimately changes the ecosystem, creating conditions in which once thriving species may now suffer declines due to the introduction of a new pathogen or a new predator. As the introduced species proliferate, the result is a lack of diversity among animal or plant species, creating more of a monoculture. As native animal populations decline in the presence of a newly introduced, highly efficient predator, for example, the impact can have an ripple effect on human activity, livelihood, and health. If we just look at it from a financial perspective, invasive species cost our planet an estimated $1.4 trillion annually.[11]

In 1988, the zebra mussel, native to the Black Sea, appeared in Lake St. Clair, Ontario. These mussels are very prolific and accumulate in large masses, growing upon rocks, ship bottoms, pipes, other animals, even each other — upon anything. Within two short years the mussels covered the Great Lakes, blocking intake pipes to utilities, factories, and municipal facilities, forcing some businesses to close and hindering ship navigation. The zebra mussel filters up to a quart of water per day and consumes animals and algae that would have been food for larval fish or other native species, which can result in the decline in native fish, mollusks, and birds. They can grow on native mussels, clams, crayfish, and turtles, threatening their populations. Even though many native animals eat zebra mussels, a positive benefit, they cannot keep the mussel population from growing. The mussels attach to the hulls of the boats, propellers, motors, and engine cooling systems. They are so prolific they sink navigation buoys. Beaches are made unattractive, cutting the feet of those who step on the shells, and the mussels negatively impact recreational fishing. Eradication of this mussel is impossible now. It is estimated that the United States and Canada lose approximately $140 million a year as a result of the zebra mussel.[12]

The introduction of invasive species can be linked to such diseases as plague (the introduction of *Yersinia pestis* into the U.S. mainland in 1900), yellow fever, malaria, and typhus, to name just a few. Of course, the introduction of invasive species can be done through standard importation channels, accidentally, or through smuggling. An example of standard importation channels is the first U.S. case of BSE in 2003 in a cow that was discovered to have been imported from Canada, resulting in billions of dollars in lost trade and production and public concern for the safety of its meat supply. An example of smuggling is that of two crested hawk eagles (*Spizaetus nipalensis*) smuggled into Europe from Thailand, both of which were positive for H5N1 avian flu.

Thanks to human activity (global commerce, travel, exploration, immigration), we are now moving species around the world faster than ever before. People have even brought canine distemper (which subsequently infected seals) and bluegrass to the Antarctic. Ornamental plants meant for our yards spread to nearby streams, choking out native plants and changing the ecology of the stream to the detriment of animals and insects. *Miconia calvescens* is a fast-growing plant from South America that has made its way around the world as an ornamental plant, taking over and displacing native plants wherever it is found. In Tahiti it has displaced two-thirds of the native forest. With a change in flora comes a concomitant impact on fauna, including humans. As miconia, with its shallow roots, displaces other plants with deeper roots, hillsides become more tenuous, and landslides more common.[12] This plant is now found on Maui, threatening Hawaii's plants and animals. As if this weren't enough, the island of Maui also contends with the quarter-size coqui, a Caribbean frog that entered on nursery plants from Puerto Rico. The coqui vocalizes at 90 decibels, about the level of a lawn mower, hampering tourism and the nursery export trade. The small frog—up to 10,000 or more per acre—has no natural enemies in Hawaii, eats the insects that native birds would have eaten, and disrupts sleep for residents and visitors, which concerns the tourism industry greatly. The frog hides during the day, hitching rides on potted plants and getting moved around the islands, and eradication seems improbable.

Not all new introductions of species are harmful. Most of the agricultural plants and animals we raise today in North America are technically aliens, coming from Europe and other parts of the world.[12] Today, however, controlling invasive species takes a monumental effort, and a monumental budget. Florida spends $50 million each year attempting to control invasive plants; states and the federal government have spent $175 million in the war against the Asian long-horned beetle. When the foot-and-mouth virus was discovered in the United Kingdom in 2001, approximately 6 million animals had to be slaughtered to contain this outbreak or for welfare reasons, halting exports of meat and livestock, putting some family farms out of business and creating physical and psychological health issues among farmers and others working to contain this disease. The outbreak cost businesses (agriculture, food, tourism, and others) at least $4 billion–$5 billion. Annually, invasive species cost the United States more than $140 billion.[12]

Another example of One Health and our ecosystem is the issue of the overuse of antibiotics and environmental contamination. Antibiotics are used extensively across the world in the human and veterinary medical fields to combat bacterial infections, and since their discovery these drugs have saved countless lives and allowed us to live longer. Unfortunately, bacteria, with their short life spans, are quite adept at evolving new traits to help them survive the pharmaceutical onslaught. These microbes can develop resistance to antibiotics, and a resistant infection often means prolonged illness, a greater likelihood of transmission of the infection to another host, a greater likelihood of dying from that infection, and the necessity of switching to a second- or third-choice drug, a drug that is often more expensive, making it less likely a patient in a poorer country can afford it and more likely they will not survive that infection.

Most antibiotics are excreted from the body unaltered, making their way into wastewater effluent from treatment plants then into our environment, particularly our aquatic ecosystems, encouraging resistance in the bacteria found there.[13,14] In fact, antibiotics have been reported in hospital wastewater, wastewater (sewage) treatment plant effluents and biosolids, surface waters (lakes, streams), sediments, biota, and drinking water. It is said that within the United States there are very few bodies of water in which antibiotics cannot be found, except for perhaps remote mountain lakes and streams before they reach urban or agricultural areas.[14] Having them in our water means we are chronically exposed to them, which likely contributes to the evolution of resistant bacteria. There are many reasons why bacteria develop resistance to a given antibiotic. Bacteria are continually adapting and changing, and resistance can develop naturally, but in the presence of antibiotics that change is accelerated. The use of the wrong drug, using a drug for too long or too short a duration, improper dosing, poor patient compliance with a doctor's instructions, and many other factors can all play a part in developing resistance. It should be noted that not all bacterial infections require antibiotics. Sometimes patients are able to clear the infections on their own. The increasing resistance of bacteria to antibiotics is an issue of concern to veterinarians, physicians, hospitals, agriculture, farmers, patients (human and animal), consumers, global trade—it is a worldwide problem. That is why finding antibiotics, antibiotic-resistant bacteria, and antibiotic-resistant genes (ARGs) from bacteria in our aquatic ecosystems (streams, lakes, sewage and agricultural runoff, and drinking water) is such a public health concern.

Bacteria in water may be indigenous or may come from soil, plants, humans, or animals. Pathogenic and potentially pathogenic bacteria are constantly released into our waterways via wastewater, and many of these bacteria harbor ARGs. The extensive use of antibiotics in human medicine and animal farming leads to antibiotic contamination of manure, which can be used as fertilizer on fields and subsequently end up in our water sources.[15] In aquaculture, antibiotics may not readily break down and will linger in the aquatic environment, selecting out susceptible microbes, leaving behind resistant ones that can pass ARGs to environmental, fish, and human microbes, ultimately contaminating fish and shellfish destined for consumption with antibiotics.[15] Antibiotic-resistant bacteria found in human sewage, animal feces, and wastewater from hospitals and intensive livestock farms very likely serve as sources for antibiotic-resistant organisms and ARGs that contaminate our environment.[15] Genes can be transferred between bacteria in many ways, passing on resistance to a particular antibiotic to bacteria that were once susceptible. Such genes can be picked up by the bacteria found in water or food, eventually ending up in people and animals. Indeed, environmental bacteria act as an endless source of genes that could serve as resistance genes in pathogenic microbes.[15] We know ARGs are a public health concern, but their full impact in our waterways has not yet been fully deciphered. We also know that as more and more antibiotics, detergents, disinfectants, industrial pollutants, and heavy metals enter our water that these contribute to the evolution and spread of resistant bacteria in the aquatic environment.[15]

How do we reduce the possibility of antibiotics and ARGs entering and spreading in our environment? There are no easy answers. We may not be able to remove all ARGs, but more judicious use of antibiotics by physicians, veterinarians, and farmers is a major step in reducing antibiotic resistance and in protecting human and animal health simultaneously. New, effective wastewater treatment to remove ARGs and antibiotics should be investigated, and the use of human and animal waste or wastewater as fertilizer should be evaluated in light of the possibility of introducing ARGs to soil and water sources.[14,15] Research and health risk assessments of ARGs should also be done, and such findings should be a foundation for regulatory guidelines developed by human and veterinary medical experts, along with input from agricultural, environmental, and water treatment experts.

Antibiotics and ARGs are just some of the public health concerns that are connected to our environment. Researchers have found hormones, caffeine, heavy metals, and other compounds in our water, all indicative of human impact, which should make us reflect on One Health—how we treat our environment eventually comes to impact our health.

WORKING TOGETHER TO TACKLE ONE HEALTH

So how do we make One Health a reality? How can we bring together veterinarians, physicians, ecologists, environmental health experts, conservationists, and other health and scientific professionals to make One Health more than just a great idea? Most important, how can we put One Health into action—actually do things that will make a difference in our everyday lives, reducing illness, reducing death, improving the food we eat, the air we breathe, the water we drink, while simultaneously bettering the health of animals, plants, and our ecosystem as a whole? How will we do all this in the face of climate change? Taken together, that all seems out of reach. One way to accomplish all of this is to start thinking beyond a job description.

12.1. DID YOU KNOW?

The consequences and impact of climate change depend on the eco-geographic response of a given region, which, in the face of accumulating greenhouse gases, might see higher or lower temperatures, humidity, rainfall, and snowfall. These changes can create such severe weather outcomes as heat waves, floods, and droughts and influence the distribution of infectious disease pathogens and the insects that may carry them. Such weather extremes can also influence the frequency and magnitude of disease outbreaks, which in turn affect human and animal health, livelihoods, and the economy.

Most people are familiar with the basics of what a veterinarian does: They provide medical and surgical care for farm animals, pets, exotic animals, and wildlife. But in addition to safeguarding the health of animals, veterinarians play a crucial role in public health and swear to promote public health as part of their oath upon graduation. They are experts on zoonotic diseases and educate animal owners daily about these risks. Across the nation and across the world we can find veterinarians working in many fields of public health, including meat inspection, research, epidemiology, infectious diseases, chronic diseases, occupational health, vaccine research, and environmental health, even in fields dominated by human health professionals, such as HIV/AIDS and obesity.

In some regions of the world, getting care to the people can be a daunting task. People may be located in remote villages or nomadic camps, far from the nearest health-care clinic, and getting care to such populations requires extraordinary effort and travel over great distances, putting lives in danger and medical supplies in jeopardy. Veterinarians too may have a difficult time reaching livestock herds, but are often more mobile than some human health-care workers, and may be the most highly educated human resource available in African rural areas. As a consequence of these realities, both the livestock and the families that own them may have very low vaccination rates and suffer illnesses or deaths that might otherwise have been prevented if care had been close by. Partnering human health care with a mobile veterinary infrastructure, as demonstrated in a program in Chad,[9] can successfully increase the vaccination rates of children and livestock simultaneously, saving lives, safeguarding livelihoods and food sources, and doing all of this at a reduced cost because of the sharing of resources, finances, and people between the veterinary and human health professions. The joint effort of professions also builds trust between the families and health workers, ensuring that a successful ongoing program can be maintained in populations that have been described as being "marginalized from development processes and vulnerable to exclusion from health services because of their geographical, social, and cultural environment."[9] In another example, in Sudan, the Expanded Programme on Immunization shared cold chain equipment (coolers designed to keep vaccines cold so they do not spoil) with veterinary services; and the Red Cross has used veterinarians' vehicles in their vaccination campaigns, with similar collaborations occurring during times of civil war or other crises. The success of all these programs hint at a new model for other governments to reach remote populations.

Bringing together various disciplines, or sectors—what is known as intersectoral collaboration—holds the key to One Health success. However, barriers between disciplines exist, and it is difficult to remove these barriers so as to reach maximum efficiency in cooperation. Some services, for example, may be the domain of one or two discipline sectors, or the barriers could be due to existing legislation, budget restraints, unequal institutional capabilities, limited communication, cultural issues, or some other reason. Sharing people, territory, vehicles, coolers, buildings, radios, money, ideas . . . these are the things that will bring about a One Health revolution, but such daring change requires governmental support, acceptance of change and the initial discomfort that accompanies it, and the support of international agencies. Organizations with broad reach and support such as the World Health Organization, the Food and Agriculture Organization, the United Nations Children's Fund, the World Bank, and others are now openly endorsing such collaboration among sectors and recognizing that a "multidisciplinary [veterinarians, physicians, nurses, ecologists, wildlife experts, environmental health experts, plant experts], multinational, and multisectoral approach" is required.[16]

Improved disease surveillance is an area where human and veterinary professionals can work together, gathering and sharing human and animal data, improving communications and community involvement, enhancing the understanding of diseases, water quality, and the impact on the environment. And the focus should not be just on infectious diseases. The importance of addressing noncommunicable diseases will grow over the next two decades. By 2030, the percentage of deaths due to infectious diseases is expected to decline while those due to noninfectious diseases (such as heart disease, cancer, strokes, diabetes) will reach an estimated 75 percent of all deaths.[2]

As veterinarians may be the only health professional in a remote region, it also makes sense to provide them with training to provide basic human health care. In 2005, 99 percent of the women who died in pregnancy and childbirth were from developing countries, with just over half occurring in sub-Saharan Africa.[3] A veterinarian trained in basic human medicine could improve maternal and neonatal care and reduce mortality rates in these groups. Dual-trained veterinarians could be enlisted to fight HIV, tuberculosis, and malaria, enhance childhood vaccination coverage, increase use of family planning, recognize and report new diseases or new health concerns, investigate disease impacts, offer basic medical/surgical procedures, empower women, provide health education to communities, and much more. The use of such a dual-trained individual does not have to be limited to remote, poor regions of the world; we could use them in the United States in medically underserved rural areas that cannot support the cost of a full-time medical professional, because it is in these regions where the food animals are raised and where veterinarians are also needed. In light of an expected shortage of 125,000 physicians over the next 15 years, this unique solution could work in some areas. Maintaining the good health of animals, as it turns out, provides an avenue for supplying both human and veterinary care.[9]

With 7 billion people on the planet, there is more opportunity than ever before for human-animal contact. Domestic animals, wildlife, and humans share the environment, including all of its risks (pesticides, antibiotic-resistant genes, pollution), and leave behind an impact, good or bad. Our health, our exposures, risks, diseases, even our prosperity, overlap.

This convergence of people, animals, and our environment has created a new dynamic, wherein the health of each is inextricably connected, impacting one another and creating new challenges to health and well-being.[4] Meeting these new challenges requires a new way of thinking and a new way of delivering health care, a new model in which human health-care professionals and veterinary health-care professionals join forces, share resources as well as knowledge and skills, and incorporate such experts from other disciplines as environmental and social sciences in finding solutions—this is known as One Health. The focus of One Health must not be solely on research, but heavy on the delivery of solutions that work on the ground. It must not focus on one disease, but must be encompassing, adaptable, and malleable. Throughout the 20th century, the human and veterinary medical fields became increasingly more fragmented, more specialized, growing ever more distant from each other. It is time to tear down the walls between professions and disciplines and recognize that the health of humans, animals, and our environment can be better than it has ever been if we are willing to break down barriers, make alliances, and try the unthinkable of taking a One Health view of our world.

FURTHER READING

Food and Agriculture Organization of the United Nations. The state of food and agriculture: Livestock in the balance, 2009. Available at: http://www.fao.org/publications/sofa-2009/en/.

International Office of Epizootics. Climate change: Impact on the epidemiology and control of animal diseases. *Revue scientifique et technique* 2008;27. Available at: http://www.oie.int/publications-and-documentation/scientific-and-technical-review-free-access/list-of-issues/.

International Office of Epizootics. Invasive species. Part 1 and Part 2. *Revue scientifique et technique* 2010;29(1)(2). Available at: http://www.oie.int/publications-and-documentation/scientific-and-technical-review-free-access/list-of-issues/.

One Health Commission. Main website for the call to action and collaboration for organizations, professions, industries, and others in the area of One Health. Available at: http://www.onehealthcommission.org/.

One Health Initiative. Broad movement supporting One Health and detailing what is currently happening in area of One Health. Available at: http://www.onehealthinitiative.com/mission.php.

One Health Newsletter. Quarterly newsletter on the topic and application of One Health. Available at: http://www.doh.state.fl.us/environment/medicine/One_Health/OneHealth.html

World Bank. People, pathogens and our planet. Volume 1: Towards a One Health approach for controlling zoonotic diseases. 50833-GLB. Washington, DC; 2010. Available at: http://siteresources.worldbank.org/INTARD/Resources/PPP_Web.pdf.

REFERENCES

1. Association of Schools of Public Health. Available at: http://www.whatis publichealth.org/. Accessed February 20, 2010.
2. Beaglehole R, Bonita R. Global public health: a scorecard. *Lancet* 2008;372: 1988–96.
3. World Health Organization. World Health Statistics 2008. Geneva, 2008. Available at: http://www.who.int/entity/whosis/whostat/2008/en/index.html. Accessed February 20, 2010.
4. American Veterinary Medical Association. One Health: a new professional imperative. One Health initiative task force: final report, 2008. Available at: http://www.avma.org/onehealth/default.asp. Accessed February 16, 2010.
5. Kahn LH, Kaplan B, Monath TP. One Health Initiative. Available at: http://www.onehealthinitiative.com/mission.php. Accessed February 24, 2010.
6. Kahn LH, Kaplan B, Steele JH. Confronting zoonoses through closer collaboration between medicine and veterinary medicine (as "one medicine"). *Veterinaria Italiana* 2007;43:5–19.
7. Braun C, Stangler T, Narveson J, et al. Animal-assisted therapy as a pain relief intervention for children. *Complimentary therapies in clinical practice* 2009;15:105–9.
8. Walsh F. Human-animal bonds I: The relational significance of companion animals. *Family Process* 2009;48:462–80.
9. Schelling E, Wyss K, Bechir M, et al. Synergy between public health and veterinary services to deliver human and animal health interventions in rural low income settings. *British Medical Journal* 2005;331:1264–7.
10. Anonymous. Pathologist's Vaccine Conquered Scourge of Cattle. Available at: http://online.wsj.com/article/SB10001424052748704479404575087853233620996. html?KEYWORDS=rinderpest. Accessed February 26, 2010.
11. Global Invasive Species Programme (GISP). Annual report, 2009. Available at: http://www.gisp.org/. Accessed March 18, 2010.
12. McGrath S. Attack of the alien invaders. *National geographic*. Available at: http://environment.nationalgeographic.com/habitats/attack-alien-invaders/#page=1. Accessed March 18, 2010.
13. Choi CQ. Pollution in solution: Drug-resistance DNA as the latest freshwater threat. *Scientific American* 2007;291:22–3.
14. Zhang X, Zhang T, Fang HHP. Antibiotic resistance genes in water environment. *Applied microbiology and biotechnology* 2009;82:397–414.
15. Baquero F, Martinez JL, Canton R. Antibiotics and antibiotic resistance in water environments. *Current opinion in biotechnology* 2008;19:260–5.
16. United Nations. Contributing to one world, one health: A strategic framework for reducing risks of infectious diseases at the animal-human-ecosystems interface, 2008. Available at: http://un-influenza.org/files/OWOH_14Oct08.pdf. Accessed July 1, 2009.

Chapter 13

The Future: Modern Animal Biotechnology

Larisa Rudenko, PhD, DABT, Jeffery Jones, DVM, PhD, and Evgenij Evdokimov, PhD

INTRODUCTION

Animals have been a part of our lives since prehistoric times. They have provided us with nourishment and medicines, shelter and clothing, protection and companionship. As we moved from being primarily hunter-gatherers and settled into a more agrarian existence, the domestication of animals followed suit. We do not know how the earliest wild animals became domesticated. Perhaps wolves followed nomadic tribes, and pups with docile temperaments were adopted and bred with others possessing similar traits until what we think of as dogs resulted, which could sound early alarms, protect the young, elderly, and infirm, and help with the hunt or herding. Likewise, perhaps cats followed people as stored grain attracted rats and mice, and the most docile mousers learned to tolerate people (some might say that even now the most domesticated cats only tolerate people). What we do know is that about 13,000 B.C.E. (before the Common Era), records indicate that dogs were domesticated from wolves somewhere in China; there are records of goats being raised by humans in the Middle East about 10,000 B.C.E., followed by the domestication of swine from wild boars in the steppes of Central Asia sometime around 8,000 B.C.E. Records of cattle domesticated from the wild auroch have been found in Anatolia dating from about 7,000 B.C.E., and chickens from wild jungle fowl in Southeast Asia about a thousand years later.

Each of these domestication events must have involved identifying animals with desirable traits, and breeding those animals with others possessing similar or other desirable traits—perhaps breeding a particularly docile bull with a cow that produced a large amount of milk. This technique, which is still practiced today, is referred to as selective breeding, and marks the beginning of what we now refer to as animal biotechnology. Similar selective breeding was applied to wild plants, until agriculture as we now broadly interpret it, became the source of food and medicinal substances.

Over time, humans have developed various approaches to make our environment less hostile and improve our living conditions. The application of technology to biology, what we call biotechnology has been responsible for development of most of the plants and animals with which we surround ourselves today. The most advanced of these are often referred to as modern biotechnology and often involve very specific alterations involving recombinant DNA techniques. Three examples have agricultural and biomedical applications in use today and great implications for the future: animal cloning, genetic engineering, and xenotransplantation.

ANIMAL CLONING

As with all new technologies, animal cloning, the production of multiple genetically identical individuals, is an area of animal biotechnology that has shown great potential and raised some concerns. Animal cloning allows for the rapid dissemination of naturally occurring desirable traits in herds of animals by reproducing those animals. The 1996 first use of somatic cell nuclear transfer (SCNT, discussed further below) to produce Dolly the sheep marked the transition from animal cloning as a relatively minor area of academic research to a topic of high public visibility and interest.[1]

Assisted reproductive technologies (ARTs) are methods in which humans help along reproductive functions. In vitro fertilization may be the best known of these in both humans and animals. Artificial insemination (AI) is another frequently used ART, especially in agriculture. In fact, most dairy cows are bred via AI.

Traits that are desired in animal agriculture include adaptability to environmental conditions, efficient conversion of feed (improved production), increased docility, improved meat, milk, or egg quality or quantity, and disease resistance. Sometimes animals are important simply because they are rare or unusual. Breeders have developed elaborate genealogies and other predictive methods to identify and increase the proportion of these naturally occurring desirable traits in animal populations, but because all of these approaches rely on sexual reproduction, it is not possible to ensure that the resulting offspring will bear the characteristic(s) of interest.

Cloning and Other Assisted Reproductive Technologies

Animal cloning is the most recent advance on the continuum of ARTs. Humans have long understood that traits are hereditary—that is, they are passed from parent to offspring. Animals with desirable traits are identified and selectively bred in the hopes of passing those desirable traits to their offspring. Offspring that display those traits are again selected for breeding, over and over. This selective breeding process has been used for centuries to increase the frequency at which these traits are passed on, thereby expanding the range of what were initially rare traits. The power of selective breeding can be seen by comparing the physical appearance of wild canines (wolves) to that of various domestic dog breeds from Chihuahuas to Great Danes—all developed by selective breeding.

Artificial insemination (AI) has been used for centuries in a wide variety of species and is widely used in modern animal agriculture. It involves collecting semen from genetically desirable males, dividing it into small units, and often freezing that semen for storage in small plastic straws and subsequent use. This allows for long-term use of such genetics, as well as ease of transport and storage of genetic material (semen from some species can be frozen and stored indefinitely in liquid nitrogen or shipped on dry ice or in liquid nitrogen). Because one semen collection can be diluted and divided, it allows for the ability to inseminate many more females than would be possible through natural mating. It also allows for using genetics in a herd from a wider variety of males than would be practical using natural mating. It reduces physical risk to both male and female animals during mating. Physical risk to the human handlers is also reduced because it is not necessary to maintain large numbers of aggressive male animals (especially bulls). It also reduces the risk of transmitting infectious disease because semen can be tested prior to transfer. Finally, it allows for the introduction of genetics from animals that have difficulty mating or that no longer exist.

In vitro fertilization (collecting eggs and sperm and fertilizing the eggs in tissue culture dishes); embryo splitting (collecting an early embryo and dividing it to form several twin embryos); and embryo transfer (mating high quality male and female animals and then collecting the embryos and transferring them to surrogate dams) are newer and more expensive techniques.

The most commonly used technique in animal cloning is referred to as somatic cell nuclear transfer (SCNT). Cells from the animal to be copied are harvested from the animal (often from an ear punch) and grown in culture. These cells are differentiated, that is, they have assumed a particular form and function in the animals. Scientists then introduce either the nucleus from these cells, or, more often, the entire cell into an oöcyte (a developing egg cell) from which the nucleus has been removed, in a special culture medium. The cell is stimulated with a small electrical current, and the contents of the egg cell in effect reprogram the differentiated nucleus and the cell becomes an embryo. Healthy appearing embryos are transferred into surrogate dams (exactly as would be the case with in vitro fertilization), and in successful cases, implanted into the uterus to develop into a pregnancy. Although the description of the process is simple, because of the many unknowns in the process, in some species, particularly cattle, the number of nuclear transfers that result in live births can be lower than the percentage of in vitro fertilized embryo transfers.

Commonly Encountered Clones

Clones are virtually identical genetic copies of organisms—identical, or monozygotic, twins, separated in time. We encounter a variety of different types of clones in the course of our daily lives, most of which naturally, including some plants like strawberries that send out shoots or runners to form babies that can later separate to form new plants. These babies are clones of the parent, because they are produced asexually. Asexual reproduction involves producing a new copy of an existing parental organism without the reshuffling of parental genomes that occurs during sexual reproduction—in other words, it copies the "parent" organism. This ability of plants to reproduce asexually can also be manipulated by taking a cutting of a plant and either rooting or grafting that cutting to make new plants. Many of our ornamental plants, including many rose varieties, and such important food crops as citrus, grapes, and potatoes are clones.

We frequently come into contact with animals that are clones, although we tend to call them twins and not clones. Identical twins occur naturally, but relatively infrequently and with limited predictability (although twinning does appear to have a genetic component). Identical or monozygotic human twin births occur at a rate of about 3 in 1,000 live births; the rate of identical twins among certain breeds of cattle is about 1-4 percent.

Potential Applications of Animal Cloning

Animal cloning allows for reproducing, more or less exactly, animals whose traits are well known and desirable. An important difference between conventional breeding and animal cloning is that conventional breeding (i.e., sexual reproduction) requires that both parents contribute part of the genetic material to the offspring. These offspring do not receive every gene from each parent and so may not have the exact genes needed to express the desirable trait (sometimes referred to as phenotype). This limitation of sexual reproduction becomes apparent if the desired traits require multiple genes—these may not be passed to progeny as a linked unit. Animal cloning avoids this issue because it allows the production of animals with the exact genome of the animal with desired traits.

Cloning also allows for the reproduction of elite animals whose reproductive function is limited. Reproductive ability may be limited in desirable animals for many reasons. Animals can be infertile due to age, disease, accident, or surgical procedures (e.g., castration). Endangered or extinct animal species may have limited access to mating partners, and may be so limited in numbers that sufficient breeding stock may be generated via cloning.

Finally, animal cloning does not rely on the reproductive capacity of the animal, so it provides the opportunity to greatly expand the numbers of animals with highly desirable traits, which can then serve as breeding stock. For example, although female cattle can produce one or (in the case of twins) two offspring per year, in theory, if that highly desirable animal were cloned, she could produce many multiples of offspring in any one year, thereby increasing the prevalence of desirable animals in the herd.

13.1. DID YOU KNOW?

Saving Endangered Species through Cloning

Audubon Nature Institute is using cloning technology to study the reproductive biology and behavior of African wild cats. This conservation program also includes a Frozen Zoo, a collection of biologic materials from various endangered species that can be used to restore the population of many of these species.

It is important to note that for food production purposes, clones are intended to be used as elite breeding animals and not as food production animals. Part of the reason is that producing clones is so expensive that it would not be practical to use these animals as sources of steak or pork chops. Second, clones will likely be incorporated into breeding programs in the same way as other elite breeding animals—they introduce desired characteristics in production herds but are not considered production animals themselves.

Application of Cloning Technology

The birth of Dolly brought the reality of animal cloning to the public. Despite science fiction portrayals of legions of automatons, Dolly was hardly scary. She was simply a sheep, who lived her life in the public eye, and died of a viral disease of the lung that swept the facility in which she was housed when she was middle-aged for a sheep. (Despite various press reports, Dolly did not die of an early old age). Since then, cloning has been used to produce various research, agricultural, companion, and endangered animals (see Table 13.1 for a list of animals that have been cloned). Not long after the announcement of Dolly's birth, cattle clones were born. Mice, the workhorses of laboratory research, were cloned soon thereafter, although it took considerably longer for rats to be cloned. Four years after the birth of Dolly, scientists cloned a pig, followed soon thereafter by

Table 13.1

Animal Species That Have Been Cloned

Species	Year Reported
Sheep	1997
Cow	1998
Mouse	1998
Gaur	2000
Pig	2000
Mouflon Sheep	2001
Cat	2002
Goat	2002
Rabbit	2002
Deer	2003
Horse	2003
Mule	2003
Rat	2003
Wildcat	2003
Dog	2005
Banteng	2005
Ferret	2006
Swamp Buffalo	2006
Gray Wolf	2007
Camel	2009

more cattle and goats. Cloning of companion animals has also received a lot of attention in the news in the past decade. Successful cloning of a cat and a dog led to commercial offers to clone pets.

Limitations of Animal Cloning

As cloning is attempted in more species, one of the key factors limiting the success of the process is the basic reproductive biology of the individual species. For example, domestic cats ovulate every 21 days, but most dog breeds only ovulate twice a year. These biologic differences affect the ease with which oöcytes can be acquired as well as preparing surrogate dams to carry the embryos to term.

There are other issues with the technology as well. Because the process of reprogramming is poorly understood, early attempts at animal cloning required many hundreds of transfers to result in one live birth, especially as attempts are made to clone species for the first time. In addition, similar to other assisted reproductive technologies such as in vitro fertilization that require culturing the developing embryo outside the body for a considerable period of time, some developmental abnormalities have been observed, particularly in cattle and sheep. These are referred to as large offspring syndrome. As the experience with the technology has increased, efficiencies continue to improve and the frequency of abnormalities in animal clones continues to decline.

In addition to success rates, expectations for clones remain difficult to keep realistic. Many people expect clones to be the same as the animal from which they are derived in every way, including behavior. In fact, although the genetic makeup of an animal may predispose it to exhibit certain traits, developmental and environmental factors also have a great influence on how that animal matures and develops. Even though an animal clone may have superior genetics, if it is raised in poor conditions—limited nutritional support or with poor hygiene—it will likely not achieve its genetic potential. Conditioning is also important. For example, the clone of a highly trained animal (such as a barrel racing horse) would have the genetics of its nuclear donor, but without training would be unlikely to either carry a rider or win a barrel race.

The strength and goal of animal cloning is also a limitation—the production of additional genetically identical individuals with the same desired trait(s) as the original animal is just that. Sexual reproduction remains the way to reshuffle the genetic deck and provide an opportunity to generate new combinations of genes that result in unique individuals. Without sexual reproduction, populations of animals would freeze in time and stop improving. The use of sexual reproduction and cloning together, on the other hand, may provide a mechanism by which such naturally arising traits as disease resistance, can be propagated among populations of resulting animals to improve their health more rapidly than would be expected by using sexual reproduction alone.

Safety of Food from Animal Clones

A science-based review (a risk assessment) of the available information on cloning in species traditionally used for food (i.e., cattle, swine, sheep, and goats) was conducted by the Center for Veterinary Medicine at the U.S. Food and Drug Administration to determine the safety of food produced by animal clones and their sexually reproduced offspring.[2] That risk assessment concluded that edible products from cattle, goat, and swine clones (the species from which appreciable data and information was available) and the progeny of clones pose no additional food consumption risk(s) relative to corresponding products from contemporary conventional comparators. Analyses by other countries and international bodies (e.g., France, New Zealand, Japan, the European Food Safety Authority) have come to similar conclusions.

GENETIC ENGINEERING

Genetic engineering (GE), the use of recombinant DNA (rDNA) technology (also referred to as modern biotechnology) to splice together pieces of DNA in new ways to introduce new traits or alter existing traits, has great potential to improve and enrich lives. It can aid in developing organisms that are resistant to diseases or pests; grow larger or faster or in inhospitable environments; have lower nutrient requirements; and produce more nutritious foods or novel therapeutics or other products. Although genetic engineering may sound exotic, genetic engineering of organisms is commonly used in pharmaceutical manufacturing and plant agriculture. For example, rDNA technology is widely used in microbial systems by the pharmaceutical industry to make an array of medicines. Humulin, the most commonly administered insulin to diabetics, is a recombinant human insulin produced in genetically engineered bacteria. In plant agriculture, many plants have been genetically engineered to exhibit desirable traits, including insect and herbicide resistance. In fact, most of the soybeans, corn, cotton, and canola grown in the United States are GE varieties that are resistant to damage from insect pests or resistant to herbicides applied to kill weeds (or both) and so improve productivity and decrease the use of pesticides.

Commonly Encountered Genetically Modified Animals

As previously described, a variety of ARTs have been used to expand the numbers of animals with desirable traits. Although cloning can be used for asexual reproduction of animals that have a desirable phenotype, conventional reproductive techniques, and even cloning, are limited to improving existing traits incrementally or expanding traits that arise spontaneously. In contrast, genetic engineering is the use of rDNA technology (also referred to as modern biotechnology) to introduce new traits rapidly that would only arise very slowly, or more likely would not arise spontaneously, into plants or animals. Genetic engineering is best thought of in the context of the many genetic modifications that people have been consolidating in our domestic species for millennia through selective breeding and the other ARTs. Similar to selective breeding that has led to the development of current domestic dog breeds from wolves, comparable approaches have been used to develop most domestic species. Domestic turkeys have been bred from wild turkeys, as have modern dairy and beef cattle from their now extinct ancestors, the aurochs. To clearly distinguish between genetic modification through selective breeding and the use of rDNA technology, we refer to the organisms derived using rDNA technology as genetically engineered.

Potential Applications of GE Animals

The range of potential applications for the use of rDNA technology to genetically engineer animals is very broad. Although the tendency to categorize these applications is strong, it limits the way the technology is considered. Specific GE animals may initially be intended for particular uses, but they likely will have utility in more than one of these categories. For example, it is fairly common to divide GE animals into groups that contain biomedical applications, improved agricultural traits, and improved quality of life traits for companion animals.

Biopharming

Biopharming is a term used to describe the use of animals to produce therapeutic substances. Because eggs and milk can be harvested easily without harm to the animals, genetically engineering animals to produce therapeutically important proteins (or other substances) in eggs or milk can be a very effective way to produce medical substances.

Some of these medically important substances have previously been purified from human donors, including cadavers. These sources have always been limited, and always carry the risk of transmitting a previously silent human disease. As an alternative, animals can produce large quantities of these substances without the risk of transmitting human diseases. Because these substances are produced by animals whose physiologies resemble ours, our bodies tend to tolerate them more easily, which has the benefit of potentially improving function and slowing the elimination of the substance by our immune systems. Proteins that could be produced easily via biopharming include many blood clotting proteins, enzymes, and peptide hormones. In fact, one such protein has been approved by the FDA, as has the goat that produced it in its milk.[3]

Agricultural Uses

The range of improved agronomic traits that could be enhanced by genetic engineering is very broad, including disease resistance, improved food quality, and the ability to flourish on lower quality feed or in harsh environments. Agronomic traits could include improved food quality or altered nutrient composition of food. For example, some researchers have genetically engineered pigs to produce omega-3 fatty acids normally found in fatty, cold water fish and thought to be important in protecting cardiovascular health. Other uses could include the production of food with a longer shelf life. Milk that is resistant to bacterial growth (without additional processing), and that could be held at room temperature for extended periods without souring would again be useful in parts of the world in which refrigeration is at a premium. Here again, cases in which apparent benefits to animal health also benefit human health: Milk produced by dairy animals engineered to be resistant to mastitis (infections of the udder caused by bacteria) might also be resistant to bacterial spoilage, and could reduce bacterially induced diarrheal diseases in animals (or humans) consuming the milk.

Although we tend to think of disease resistance as being a benefit to animals, it can be a benefit to both animals and humans. A key example is the recent concern about pandemic flu, or any of the recently arising swine or bird flus. Poultry and swine are susceptible to, and reservoirs of, viruses causing these influenza epidemics; they also can play a role in the emergence of new strains, leading to proposals to genetically engineer flu-resistant chickens and pigs.

Food security is another example of disease resistance in animals providing a benefit to humans. Foot-and-mouth disease is extremely infectious and largely untreatable. Outbreaks of this disease have led to wholesale destruction of herds of animal on infected farms, and even those neighboring the sources of infection. This results in removing the potential food from those animals for at least one animal generation and possibly longer if breeding animals are also destroyed. Although costly in developed countries, in areas of the world in which animal protein is at best scarce, and often beyond the economic reach of many individuals, such herd destructions can be catastrophic. Development of animals resistant to foot-and-mouth disease could have an immediate impact on animal health, but could also help provide food security and improve human health by ensuring a steady source of high quality protein.

Companion Animals

GE companion animals would probably most often be engineered to improve their health and enhance their interactions with humans. Health improvements could include resistance to infectious diseases common in pets such as feline leukemia virus and correcting predispositions to metabolic diseases such as cancer. Healthier, longer-lived companion animals would enhance the human-animal bond through longer and higher quality of life benefits to both the human and the companion animal. Another class of engineered traits that could enhance the human-animal bond might be alterations that minimize undesirable traits. These include reduction of the secretion of scents or allergens. As discussed in chapter 1, many people are allergic to various pet animals, so GE house cats (or rabbits or dogs) that do not secrete the proteins responsible for the allergic reaction could allow many more households to have pets.

Selective breeding has been used to develop many breeds of companion animals better at such specific tasks as hunting or herding. Many animals have been selectively bred for what some people consider beauty, resulting in unusual pet birds, fish, and toy breed dogs. Genetic engineering may provide the opportunity to avoid the undesirable traits often caused by inbreeding in selective breeding programs. For example, GE animals that have new or additional colors have been marketed as a type of exotic pet (see GloFish below).

How Genetically Engineered Animals Are Produced

Genetic engineering is one of the tools of modern biotechnology that allows us to make specific changes in the genome of an animal. In order to do so, we use laboratory methods to take pieces of DNA that have specific functions and reassemble them. Because we have made new combinations of the pieces of DNA, we call them recombinant DNA or rDNA for short. A specific rDNA is often called a construct. Constructs are introduced into the genomes of animals to make what are referred to as genetically engineered or GE animals.

The goal of inserting an rDNA construct into an animal genome is to alter some function or trait of that animal. Traits can be altered by adding a new function (often referred to as gain of function) or by disrupting an existing function (often referred to as loss of function or knockout or knockdown). Gain of function traits, such as addition of a construct that results in the expression of a protein, are relatively easy to detect. Loss of function or knockout traits can be more difficult to detect, as the goal of the construct is to get a specific gene in the chromosome of the animal to stop functioning.

When an rDNA construct is introduced into germ line cells, it is passed from generation to generation, and is referred to as a heritable construct.

Animals with heritable constructs are often called transgenic animals. Alternatively, when a construct is inserted in somatic cells (cells of the body that do not make cells that become eggs or sperm), it is not passed from one generation to the next and is referred to as nonheritable. Gene therapy, the introduction of an rDNA construct to treat a disease in a specific patient, is an example of the introduction of a nonheritable construct.

Demonstrated Uses of GE Animals

Genetic engineering of animals has been performed for decades. Mice were the first genetically engineered animals, and were produced in the 1970s, more than 40 years ago. Today, thousands of different genetically engineered mice carrying various constructs and displaying various traits exist in academic research facilities. Although progress in genetically engineering large animals has been slower, numerous examples of genetically

Figure 13.1
GE and non-GE goats at a water station. Female offspring of these GE goats are designed to express spider silk proteins in their milk. These proteins can then be used to spin fibers that have many applications, including artificial ligaments and bulletproof vests

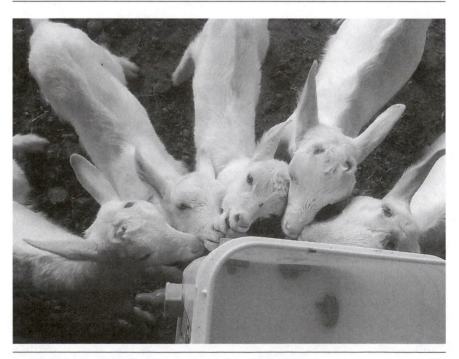

Source: Photo courtesy of Dr. R.V. Lewis. Photographer Holly Steinkraus.

engineered domestic animals have been reported in the scientific literature and the popular press. In the following section, we present a few
examples of such animals.

Mastitis-Resistant Dairy Cows

Mastitis (inflammation of the mammary gland caused by microorganisms, usually bacteria that invade the udder) is an important problem in
dairy cattle. Clinical mastitis compromises milk production and use of
the milk from affected animals and can cost the U.S. dairy industry $1.7 bil-
lion a year. In addition to the economic effects, mastitis can be a devastating disease for the dairy cow. It is extremely painful, difficult to treat,
and in severe cases can result in gangrene leading to the death of the
animal. Several research groups are employing genetic engineering to
prevent or reduce the incidence and severity of mastitis in dairy cattle.
At the USDA's Agricultural Research Service, researchers have inserted a
gene from a nonpathogenic species of Staphylococcus bacteria (lysostaphin)
into the genome of Jersey cows.[4] The lysostaphin is secreted into milk,
where it kills pathogenic bacteria (S. aureus) and protects the cows from
becoming infected. Three genetically engineered cows have been tested
and shown to express lysostaphin in their milk and resist S. aureus infection of the mammary gland.

Bovine Spongiform Encephalopathy–Resistant Cattle

Cattle that are resistant to bovine spongiform encephalopathy (BSE),
commonly referred to as mad-cow disease, have been produced by blocking the synthesis of the normal cellular prion proteins causing the disease.
When tested at about 20 months of age, these GE cattle did not contract
the disease, but otherwise appeared normal.[5] Here again, improving
the health of animals has a direct impact on improving human health.
Humans can become infected with BSE from cattle and their products
(including medicinal products derived from cattle such as gelatin), developing devastating neurological symptoms that eventually result in death.

Pigs with Altered Omega Fatty Acid Composition

The muscle tissue of fish is an excellent dietary source of omega-3 fatty
acids, whereas terrestrial animals tend to have high levels of omega-6,
but low levels of omega-3 fatty acids. Cold water fatty fish provide the
best source of omega-3 fatty acids, but many species have been overfished.
Genetic engineering has allowed development of pigs that express a gene
(fat-1 from the flatworm Caenorhabditis elegans) that converts omega-6 fatty
acids into omega-3 fatty acids so that the GE pigs produce high levels
of omega-3 fatty acids.[6] These animals again demonstrate the multiple

Figure 13.2
Genetically engineered calves. These GE Holstein bull calves are GE animals produced to be resistant to developing bovine spongiform encephalopathy (BSE) or mad-cow disease

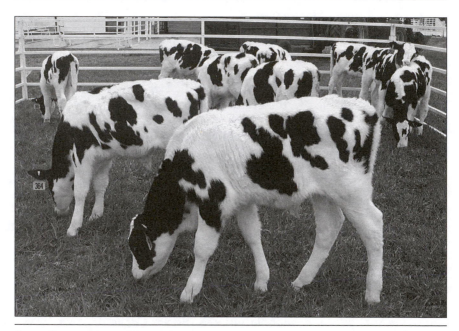

Source: Photo courtesy of Hematech Inc.

category concept introduced earlier. The altered omega fatty acid composition pigs were first developed as a research model for human cardiovascular disease, but could also be used to make heart-healthy bacon.

Marketed GE Animals or Products

GloFish

GloFish are freshwater ornamental fish (*Zebra danio*) genetically engineered to express proteins that give color to the fish; the color is enhanced because the proteins fluoresce when the fish are viewed under a black light. Several different lines have been developed that express different colors. These fish also illustrate the multiple category concept—although GloFish are currently sold across the United States (but not in California) as ornamental companion animals, they were initially intended to detect environmental pollutants in fresh water, and to be a research model for study of growth and development.

Goats Producing a Therapeutic Protein

Goats have been genetically engineered to produce human antithrombin in their milk. Antithrombin naturally occurs in the blood of healthy individuals and helps to keep blood from clotting inappropriately. Patients with a rare disease known as hereditary antithrombin (AT) deficiency, clot inappropriately, particularly during surgery and at childbirth, often with fatal results. Purification of the antithrombin from the goat milk and other manufacturing steps result in production of ATryn, an anticoagulant used for the prevention of blood clots in affected individuals. ATryn and the GE goats that produce the recombinant human antithrombin in their milk were approved by the U.S. Food and Drug Administration in February 2009.[3]

Limitations and Regulation of GE Animal Technology

Although GE animals have the potential to greatly improve human and animal health, the technology is not without its limitations. We still do not fully understand the basic science that is at the root of how genomes of the animals function. General expansion of our scientific knowledge and specific scientific initiatives (for example, the genome projects for several species) have led to exponential advances in our level of understanding and technical abilities and progress in GE animal technology has followed. Nevertheless, we have not yet achieved sufficient understanding to predict the precise effect of the addition of a specific rDNA construct to a GE animal. Because of this lack of predictability, production and verification of the traits of new GE animals can be a slow and costly process. GE animals are regulated by the U.S. Food and Drug Administration under the Federal Food Drug and Cosmetic Act, which requires the demonstration of safety and effectiveness prior to introduction into commerce. Applications for approval must also comply with the requirements of the National Environmental Policy Act.[7]

Concerns about Biotechnology

Some people are uncomfortable with the idea of genetically engineering plants or animals, especially for food uses. Concerns can range from food and environmental safety (which can be addressed with empirical studies) to a more general unease that sometimes is expressed as concerns with the unnaturalness of the technology, and economic concerns about where the benefits of the technology end up. Often, if biotechnology is used to make products that directly benefit people, such as medicines, these concern levels are lower than if the technology is used to make food, or products that some may considered more frivolous. These concerns cannot be dispelled with scientific evidence.

Various approaches have been suggested for accommodating these discomforts, which range from more education about the technology and its uses and benefits to banning it entirely. Some have suggested mandatory labeling of food from GE organisms (as is the case in some countries but not in the United States); others make the argument that if there are no differences in the food itself, that it doesn't matter that it was produced via modern or more classical biotechnologies. (It is important to remember that selective breeding, a classical biotechnology, has been used to modify organisms, from bacteria to large animals, for millennia. As this chapter has attempted to demonstrate, what is objectively different about modern biotechnology is the speed and precision with which those changes can be made.) Other people prefer to eat organic food, which tends to consider modern biotechnology as incompatible with the organic philosophy and therefore excludes foods from GE organisms. Although there are no easy resolutions to these disparate points of view, perhaps the attempts to find common ground by holding respectful, constructive dialogs will be the most useful outcome in allowing apparently opposing sides see that their concerns may not be as irreconcilable as they may appear.

XENOGRAFTS AND XENOTRANSPLANTATION

The use of materials from animals, including the transplantation of cells, tissues, and organs to replace damaged or nonfunctional counterparts in humans has improved or saved the lives of hundreds of thousands of patients. Defective heart valves can be replaced with valves from cows or pigs. People with injuries, end-stage organ failures, diabetes and various life-threatening metabolic hereditary disorders whose fates would have been very uncertain in the past, can now be treated, and in many cases cured, using human-to-human organ transplantation.

Although the transplantation of human organs has become a relatively routine procedure, every success comes at a price. The increasing number of patients who need transplants exceeds the number of available donor organs. Various educational programs and campaigns promoting kidney, liver, and pancreas transplantation from living donors have helped improve the situation, but the demand for donor organs still far exceeds availability. According to the United Network Organ Sharing organization, over 110,000 people require transplants in the United States alone; many of these people may not get a life saving organ in time. Biomaterials and tissue engineering using stem cells to grow functional organs are elegant ideas under development but are not yet available. Xenotransplantation, or the use of animals as a source of organs for transplantation, is considered one of the possible pragmatic solutions to organ shortage.

Historical Uses of Animal Tissues in Humans

What is xenotransplantation and is it really possible? The term xeno-transplantation comes from the Greek *xeno* meaning strange or foreign, and is used to describe a surgical procedure during which cells, tissues, or organs are transferred from one species to another, for example from pigs to humans. The transplanted material is often called a xenotransplant or a xenograft.

The concept of xenotransplantation is not new; the idea of using animal organs to replace damaged or diseased organs has been viewed as a potential approach to saving a human life for centuries. Until recently, however, it was a very remote possibility. The first documented accounts of transferring blood between humans and animals date to the 17th century. Although heroic in intent, these attempts were unsuccessful due to medicine's lack of understanding of the function of immune systems, including rejection. Later attempts to replace entire organs did not fare better, and over time the medical profession abandoned the idea of xeno-transplantation.

The first successful human-to-human transplants of kidney (1954), pancreas (1966), liver, and heart (1967) renewed the interest in xenotrans-plantation. Xenotransplantation studies mainly focused on the transfer of kidney, liver, and heart xenografts. Most of the recipients survived for only for a few days or weeks due to rejection of the xenografts by the recipients' immune systems, although the survival of one patient with a kidney xenograft for nine months indicated that xenotransplantation could be possible.[8] A significant advance in xenotransplantation came with the introduction of the immunosuppressant cyclosporine, a drug used to reduce the activity of the immune system, which decreased the risk of organ rejection. One of the most famous xenotransplantation procedures was the transfer of a baboon heart to a 12-day old newborn; the heart xenograft functioned for 20 days before it was rejected by the infant's immune system.[9]

Medicine was more successful in using acellular grafts from animals in humans. An acellular graft is a tissue, such as a heart valve, from which all live cells have been removed by chemical treatment to remove any material that could trigger immune rejection. Heart valves from pigs and cows have routinely been used as replacements for defective valves in human hearts since the 1960s. Valve replacement is now a relatively routine surgical procedure, and patients and their doctors may choose between pig, cow, and mechanical heart valves. A similar approach is used for making skin grafts from acellular matrices from pig skin, which are used as temporary covers to preserve sterility and to provide pain relief and protection from further damage in patients with severe burns or wounds who can not regrow their own skin. Although these procedures are not considered to be xenotransplantation because there are no cellular materials involved, their use paves the road for the future xenotransplantation procedures and demonstrates that animal products can be used as one of the tools to save human lives.

Animal organs are also used to maintain the physiologic function of patient's organs without going through a xenotransplantation procedure. The first successful extracorporeal (from the Latin *extra,* meaning outside, and *corporeus,* meaning body) procedures were carried out in the1960s, in which the blood of patients with liver failure was pumped through pig livers located outside of the patient's body. Although the patients' vital signs improved markedly, they later died because of the advanced stage of their disease. Nevertheless, these experiments showed that extracorporeal use of animal organs can successfully be used as a bridge to maintain the physiologic function of patient's organs until a suitable organ is available for transplantation. Since then, the bridging approach has been used successfully to stabilize a number of patients with liver failure. Patients who later on received a human-to-human liver transplant made a full recovery.[10] The bridging approach has also successfully extended to other organs such as the spleen.

The idea of bridging animal organs has led to the development of various bioartificial liver assisted systems (BLA). BLA systems may be described as bioreactors that contain metabolically active pig liver cells capable of maintaining regulatory and detoxification functions. A real advantage of these bridging systems is that they do not require a patient to commit to a complete xenotransplantation procedure. The whole procedure is minimally invasive and can be interrupted at any time in case of any adverse side effects. In preliminary studies, patients with liver failure that used BLA systems have made complete recoveries after receiving a human-to-human liver transplant.[11] Currently, a number of these systems are in clinical trials.

The use of animal cell grafts also found a successful application in the treatment of the Type I diabetes. Patients with Type I diabetes are unable to control the level of sugar in their blood because they do not produce enough insulin, a hormone essential for the regulation of the glucose uptake from blood and regulation of lipid metabolism. Islet cells found in the pancreas are responsible for insulin production; these cells are selectively destroyed by an autoimmune response in Type I diabetes. Replacing the destroyed cells has been a goal of many researchers. One new approach that has been used in some clinical trials uses pig islet cells that are protected from the host immune response by encapsulation in membranes that allow nutrients and insulin to flow to and from the cells, but keeps the cells isolated from large antibody molecules. Insulin produced by the pig islets only differs from human insulin by a single amino acid, and functions identically (prior to the approval of Humulin, most diabetics were treated with a mixture of porcine and beef insulin). This approach has been used successfully in recent clinical trials in several countries and may be developed as a commercial product in the near future.

But why would scientists choose pigs over other animals as a source of organs for xenotransplantation? Early on, a variety of different species were suggested as sources of organs. Although nonhuman primates were considered to be the most appropriate choice due to genetic, physiological, and immunological similarities with humans, they are not the best choice for several reasons. Xenografts from primates are still immunologically rejected by human hosts; their size is too small to provide adequate function in human hosts; and the use of the nonhuman primates raises serious concerns about the possibility of infectious disease transmission to human hosts. Because the primates are genetically very close to humans, there is a significant risk that primate viruses present in the xenografts may infect human organ recipients. The use of primates for xenotransplantation also poses profound ethical questions for some.

Although genetically more distant from humans than primates, pigs are considered a good compromise species. Because the physiology and size of pig organs are similar to those of humans, it is thought that they will be able to provide adequate substitutes for human cells, tissues, and organs. Pigs are sufficiently different from humans that infectious agents generally do not pass between the species. In addition, pigs are easy to breed, and could provide a steady source of organs. Although there are ethical concerns regarding the use of pigs as sources of materials for transplantation to humans, they tend not to be as profoundly felt as with nonhuman primates. Nonetheless, pigs still present a formidable immunorejection hurdle.

Genetically Engineered Animals as Sources of Xenotransplant Materials

Genetic engineering may be able to address one of the biggest hurdles in xenotransplantation—the rejection of animal organs by the human recipient's immune system. Rejection occurs when the recipient's immune system identifies the xenograft as foreign, or non-self and unleashes a complex series of defensive mechanisms against it.

The initial rejection response is triggered by the presence of antibodies that recognize foreign structures on the cell surface of the xenograft. These antibodies are primarily directed against sugar molecules (αGal carbohydrates) present on the surface of pig cells. These carbohydrates are synthesized by an enzyme (α-1,3-galactosyltransferase, αGalT)) present in all vertebrates except humans, apes, and Old World monkeys. Because humans do not synthesize these molecules, they produce antibodies against them, which then serve to trigger the initial rejection response that eventually leads to the destruction of the entire xenograft.

One of the proposed strategies to avoid xenograft rejection is the production of genetically engineered (GE) pigs that lack the enzyme that produces αGal carbohydrates to avoid initiating the rejection response. In fact, during the past decade, GE pigs lacking αGal carbohydrates have been developed and are beginning to be used in early xenotransplantation studies.[12] Although the use of αGal-deficient pigs helps to evade the initial rejection response, additional modifications may need to be made to help evade the additional responses that the human immune system recruits that lead to a gradual destruction of xenografts.

In addition to serving as a source of replacement organs, other products from GE animals have the potential to be used in medical applications. GE animals that are more immunocompatible with humans can

Figure 13.3
These sleeping (and one curious) genetically engineered piglets lack the aGal enzyme. Developing these pigs will contribute to our understanding of immune responses in transplantation and possibly a source of cells, tissues, and organs for xenotransplantation

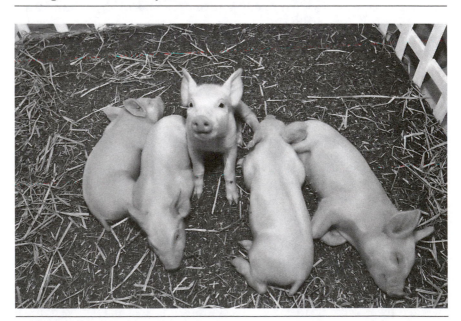

Source: Photo courtesy of Revivicor® Inc.

serve as sources of cells or tissues that can produce replacement proteins or other substances for individuals with hereditary metabolic disorders. For example, immunocompatible porcine islet cells could be infused into the pancreas of humans with Type I diabetes to provide insulin.

Xenotransplantation Concerns

Although human-to-human organ transplantations are relatively common nowadays, there are residual risks of infectious disease transmission between donors and recipients. Donor organs come from people with diverse medical histories, and though they are carefully screened, there is a possibility that cryptic (silent) viruses may slip through undetected. Xenotransplantation is thought to lessen this risk. Xenotransplantation does, however, raise potential concerns about the transmission of diseases present in the xenografts to human recipients, especially as immunosuppression will likely continue to be a part of the transplant protocol. Such viruses may mutate and spread into the larger human population. Any xenotransplantation study in humans would require approval from the FDA after rigorous review of the proposal to ensure safety and limit the potential for such concerns.

Animals and humans have lived side by side for thousands of years, and, in general, humans and animals do not share many diseases. There are, however, examples of viruses that do cross species boundaries such as the recent bird and swine flu epidemics. Much of the risk of these diseases, as well as otherwise silent porcine viruses, can be managed by raising the animals in controlled, biosecure conditions, and careful screening. Nonetheless, these are concerns that will need to be addressed if the field of xenotransplantation continues to show promise.

CONCLUSION

Human and animal lives have been closely intertwined for millennia. We have depended, and continue to depend, on animals for food, medicinal products, and comfort. Biotechnology has shown us that not only can we improve the lives of animals, but in doing so, we may improve our own lives as well. Nonetheless, these technologies must always be introduced and used carefully to ensure safety and to strengthen and improve the quality of both sides of the human-animal bond.

FURTHER READING

Committee on Xenograft Transplantation. Ethical issues and public policy. *Xenotransplantation: Science, ethics, and public policy.* Washington, DC: National Academy Press; 1996.

Cooper DKC, Lanza RP. *Xeno: The promise of transplanting animal organs into humans.* Oxford: Oxford University Press; 2000.

Fedoroff NV, Brown NM. *Mendel in the kitchen: A scientist's view of genetically modified foods.* Washington, DC: Joseph Henry Press; 2004.

Houdebine LM. *Animal transgenesis and cloning.* Hoboken, NJ: John Wiley and Sons; 2003.

Ronald PC, Adamchak RW. *Tomorrow's table: Organic farming, genetics and the future of food.* New York: Oxford University Press; 2008.

U.S. Food and Drug Administration Center for Veterinary Medicine. *Animal cloning and food safety.* Available at: http://www.fda.gov/ForConsumers/Con sumerUpdates/ucm148768.htm.

U.S. Food and Drug Administration Center for Veterinary Medicine. *Myths about cloning.* Available at: http://www.fda.gov/AnimalVeterinary/SafetyHealth/ AnimalCloning/ucm055512.htm.

U.S. Food and Drug Administration Center for Veterinary Medicine. *Regulation of genetically engineered animals.* Available at: http://www.fda.gov/ForConsum ers/ConsumerUpdates/ucm048106.htm.

Wheeler MB. Production of transgenic livestock: Promise fulfilled. *Journal of Animal Science* 2003;81:32–7.

REFERENCES

1. Wilmut I, Schnieke AE, McWhir J, et al. Viable offspring derived from fetal and adult mammalian cells. *Nature* 1997:385;810–13.

2. U.S. Food and Drug Administration Center for Veterinary Medicine. *Animal cloning: A risk assessment.* Available at: http://www.fda.gov/AnimalVeterinary/ SafetyHealth/AnimalCloning/ucm055489.htm.

3. U.S. Food and Drug Administration Center for Veterinary Medicine. *FDA approves orphan drug ATryn to treat rare clotting disorder.* Available at: http://www. fda.gov/NewsEvents/Newsroom/PressAnnouncements/2009/ucm109074.htm.

4. U.S. Department of Agriculture, Agricultural Research Service. *Scientists develop first transgenic cow clone for mastitis disease resistance.* Available at: http:// www.ars.usda.gov/is/pr/2001/010110.2.htm.

5. Richt JA, Kasinathan P, Hamir AN, et al. Production of cattle lacking prion protein. *Nature Biotechnology* 2007:25;132–8.

6. Lai L, Kang JX, Li R, et al. Generation of cloned transgenic pigs rich in omega-3 fatty acids. *Nature Biotechnology* 2006:24;435–6.

7. U.S. Food and Drug Administration Center for Veterinary Medicine. *Guidance for Industry 187: Regulation of genetically engineered animals containing heritable recombinant DNA constructs.* Available at: http://www.fda.gov/downloads/ AnimalVeterinary/GuidanceComplianceEnforcement/GuidanceforIndustry/ UCM113903.pdf.

8. Starzl TE, Marchioro TL, Peters GN, et al. Renal heterotransplantation from baboon to man: Experience with 6 cases. *Transplantation* 1964:2;752–76.

9. Bailey LL, Nehlsen-Cannarella SL, Concepcion W, Jolley WB. Baboon-to-human cardiac xenotransplantation in a neonate. *Journal of the American Medical Association* 1985:254;3321–9.

10. Chari RS, Collins BH, Magee JC, et al. Brief report: Treatment of hepatic failure with ex vivo pig-liver perfusion followed by liver transplantation. *New England Journal of Medicine* 1994:331;234–7.

11. Rozga J, Podesta L, Lepage E, et al. A bioartificial liver to treat severe acute liver failure. *Annals of Surgery* 1994:219;538–46.

12. Bas-Bernardet SL, Anegon J, Blancho G. Progress and prospects: Genetic engineering in xenotransplantation. *Gene Therapy* 2008:15;1247–56.

Index

Abortion, spontaneous: and *Brucella* infection, 131; and *Chlamydophila abortus,* 130

Abuse, 65

Acellular grafts, 255

Acquired immunity, 120–21

Acquired immunodeficiency syndrome (AIDS), 72; and zoonoses, 126–27

Adenovirus-2, 159

Aedes mosquitoes: and Rift Valley fever, 89; and yellow fever, 82

Africa: cholera epidemic, 77; Ebola and Marburg viruses, 91; monkeypox in, 87–88, 107, 192; plague cases, 79; Rift Valley fever in, 89; and rinderpest, 228; simian retroviruses in, 111; and SIV-infected chimpanzees, 109; yellow fever in, 82

African buffaloes (*Syncerus caffer*), 101

African dwarf frogs, and salmonella, 122

African frogs, 112

African pygmy hedgehogs, 112; as pets, 181; and salmonella, 188

African rodents, and monkeypox virus, 88, 107

African spurred tortoise (*Geochelone pardalis*), 113

African wild cats, cloning technology, 243

Aggression, types of in dogs, 37–38

Agronomic traits, and genetic engineering, 248

Ahimsa House Safe Havens Directory, 67

AIDS. *See* Acquired immunodeficiency syndrome

Alabama, lymphocytic choriomeningitis epidemic (1973–1974), 191

Allergens, 3, 4; and antibodies, 8

Allergies: defined, 2–3; and hypersensitivity, 2–3; and pets, 1–12; to small mammals, 198

Allergy testing, 8–9

Alligators, and viral encephalomyelitides, 213

α-1,3-galactosyltransferase (αGalT), 257

α-Gal carbohydrates, 257, 258

Alveolitis, allergic, 6

Amblyomma tick, 113

American Humane Association: "The Link," 51; Pets and Women's Shelters Listing, 67

American Humane Society, 66
American Kennel Club (AKC), 19, 31
American Medical Association, and One Health, 223
American pit bull terrier, 58
American Plague of 1793–1798 (yellow fever), 81–82
American Society for the Prevention of Cruelty to Animals (ASPCA), 54, 67; and dogfighting, 40
American Veterinary Medical Association (AVMA): and One Health, 222, 223; pet therapy guidelines of, 14; on rabies vaccine, 48; Task Force on Canine Aggression and Human-Canine Interactions, 39
Amphibians: and *Coxiella burnetti*, 172; and salmonella, 122–23, 154; and viral encephalomyelitides, 213
Amphotericin B, 211
Anaphylactic reactions, 198
Ancylostoma braziliense, 146–47
Ancylostoma caninum, 146
Ancylostoma duodenale, 146
Animal abuse: history of and definition, 52, 54, 55–56; and human violence, 51–52, 53; recognizing, 57–58; reporting, 59–61. *See also* Bestiality
Animal and Plant Health Inspection Service (APHIS), 43
Animal-assisted activities (AAA), 15, 225
Animal-assisted intervention (AAI), 15, 17, 21–24; guidelines for visits to health-care settings, 20–29; and infection control, 16; laws and regulations for, 20; and mental illness, 18; programs, 19–20; and service animals, 16
Animal-assisted therapy (AAT), 15, 223–24
Animal biotechnology, 240
Animal bites, costs of, 35
Animal cloning: and food safety, 246; limitations on, 245–46; potential applications of, 242–43

Animal cruelty, 51; history and definitions of, 54–55; investigation and prosecution of, 62–63. *See also* Bestiality
Animal exhibits, and illnesses, 125
Animal Fighting Prohibition Enforcement Act (2007), 40
Animal handlers: and animal-assisted intervention, 24–25; and therapy animals, 21, 22
Animal hoarding, 57
Animal influenza viruses, 77
Animal Legal Defense Fund, 67
Animal neglect, 55–56
Animals, and One Health, 222
Animals, genetically engineered, 246–54; regulation of, 253; and xenotransplant material, 257–59
Animals, transgenic, 250
Animals and Society Institute, 66
Animals Asia Foundation, 111
Animal shelters, and One Health, 225–26
Animal Welfare Act, 43
Anthrax, 75–76
Antibiotic contamination, 233–34
antibiotic-resistant genes (ARGs), 233–34
Antibiotics, and bacteria resistance, 232–33
Antibodies, 121, 177; and allergens, 2, 8; and plague, 170; in pregnant women, 127; and xenografts, 257–58
Antigens, 2
Antihistamines, 9
Antimicrobial-resistant infections, 82
Antithrombin deficiency, 253
Anxiety, and pet therapy, 17
Apes, Great, 44, 46
Aquaculture, and antibiotic contamination, 233
Arboviruses, 92–93, 94
Arenavirus, 189
Argentina, *Histoplasma* in, 210
Arthropod parasites, and lymphocytic choriomeningitis virus, 191

Arthropod vectors, and viral encepha-
lomyelitides, 213
Artificial insemination (AI), 240–41
Asexual reproduction, 242
Asia: and H1N1 influenza, 108; and
H5N1 virus, 212; and hantavirus,
193; and live reptile trade, 111;
SARS outbreak in, 113; simian retro-
viruses in, 111
Asian long-horned beetle, 232
Assisted reproductive technologies
(ARTs), 240–41, 246–47
Association for Professionals in Infec-
tion Control and Epidemiology
(APIC), pet therapy guidelines,
14
Asthma, and pet allergies, 5, 9
Athens, Greece, 222
Atopy, 2
ATryn, 253
Audubon Nature Institute, 243
Aurochs, 247; domestication of, 240
Australia: and Hendra virus, 86; and
Q fever, 172
Avian illness. *See* Zoonoses: from pet
birds
Avian influenza virus (H5N1), 79, 104,
108–9, 189, 203, 211–13, 229
Avian medicine, 203
Avian tuberculosis, 209–10
Aviaries, maintenance of, 204, 206

Baboons, 46
Bacillary angiomatosis, 163
Bacillus anthracis, 75
Bacterial zoonoses, and birds, 206–10
Badgers, and plague, 170
Bait animals, 40
Banded mongooses, 101
Bangladesh, Nipah virus in, 88
Banteng clones, 244
Bartonella henselae, 162, 163, 164
Bartonellosis, 162–63
Batrachochytrium dendrobatidis, 112
Bats: bans on, 115; and rabies, 140,
142, 227; and SARS, 107; in wildlife
trade, 107; as zoonoses hosts, 107
Battered victims, 65

Baylisascaris, 84–85, 196
Baylisascaris porcinis, 84
Baylisascaris proecyonis, 195
B cells, 121; in pregnant women, 127
Bedlington terrier, 4
Belgium, and illegal bird trade, 108,
110
Bell's hingeback tortoise (*Kinixys bel-
liana*), 113
Benzyl benzoate, and pet allergies,
10
Bergh, Henry, 54
Berkowitz, David, 53
Bestiality, 56
Beta-lactams, 83
Bichon frise, 4
Bioartificial liver assisted (BLA) sys-
tems, 256
Biocontainment, 204
Biodiversity, and invasive species,
230–31
Biopharming, 247–48
Biosecurity, 94, 204
Biotechnology, 240; concerns about,
253–54
Biotechnology, modern. *See* Recombi-
nant DNA (rDNA) technology
Bioterrorism, 94; and anthrax, 75
Biphasic fever, 190
Bird flu. *See* Avian influenza virus
(H5N1)
Birds, 181; and allergies, 3, 6; and
avian tuberculosis, 209–10;
and bacterial zoonoses, 206–10;
and *Campylobacter*, 153; and children, 124; and *Coxiella burnetti*, 172;
and fungal zoonoses, 210–11; and
giardiasis, 215; health and illness
basics, 202–3; and influenza
viruses, 108; and parasitic zoonoses, 214–15; pet birds, 201; and red
fowl mites, 214–15; and *Salmonella*,
112, 154, 208; trade in, 103; and viral
encephalomyelitides, 213; and viral
zoonoses in, 211–14; and West Nile
virus, 92; and zoonoses, 201–16
Birthing fluids: and *Brucella*, 130; and
Coxiella burnetii, 129–30, 172–73

Black Death (1347–1400), 79, 170
Blood clotting, and antithrombin, 253
Blood tests, for pet allergies, 8–9
Bluegrass, 231
Bobcats, and plague, 170
Bordetella bronchiseptica, 159, 187
Borelia burgdorferi, 87, 132, 187
Bovine spongiform encephalopathy (BSE), 90, 94; losses from 2003 outbreak, 231; and resistant cattle, 251, 252;
Bovine tuberculosis, 101
Brain damage, from rabies, 140, 143
Breathing difficulties, and pet allergies, 5, 6, 7, 9
Breeding aviaries, 204, 206
Breed-specific legislation, and dog attacks, 39–40
Brucella canis, 130–31, 157
Brucellosis, 101, 125, 157
Brushtail porcupines, 107
Brushtail possums, 115
Buboes, 80, 94, 171, 185
Bubonic plague, 80, 171, 185
Buffalo: African, 101; swamp, 244
Bundy, Ted, 53
Bushmeat: smuggling of, 116; and STLV, 110; trade in, 103–4, 109

Camel clones, 244
Cameroon: HTLV and STLV in, 110; SIV in, 109
Campylobacter (multiple species), 124, 187; fluoroquinolone-resistant, 82–83; and Q fever, 172; and zebra mussel, 231
Campylobacter coli, 82, 153
Campylobacteriosis, 153, 187
Campylobacter jejeuni, 82, 153, 208–9
Canada: Q fever in, 172; and zebra mussel, 231
Cancer patients, and pet therapy, 17
Canine adenovirus-2, 159
Canine distemper virus, 159, 231
Canine Good Citizen (CGC) Program, 19–20, 31
Canine parvovirus, 159

Canine rabies virus, 141, 142
Capnocytophaga canimorsus, 34, 41–42
Capuchins, 46
Cardiac disease, and pet therapy, 17
Carneal, Michael, 53
Carnivores, and plague, 79–80
Carp, 112
Carpets, and pet allergies, 10
Caseous lymphadenitis, 184
Cat food, and human salmonellosis, 134
Cat scratch disease (CSD), 162–63
Cats, 161; African wild, 243; and allergies, 3, 4; as animal-assisted intervention animals, 23; and bartonellosis, 162–63; bites, 34, 168–69; clones, 244, 245; and *Coxiella burnetii,* 129, 172, 173; dermatophyte infections in, 167–68; domestication of, 239; and hookworm, 146, 147; and human asthma attacks, 5; large, 43–44; and *Pasteurella multocida,* 168–69; litter boxes, 4; and plague, 80, 170, 171, 172, 185; and prevention guidelines, 176–77; and rabies, 143, 173–75, 227, 228; and ringworm, 156; roundworms in, 144; and *Salmonella,* 133; and *Toxoplasma gondii,* 127–29; and toxoplasmosis, 163–66; and tularemia, 176; and viral encephalomyelitides, 213; zoonoses from, 161–77
Cattle: and bovine spongiform encephalopathy, 90, 251, 252; and bovine tuberculosis, 101; and cloning, 244, 245; and *Coxiella burnetii,* 129, 172; and cryptosporidia, 155, 194; domestication of, 240; and *E. coli,* 86; and *Escherichia coli* 0157:H7 infection, 158; and genetic engineering, 247, 251, 252; and *Leptospira,* 131, 149, 150; and rabies, 227; and rinderpest, 228; and somatic cell nuclear transfer (SCNT), 242; twins of, 242. *See also* Dairy cattle
C-BARQ (Canine Behavioral and Research Questionnaire), 22, 31

CD4+ T cells, 126; in pregnant women, 127

CD8+ T cells, in pregnant women, 127

Centers for Disease Control and Prevention (CDC), 31; ban on African rodents, 107; on H1N1, 105; pet therapy guidelines of, 14; *Salmonella* prevention, 123; on tularemia, 184; wildlife regulation, 114, 115

Cercopithecine herpesvirus, 1. *See* Macacine herpesvirus-1

Cestodiasis, 195

Challenge (provocation) testing, and pet allergies, 9

Chest tightness and pain, and pet allergies, 5, 6

Cheyletiella mites, 176, 196

Cheyletiella parasitovorax, 195, 196

Cheyletiellosis, 195

Chickens, 211; and campylobacteriosis, 153; domestication of, 240; and red fowl mites, 215; and *Salmonella*, 133, 188, 208

Chigger bites, and typhus, 186

Child abuse: and animal abuse, 53; defined, 65

Child-care settings, and animals, 125

Children: and age of pet exposure, 3; and animal-assisted activities, 225; and animal cruelty, 52, 53–54; and dog bites, 34, 35; and pet allergies, 6; and pet therapy, 14; and pets in classrooms, 124–25; and reptiles and amphibians, 122–23; and wolf hybrids, 48; and zoonoses, 122

Children's hospitals, and pet therapy, 15

Chimpanzees, and HIV-1, 109

China: and cryptosporidia, 194; domestication of dogs in, 239; H5N1 virus in, 212; SARS in, 90, 107, 110; turtle consumption in, 111; and wildlife exports to U.S., 114

Chinchillas: and bacterial zoonoses, 187; as pets, 181, 182

Chinese crested dog, 4

Chinese horseshoe bats, and SARS, 90

Chinese medicine, animals harvested for, 104

Chipmunks: as pets, 181; and plague, 170, 185

Chlamydophila abortus, 130

Chlamydophila felis, 176

Chlamydophila psittaci, 124, 206–7

Chlamydosis, 125

Cholera, 76–77

Chytrid fungus, 112

Chytridiomycosis, 112

CITES. *See* Convention on International Trade in Endangered Species of Wild Fauna and Flora

Civets, bans on, 115

Climate change, 234

Cloning, 246–47; animals, 241–46

Clostridium difficile, 29, 30

Clostridium piliforme, 187

Cockatiels: and giardiasis, 215; and psittacois, 206

Cockatoos, and psittacois, 206

Cockfighting, 40

Cockroaches, and mold and allergies, 7

Colibacillosis, 202

Collies, 158

Colorado, and bans on pit bull–type dogs, 40

Colorado Bar Association, 68

Companion animals, 181; and genetic engineering, 249

Conjunctivitis, *Chlamydophilia felis*, 176

Constructs, 249–50

Convention on International Trade in Endangered Species of Wild Fauna and Flora (CITES; 1973), 103, 104, 114

Coqui, as invasive species, 232

Coronaviruses, 107; SARS, 90, 107

Corvids, and West Nile virus, 214

Corynebacterium kutscheri, 187

Cow clones, 244

Coxiella burnetii, 125, 129–30, 164, 172

Coxsackie's virus, 132

Coyotes: and plague, 170; and rabies, 228; and tuberculosis, 227

Crimean-Congo hemorrhagic fever, 92
Criminals, and rehabilitation with
    animals, 225
Crows, 211; and West Nile virus, 214
Cryptococcosis, 126
Cryptococcus, 210–11
Cryptococcus gatti, 85–86, 210
Cryptococcus neoformans var. *neofor-*
    mans, 210
Cryptosporidia, 193–94
Cryptosporidiosis, 126, 155–56,
    193–94, 195
Cryptosporidium, 124, 125, 155
Cryptosporidium canis, 155
Crytosporidium parvum, 193, 195
Culex mosquito, West Nile virus, 92
Culture, 177
Customs and Border Protection, 116
Customs and Border Protection Agri-
    culture Specialists, 116
Cutaneous infections, anthrax, 76
Cutaneous larva migrans, 147–48, 175
Cyclosporine, 255

Dahmer, Jeffrey, 53
Dairy cattle: mastitis-resistant, 251;
    and tuberculosis, 227
Dairy products, and *Brucella,* 130–31
Dander, 1; and allergies, 3, 9, 10, 11;
    and dog breeds, 4
Day-care centers, and *Giardia* out-
    breaks, 152
Deaths: causes of in humans (1900),
    220; causes of in humans (2030),
    221; from dog bites, 35
Decongestants, for pet allergies, 9
Deer: clones of, 244; and *Ixodes* ticks,
    87
Deer fly fever. *See* Tularemia
Deer mouse: and hantavirus, 193; and
    Sin Nombre virus, 91
Deforestation, and disease transmis-
    sion, 102
Degus, as pets, 181, 182
Delta Society Pet Partner Program,
    19, 31
Dementia, and pet therapy, 18
Dengue fever, 92

Denver, Colorado, and bans on pit
    bull–type dogs, 40
Department of Homeland Security,
    116
Depression: and animal-assisted
    activities, 225; and pet therapy, 17
Dermanyssus gallinae, 214–15
Dermatitis, allergic, 5
Dermatophyte infection, 197
Dermatophytosis, 166–68
DeSalvo, Albert, 53
Diabetes, Type I, and cell grafts, 256,
    259
Diarrheal diseases: campylobacte-
    riosis, 153; cryptosporidiosis, 155;
    giardiasis, 152–53; salmonellosis,
    153–55
Dipylidium caninum, and cats, 175
Disease ecology, 102
Disease reservoirs, humans as for
    wildlife, 101
Disease resistance, and genetic engi-
    neering, 248
Diseases: emerging, 72–93, 221; his-
    torical, and reemergence of, 75–82
Disease transmission (exchange):
    across species, 105; from livestock
    to wildlife, 101; preventing, from
    birds to humans, 203–6; from wild-
    life to humans, 100–101
disseminated intravascular coagula-
    tion (DIC), 41
Distemper, 159, 231
DNA. *See* Recombinant DNA (rDNA)
    technology
Dog aggression, 37
Dog bites, 33, 34–43, 169; causes of,
    36–38; diseases from, 41–43; inju-
    ries from, 34–36; laws concerning,
    39; prevention of, 38–39; and
    rabies, 141; treatment for, 36; warn-
    ing signs of, 37
Dog breeds, and bites by, 35–36
Dog fighting, 40, 58; in Chicago, 61
Dog food, and human salmonellosis,
    134
Dogo Argentinos, 40, 58
Dog rabies vaccination programs, 140

Dogs: and allergies, 3, 4; animal-assisted intervention animals, 23; breeds and allergens, 4; and breed-specific legislation, 39–40; and *Brucella canis,* 157; and campylobacteriosis, 153; clones of, 244; and *Cryptosporidium,* 155–56; dermatophyte infections in, 167–68; domestication of, 239; and *Giardia* infections, 152; health benefits of for owners, 139–40; and hookworm, 146–47; and *Leptospira,* 149, 150–51; and leptospirosis, 131; and methicillin-resistant *Staphylococcus aureus* infection, 157; with nonshedding coats, 4; and pet therapy, 14, 17; and plague, 79–80, 170; and prevention of disease transmission, 159; and rabies, 140–44, 174, 227–28; and ringworm, 156; and roundworm, 144–46; and *Salmonella,* 133, 154, 155; and scabies, 158; short-haired, and allergies, 3–4; and tuberculosis, 158–59; and wolf-dog hybrids, 47–48; zoonoses from, 139–59. *See also* Therapy dog
Dolly the sheep, 240, 244
Domestic abuse/violence, 65
Domestic animals, and wildlife, 100
Domestic violence, and animal abuse, 52
Dormice, 106, 107
Drapes and curtains, and pet allergies, 11
Droppings, bird, and allergies, 3
Ducks, and avian influenza, 211
Dumb rabies, 142; in cats, 174
Dwarf tapeworm, 194

East Africa, *Histoplasma* in, 210
Eastern equine encephalitis (EEE), 93, 213, 214
Ebola-Reston virus, 91
Ebola virus, 91
Ecology, and One Health, 230–34
Ecosystems: alteration of, 101–2; and invasive species, 230–31
Edema, 94; and anthrax, 76

Eden Alternative homes, 20, 31
Education, and prevention of animal cruelty, 63–64
Eggs: and biopharming, 247; and *Salmonella,* 134
Elder abuse, 65
Elderly: and dog bites, 34; and pet therapy, 14, 18; immunosenescence and animals, 132–33
Embryo splitting, 241
Embryo transfer, 241
Emerging diseases, 72–93, 221; and wildlife trade, 105
Encephalitis, 94
Encephalitozooan cuniculi (EC), 195, 197
Encephalitozoonosis, 195
Endangered populations, conservation agreement (1973), 103
Endangered species, and Frozen Zoo, 243
Endangered Species Act, 114
Endocarditis, 177; in cats, 162; and *Pasteurella multocida,* 169
Environment, and One Health, 222, 230–34
Epidemic: cholera, 76–77; defined, 94; typhus, 186
Equine animals, 181
Equine influenza (H1N1), 189
Erysipeloid, 202
Erythema migrans, 87, 94
Eschars, 94; and anthrax, 76
Escherichia coli, 29; in petting zoos, 125; and stillbirths, 132
Escherichia coli 0157:H7 infection, 86, 124, 157–58
Europe: and hantavirus, 193; and rinderpest, 228
Exotic pets, 33, 43–45; and salmonellosis, 188
Exotic small mammal specialist, 182
Extensively drug-resistant tuberculosis (XDR-TB), 81
Extracorporeal procedures, 256
Eyes, and ocular larva migrans, 145

Feathers, and allergies, 3
Fel d 1 protein, 4

Fennec foxes, 181
Ferrets: and bacterial zoonoses, 187; and children, 124; clones of, 244; and influenza, 188; parasitic zoonoses from, 195; as pets, 181; and rabies vaccination, 143; and salmonella, 188; and viral zoonoses, 189
Fila Brasileiros, 40, 58
Fish: and GloFish, 252; omega-3 fatty acids in, 251; trade in, 103
Fish diseases, and wildlife trade, 112
Flaviviruses, 213, 214
Fleas: and animal-assisted intervention animals, 23; and bacterial zoonoses, 187; and *Bartonella*, 162, 163; from cats to humans, 176; and plague, 79, 170, 185, 186; and typhus, 186
Flora, 177
Florida: Class I wildlife regulations, 43; and invasive plants, 232
Florida State University Institute for Family Violence Studies, 67
Flu. *See* Influenza
Flu season, 188
Flu viruses, and genetic engineering, 248
Fluoroquinolone-resistant *Campylobacter* species, 82–83
Fluoroquinolones, 83
Flying foxes. *See* Fruit bats
Flying squirrel, and typhus, 186
Fomites, 94
Food and Agriculture Organization: and One Health, 223, 236; and rinderpest eradication, 228–29
Food animals, 181
Food production, and clones, 243
Food security, and genetic engineering, 246, 248
Foot-and-mouth disease, 112–13, 115; and disease-resistant animals, 248; in United Kingdom, 232
Fowl red mite. See *Dermanyssus gallinae*
Fowl typhoid. *See* Salmonellosis
Foxes: parasitic zoonoses from, 195; and rabies, 125, 140, 227, 228

Francisella tularensis, 176, 183, 187
Frogs: African, 112; and salmonella, 110, 122
Frozen Zoo, 243
Fruit bats (flying foxes): Hendra virus, 86; Nipah virus, 88
Fungal meningitis, 210
Fungal zoonoses: in birds, 210–11; ringworm, 197–98
Fur. *See* Dander
Furious rabies, 141, 142; in cats, 174

Gambian giant pouched rat, 106, 107; and monkeypox, 192; and viral zoonoses, 189
Gastrointestinal anthrax, 76
Gastrointestinal tract, and immune system, 120
Gaur clones, 244
Geese, and avian influenza, 211
Gene therapy, 250
Genetic engineering, 246–54; regulation of technology, 253
Georgia, dog bite prevention, 39
Gerbils, 4, 181
Ghana, and monkeypox virus, 105
Giardia (multiple species), 195
Giardia intestinalis, 152
Giardia lamblia, 215
Giardiasis, 152–53, 195, 215
Global health threats, 104
Global public health, 220–21
GloFish, 252
Goats: antithrombin production in, 253; clones of, 244; and *Coxiella burnetii*, 129, 172; domestication of, 239–40; genetically engineered, 250, 253; and Orf virus, 125
Golden, Andrew, 53
Gray squirrels, *Ixodes* ticks on, 87
Gray wolf, clones of, 244
Great Apes, 44, 46
Great Lakes, and zebra mussel, 231
Great Plague of London (1665), 170
Green monkeys, 109
Ground squirrels, and bacterial zoonoses, 187

Guangdong Province, China, SARS
    in, 107
Guillain-Barré disease, 153
Guinea pigs, 4; and bacterial zoo-
    noses, 187; and lymphocytic cho-
    riomeningitis virus, 132; parasitic
    zoonoses from, 195; as pets, 181,
    182; and plague, 185; and *Strepto-
    baccilus*, 184; and Trixacarus mites,
    195; and viral zoonoses, 189

H1N1 influenza, 212, 229; outbreak of
    1920, 188; pandemic of 2009, 77, 79,
    104–5
H3N2 virus, 212
H5N1 influenza (bird flu). *See* Avian
    influenza virus
H7N3 virus, 212
H7N3/02 virus, 189
H9N2 virus, 212
Hahn, Dr. Beatrice, 109
Hair. *See* Dander
Hamburger, and *E. coli,* 86
Hamsters, 4; and bacterial zoonoses,
    187; and children, 124; and crypto-
    sporidia, 194; and hymenolepiasis,
    195; and lymphocytic choriomen-
    ingitis virus, 132, 190, 191; as pets,
    181; and viral zoonoses, 189
Hand hygiene, and infection control,
    15
Hand sanitizers, and animal-assisted
    intervention visits, 23
Hand washing: and animal-assisted
    intervention visits, 23; and pet aller-
    gies, 11; with pet birds, 204
Hantavirus, 189, 193
Hantavirus pulmonary syndrome
    (HPS), 91–92, 189, 193
Hares: and bacterial zoonoses, 187;
    and plague, 185
Harris, Eric, 53
Hawaii, and human leptospirosis, 149
Hawk eagles, 108; and H5N1 avian
    flu, 231
Healing, and pet therapy, 17
Healthcare Infection Control Practices
    Advisory Committee, 84

Health-care settings: defined, 15;
    guidelines for animal-assisted inter-
    vention visits, 20–29; and infection
    control, 16; MRSA infections in, 84;
    pets in, 13–31; potential zoonoses
    in, 29–30
Heart xenografts, 255
Heartwater, 113, 115
Hedgehog hives, 198
Hedgehogs, 115; and bacterial zoo-
    noses, 187; parasitic zoonoses
    from, 195. *See also* African pygmy
    hedgehogs
Heliobacter (multiple species),
    187
Hemagglutinin (H), 77
Hemolytic uremic syndrome (HUS),
    86, 94
Hemorrhagic fever with renal syn-
    drome (HFRS), 193
Hendra, Australia, 86
Hendra virus, 86–87, 107
Henipaviruses, 107
HEPA (high energy efficiency particu-
    late air) filters, 10
Heritable constructs, 249–50
Herodotus, 222
Herpes, 189
Herpes B virus, 46–47
Herpes Simplex I, 189
Histamines, 3
Histoplasma capsulatum, 210
Histoplasmosis, 210–11
HIV. *See* Human immunodeficiency
    virus
HIV-1, 109
HIV-2, 109
Hives: and pet allergies, 5, 6; hedge-
    hog, 198
Hoarding of animals, 65
Hoarding of Animals Research Con-
    sortium (HARC), 57, 67
Hogarth, Thomas, 51
Homeland Security, Department of,
    116
Homing pigeons, 211
Hong Kong, wildlife exports to U.S.,
    114

Hookworm: and cats, 175; infections, 146–48
Horses: and allergens, 4; clones of, 244; and Hendra virus, 86; and Leptospirosis, 131; and togavirus infection, 213; and West Nile virus, 92
Host, 94
HTLV-1, 2, 3, and 4, 110
Human-animal bond, 1, 54, 198, 223; and genetic engineering, 249
Humane Society of the United States, 66; First Strike Campaign, 68
Humane Society University, 63
Human health, and benefits of animals, 16–19
Human immunodeficiency viruses (HIV), 72, 73, 109; and cryptosporidiosis, 155; and tuberculosis co-infection, 81; and zoonoses, 126
Humans: and avian influenza, 212; and *Baylisascaris,* 196; and cat rabies, 174–75; and cryptococcosis and histoplasmosis, 210; and giardiasis, 215; and influenza, 212; and lymphocytic choriomeningitis virus, 190, 191; and monkeypox, 192; and *Mycobacterium* infection, 209; and One Health, 222; and plague, 170–72, 185; and psittacosis, 207; and Q fever, 173; and red fowl mites, 215; and togavirus infection, 213–14; and West Nile virus, 213–14
Human salmonellosis, 134, 208
Human scabies, 158
Human T-lymphotropic virus (HTLV), 110
Human tularemia, 176
Human-wildlife interface, 100–101
Humoral immune response, 121
Humulin, 246
Hunters, and tularemia, 183, 184
Hunting, 102
Hyacinth macaw, 211
Hydrophobia, 43, 143
Hymenolepiasis, 194–95
Hymenolepsis nana, 194, 195
Hypersensitivity, and allergies, 2–3

Hypertension, and pet therapy, 17
Hyposensitization, and pet allergies, 10

IgA antibodies, 2
IgD antigens, 2
IgE antibodies, 2, 9
IgG antibodies, 2
IgM antibodies, 2
Iguanas, and salmonella, 112
Immune response, and allergies, 2
Immune system, human, 120–21; in pregnant women, 127; and xenografts, 255
Immunity, acquired, 120–21
Immunocompromised people, 121–22, 203–4; and cats, 163, 168, 177; and cryptococcosis and histoplasmosis, 210–11; and cryptosporidiosis, 193–94; and immunodeficiency viruses, 109; and microsporidiosis, 197; and *Pasteurella multocida,* 169; and rodents, 132; and *Salmonella,* 133; and zoonotic disease prevention, 135–37; and zoonotic infections, 122
Immunoglobulins. *See* Antibodies
Incidence, 94
Incubation, 94
Incubation period, 177
India: Kyanasur forest disease, 102; parakeets from, 110; and rinderpest, 228, 229
Indonesia, and H1N1 influenza, 108
Infants, and dog bites, 35
Infection control: and hand hygiene, 15; in health-care settings, 16
Infection preventionists, 16; and animal-assisted intervention, 19, 23
Infections: antimicrobial-resistant, 82; opportunistic, 126
Infectious diseases, 71–72; emerging, 72–93; historical, and reemergence of, 75–82; and wildlife trade, 104–13
Influenza, 77–79; and One Health efforts, 229–30; seasonal, 212

Influenza A and B viruses, 188–89, 211–12

Influenza pandemics, 77–78, 79, 104–5

Influenza viruses: H1N1, 77, 79, 104–5, 188, 212, 229; H3N2, 212; H7N3, 212; N3/02, 189; H9N2 virus, 212. *See also* Avian influenza virus (H5N1)

Inhalation anthrax, 76

Institute of Medicine (IOM) of the National Academy of Sciences, 94; on emerging infections, 72–73; on zoonotic diseases, 73–75

Insulin: from animals, 256–57, 259; recombinant, 246

Intestinal parasites, 144–48

Introduced species, 230

Invasive species, 230–32; and bovine spongiform encephalopathy, 231

In vitro fertilization, 240, 241

Iowa: salmonellosis outbreak (2010), 208; school and child-care settings animal restrictions, 124–25

Irish water spaniel, 4

Isolation, 204

Ivermectin, 215

Ixodes ticks, and Lyme disease, 87

Japan: and hantavirus, 193; and rat bite fever, 183

Japanese encephalitis, 92

Jays, and West Nile virus, 214

John F. Kennedy Airport, 116

Joint Commission on Accreditation of Healthcare Organizations (JCAHO), 20

Justinian's Plague, 170

Kahn, Laura H., 222

Kaplan, Bruce, 222

Kennel cough. See *Bordetella bronchiseptica*

Kenya, Rift Valley fever in, 89

Kerry blue terrier, 4

Keusch, Dr. Gerald T., 93

Kinkel, Kip, 53

Kinsey, Alfred, 56

Kittens: and *Coxiella burnetti,* 172, 173; and dermatophytosis, 167, 168; and *Pasteurella multocida,* 169; and *Toxoplasma,* 166

Klebold, Dylan, 53

Knockout (or knockdown) traits, 249

Koi herpes virus, 112

Komodo dragon, 123

Korea, and hantavirus, 193

Kruger National Park, South Africa, 101

Kyanasur forest disease, 102

Lacey Act, 114

LaCrosse encephalitis, 92

Lagomorphs: and bacterial zoonoses, 187; and *Francisella,* 183; and plague, 185

Lameness, and rabid cats, 174

Large cats, 43–44

Large offspring syndrome, 245

Larva, 94

Lassa fever,92

Latham Foundation, 67

Law, James, 223

Law enforcement, and animal cruelty cases, 62–63

Law Enforcement Management Information System (LEMIS), 114

Law Enforcement Training Institute, 63

Lentaviruses, 109

Leopard tortoise (*Geochelone pardalis*), 113

Leptospira, 187; species and subspecies, 149

Leptospira interrogans, 131

Leptospira serovars, 151

Leptospira vaccines, 151

Leptospirosis, 125, 131, 148–51, 183, 186, 187

Levinson, Dr. Boris, 14

Lice, and typhus, 186

"Link, The," 51, 53, 65

Liponyssus bacoti, 195

Listeria monocytogenes, 127, 129, 187

Listeriosis, 125, 129, 187

Litter boxes: and cat zoonoses transmission, 177; and *Toxoplasma*, 165, 166

Liver failure, and extracorporeal procedures, 256

Livestock: disease transmission from, 101; and foot-and-mouth disease, 112–13; and leptospirosis, 183; and *Pasteurella*, 42; and Rift Valley fever, 89; and tuberculosis, 227; as wealth measure, 228

Livestock-birthing exhibits, 125

Lizards, U.S. import of, 112

Long-term care facilities: and pet therapy, 14, 15, 18; and scabies, 158

Lories, and *Salmonella* infection, 208

Los Angeles, wildlife imports, 114

Louisiana, iguana regulation, 112

Lyme, Connecticut, 87

Lyme disease, 87, 132, 187

Lymph nodes, 177

Lymphocytic choriomeningitis (LCM), 189, 190; epidemic (1973–1974), 191

Lymphocytic choriomeningitis virus (LCMV), 131–32, 189–92

Lysostaphin, 251

Lyssavirus, 189

Macacine herpesvirus-1, 46–47

Macaques, and diseases, 46–47

Macrophages, 120

Madagascar hissing cockroach, 7

Mad-cow disease. *See* Bovine spongiform encephalopathy

Mail carriers, and dog bites, 34

Malaria, 132; deforestation and epidemics of, 102

Malaysia, Nipah virus in, 88

Maltese, 4

Mammals: and *Campylobacter*, 153; and *Salmonella* bacteria, 154. *See also* Small mammals

Mangabeys, sooty, 109

Manure, and antibiotic contamination, 233

Marburg virus, 91

Marmosets, 46

Masked palm civet (*Paguna larvata*), 107

Mastitis, 251

Maui, Hawaii, and miconia, 232

Mead, Margaret, 53

Meat practices, in ancient times, 222

Medical substances, and biopharming, 247–48

Medicine: human and veterinary connectedness, 222–23; and pet therapy, 19; from wildlife species, 102–3

Medicines, Mental illness, and pet ownership and therapy, 18

Methicillin-resistant *Staphylococcus aureus* (MRSA), 29–30, 83–84, 156–57; community-acquired, 83

Metronidazole, 215

Mexico, bird smuggling to U.S., 115

Miami, wildlife imports, 114

Mice: and allergens, 4; and bacterial zoonoses, 187; and children, 124; clones of, 244; genetically engineered, 250; house, and lymphocytic choriomeningitis virus, 131–32; and *Ixodes* ticks, 87; parasitic zoonoses from; as pets, 181; and pinworms, 183; and plague, 185; striped, 107; and viral zoonoses, 189

Michigan, and deer tuberculosis, 226–27

Miconia calvescens, 231–32

Microimmunofluorescence (MIF), 206

Microsporidia, 197

Microsporidiosis, 197

Microsporum canis, 156, 167, 197

Microsporum gypseum, 167

Middle East: and domestication of goat, 240; and rinderpest, 228

Migratory waterfowl, One Health monitoring, 226

Milk: and biopharming, 247; and *Brucella*, 130; and genetic engineering, 248

Milwaukee, Wisconsin, cryptosporidiosis in, 155

Mites: and bacterial zoonoses, 187; from cats to humans, 176; chey-letiella, 196; *Dermanyssus gallinae*, 214–15; *Sarcoptes scabiei*, 158; Trixa-carus, 195–96
Mold, and pet allergies, 7
Monath, Thomas P., 222
Mongooses, banded, 101
Monkey B virus, 46–47
Monkeypox virus, 87–88, 105–7, 189, 192–93
Monkeys, 44; and monkeypox virus, 192
Morbidity, 95
Mortality, 95
Mosquitoes: and togaviruses, 214; and viral encephalomyelitides, 213; and yellow fever, 82
Mouflon sheep, clones of, 244
Mouse Reovirus-3, 189
MRSA. *See* Methicillin-resistant *Staphylococcus aureus*
Mule, clones of, 244
multidrug-resistant tuberculosis (MDR-TB), 81, 95
Murine typhus, 186
Murray Valley encephalitis, 93
Mycobacteriosis, 126, 187
Mycobacterium (multiple species), 187
Mycobacterium avium, 209–10
Mycobacterium bovis, 209, 226–27
Mycobacterium tuberculosis, 45–46, 81, 158, 209–10

Nasal symptoms, and pet allergies, 5, 6, 9
National Association of State Public Health Veterinarians: and *Salmo-nella* prevention, 123; on school and child-care pets, 124
National Cruelty Investigations School, 63
National Environmental Policy Act, 253
National Research Council, on zoo-notic diseases, 73–75
Native American reservations, and plague, 170

Necator americanus, 146
Neglect, 6
Netherlands, and cryptosporidia, 194
Neuraminidase (N), 77
Neuropathy, 95
Neutrophils, 120
Newcastle disease, 202
New World monkeys, 46
New York City: H1N1 pandemic, 105; wildlife imports into, 114
New York State, West Nile virus in, 92, 213
Nigeria: and Lassa fever, 92; and wild-life exports to U.S., 114
Nightingale, Florence, 14, 223
Nipah virus, 88–89, 107
Nonhuman primates, 44–45; and immunodeficiency viruses, 109; import regulation of, 115; and mon-key B virus, 46; simian retroviruses in, 111; and tuberculosis, 46; and yellow fever, 82
North America, hantavirus in, 91
Norway rat, and plague, 80
Notoedres, 176
Nursing homes: and high-risk ani-mals, 133; and pets, 225; and pet therapy, 14, 15, 18

O1 cholera serogroup, 77
O139 cholera serogroup, 76–77
Ocular disease, in cats, 162
Ocular larva migrans (OLM), 145, 175
Ohio River and Mississippi River val-leys, *Histoplasma* in, 210
Old World apes, 46
Old World monkeys, and diseases, 46–47
Omega-3 fatty acids, 251; genetically engineered, 248
Omega-6 fatty acids, 251
One Health, 222–37; and ecology and environment, 230–34; at grassroots level, 224–26; international efforts, 228–30; on national level, 226–28
One Medicine, 223
Opossums: and bacterial zoonoses, 187; and typhus, 186

Opportunistic infections, 126
Orf virus, 125
Ornamental plants: and clones, 242; as invasive species, 231–32
Orthomyxovirus, 189
Orthopoxvirus, 189
Osteomyelitis, in cats, 162

Pacific Northwest, *Cryptococcus gatti* infections in, 85–86
Pandemic, 95
Pappaioanou, Dr. Marguerite, 93
Papules, 177
Parakeets, 110
Paralysis, and rabies, 141–42, 143
Parasites, arthropod, 191
Parasitic zoonoses: in birds, 214–15; and small mammals, 193–97
Paratyphoid. *See* Salmonellosis
Parrots, 181, 211; and avian influenza, 213; and avian tuberculosis, 209; and H1N1 influenza, 108; and psittacosis, 206; and West Nile virus, 214
Parvovirus, 132, 159
Pasteur, Louis, 140
Pasteurella multocida, 168–69, 187
Pasteurella spp., 29, 42
Pasteurellosis, 42, 202
Pathogen pollution, 104
Pediatric cancer centers, and pet therapy, 14
Peliosis hepatis, 163
Permethrin 5 percent cream, 158
Personal protection equipment (PPE), and birds, 204
Peru, cholera epidemic, 77
Pet Abuse.com, 67
Pet allergies, 1–12; symptoms of, 4–5; treatment for, 9–11
Pet dander, and allergies, 2
Pet foods: and human health risks, 133–34; and *Salmonella*, 134
Pets, 119; in classrooms, 124; and healing, 223; in health-care settings, 13–31; and owners health, 223; small mammals as, 181–82; and zoonotic disease prevention, 135

Pet therapy: history of, 13–14; physiological and psychological effects of, 17–18
Petting zoos: and *E. coli*, 86; and zoonotic pathogens, 125, 126
Philippines: Ebola-Reston virus, 91; and wildlife exports to U.S., 114
Physical abuse, defined, 66
Physician visits, for pet allergies, 6–9
Pigeons: and avian influenza, 213; and fungal zoonoses, 210; and psittacosis, 206; and *Salmonella* infection, 208
Pigs: clones of, 244; Ebola-Reston virus, 91; and genetic engineering, 248, 251–52, 258; and H1N1 pandemic, 77, 79, 104–5; and heart valve xenografts, 255; and islet cells, 256, 259; as Nipah virus reservoir, 88–89; and *Salmonella* bacteria, 153; and skin grafts, 255; and xenotransplantation, 257
Pinworms, 183
Pit bull terrier, 40, 58
Pit bull–type dogs: and injuries and deaths by bites, 35–36; and legislation, 40
Plague, 79–80, 169–72, 187, 195; and small mammals, 185–86
Plants: and asexual reproduction, 242; genetically engineered, 246
Plowright, Walter, 228
Plutarch, 222
Pneumonia: and cryptococcosis and histoplasmosis, 210; and influenza, 188, 212; and Q fever, 173; and tuberculosis, 158
Pneumonic plague, 80, 170, 185, 186
Pocks, 88, 95
Polymerase chain reaction (PCR), 177, 206; *Bartonella*, 163
Poodles, 4
Porcupines, brush-tailed, 107
Portuguese water dog, 4
Possums, parasitic zoonoses from, 195
Poultry: and avian influenza, 79, 108, 211–12; baby, and children, 124; *Campylobacter* contamination, 83; and fowl red mite, 214; H5N1 virus,

212, 213; *Pasteurella*, 42; and *Salmonella* infection, 208

Poxviruses, 106

Prairie dogs: and bacterial zoonoses, 187; and monkeypox, 88, 105–6, 192–93; as pets, 181; and plague, 170, 185; and salmonella, 188; and viral zoonoses, 189

Pregnancy: and lymphocytic choriomeningitis virus, 190, 192; and *Toxoplasma*, 165, 166

Pregnant women: and animal-related infections and diseases, 127–32; and livestock-birthing exhibits, 125; immune system in, 127

Presa Canarios, 40, 58

Prevention of zoonotic disease transmission, 134–35

Primates: and monkeypox, 192; trade in, 103

Primates, nonhuman, 44–45; and immunodeficiency viruses, 109; import regulation of, 115; and monkey B virus, 46; simian retroviruses in, 111; and tuberculosis, 46; and xenografts, 257; and yellow fever, 82

Prions, 95

Prosimians, 44

Proteins: and allergies, 2, 3; Fel d 1, 4; feline, 4. *See also* Allergens; Antigens

Psittacosis, 206–7

Public health: defined, 220; global, 220–21

Pulmonary tuberculosis, 81

Puppies: and *Brucella canis*, 157; and campylobacteriosis, 153; and *Cryptosporidium*, 156; and *Giardia* infections, 152; and hookworm, 147, 148; and salmonellosis, 154; *Toxocara* infection in, 146, 148

Puppies Behind Bars program, 225

Pygmy parrot, 211

Q fever (*Coxiella burnetii*), 125, 129–30, 172–73, 195

Quakers, and animals, 14

Quarantine, 204

Rabbit fever. *See* Tularemia

Rabbits: and allergens, 4; and allergies, 198; and bacterial zoonoses, 187; and Cheyletiella mites, 195; clones of, 244; and cryptosporidia, 194; and *Encephalitozoon cuniculi*, 197; and monkeypox, 192; parasitic zoonoses from, 195; as pets, 181; and plague, 170, 185; and salmonella, 188; and tularemia, 176, 183, 184; and viral zoonoses, 189

Rabies, 16, 42–43, 140–44, 189; and animal-assisted intervention animals, 23; and bats, 107; in cats, 173–75; in dogs, 141–42; human cases, 142–43; in large cats, 44; and One Health, 227; and petting zoos, 125; and wolf hybrids, 48

Rabies prophylaxis, post-exposure (PEP), 142–43

Rabies reservoirs, 42

Rabies vaccination, 227–28; for cats, 175; for humans, 143–44

Rabies vaccination baits, 228

Rabies vaccines, 140, 142, 143; regulation of, 48

Raccoons: and bacterial zoonoses, 187; and *Baylisascaris*, 84–85, 196–97; and *Leptospira*, 149; and plague, 170; and rabies, 125, 174, 227, 228; as rabies reservoir, 140; parasitic zoonoses from, 195; and roundworm, 84

Radioimmunoassay test (RAST), for pet allergies, 9

Rashes, and pet allergies, 6

Rat bite fever (RBF), 183, 184–85, 187

Rats: and allergens, 4; and bacterial zoonoses, 187; clones of, 244; and leptospirosis, 186; parasitic zoonoses from, 195; as pets, 181; and plague, 170; and typhus, 186

Ravens, 211; and West Nile virus, 214

Raw diets, for pets and human health risks, 133

Raw meat diet and treats, 23; health risks of, 133

Raw milk, and tuberculosis,
    227
Reactive arthritis, 153, 154
Reassortment virus, 77, 95
Recombinant DNA (rDNA) technol-
    ogy, 246, 247, 249–50
Red Cross, partnering veterinary and
    human health care, 235
Reindeer, and Orf virus, 125
Reiter's syndrome. *See* Reactive
    arthritis
Rejection, in xenotransplantation,
    257–58
Reproductive ability and capacity, and
    cloning, 243
Reptiles, 181; and human allergies, 3;
    and *Salmonella,* 16, 111–12, 122–23,
    154; and salmonellosis, 188; trade
    in, 103; U.S. pet trade, 112; and viral
    encephalomyelitides, 213
Reservoirs, 95, 177
Respiratory symptoms, and pet aller-
    gies, 6, 9
Respiratory tract: and allergies, 2, 3, 5;
    and immune system, 120
Retroviridae family, 111
Retroviruses, 111
Rhinos, 103
Rickettsia (multiple species), 187
Rickettsial bacteria, 186
Rickettsia typhi, 186
Rift Valley fever (RVF), 89–90
Rinderpest, 101, 228; eradication of,
    228; vaccine, 228
Ringworm, 156, 197–98. *See also*
    Dermatophytosis
Rodents: and allergies, 198; and bacte-
    rial zoonoses, 187; and cryptospo-
    ridia, 194; and hantaviruses, 91–92,
    193; and Lassa fever, 92; and *Lep-
    tospira,* 149, 151; and leptospirosis,
    183; and lymphocytic choriomenin-
    gitis virus, 189, 191; and monkey-
    pox, 88, 107, 192; parasitic zoonoses
    from, 195; as pets, 181; and plague,
    170, 185–86; and salmonella, 188;
    and *Trichophyton,* 197; and tulare-
    mia, 176

Rome, ancient, 222
Rope squirrel, 106, 107
Rottweilers, and injuries and death by
    bites from, 35–36
Roundworms: *Baylisacaris,* 196; and
    cats, 175; in and from dogs, 144–46;
    and raccoons, 84
Ruminants, 95, 115; and anthrax, 76;
    and *Escherichia coli* 0157:H7 infec-
    tion, 158; young, and children,
    124
Russia, and hantavirus, 193

Sadism, 66
Saliva: of dogs and allergens, 4; of
    pets and allergies, 3, 4; and rabies,
    42, 141
Salmon, Daniel Elmer, 153
Salmonella, transmission prevention,
    123
Salmonella, 16, 111–12, 140, 153–55,
    207–8; in petting zoos, 125; and raw
    meat diet and treats, 23, 133–34; in
    reptiles and amphibians, 122–23
Salmonella (multiple species), 187
Salmonella enteriditis, 208
Salmonella gallinarum, 208
Salmonella pullorum, 208
Salmonella typhimurium, 155, 208
Salmonellosis, 123, 126, 153–55,
    186–88; 2009 outbreak, 110; and
    birds, 207–9; in infants and tod-
    dlers, 140; and turtles, 111–12
Sarcoptes, 176
Sarcoptes scabiei, 158, 195
SARS. *See* Sudden acute respiratory
    syndrome
Saudi Arabia, Rift Valley fever in, 89
Scabies, 158, 195
Scales, reptile, and allergies, 3
Schizophrenia, and animal-assisted
    intervention, 18
Schnauzer, 4
Schwabe, Calvin, 223
Scrub typhus, 186
Seahorses, harvest of, 104
Seal flu virus (H3N2), 189
Seasonal influenza, 212

Selamectin, 158, 215
Selective breeding, 240, 241, 247; of companion animals, 249
Septicemia, 95, 177; and dog bites, 41
Septicemic plague, 80, 171, 185
Serology, 178; test for *Bartonella,* 163
Service animals, 16
Sexual abuse, 66
Sexuality. *See* Bestiality; Zoophilia
Sexual reproduction, and cloning, 245
Shedding, 178
Sheep: and *Chlamydophila abortus,* 130; and cloning, 244, 245; and *Coxiella burnetii,* 129, 172; and *Leptospira,* 150; and Orf virus, 125
Shiga toxin–producing *Escherichia coli* (STEC), 86, 157–58
Shiga toxins, 95
Siberian chipmunks, and cryptosporidia, 194
Simian foamy virus (SFV), 111
Simian immunodeficiency virus (SIV), 109
Simians, 44
Simian T-lymphotropic virus (STLV), 110
Simian type D retrovirus (SRV), 111
Singapore, Nipah virus in, 88
Sin Nombre virus, 91
Skin, dried. *See* Dander
Skin grafts, 255
Skin tests, for pet allergies, 8
Skunks: and bacterial zoonoses, 187; and plague, 170; and rabies, 125, 140, 173, 227
Sleep difficulties, and pet allergies, 5
Small mammals, 181–99; and bacterial zoonoses, 183–88; and nonzoonotic illnesses, 198; and parasitic zoonoses, 193–97; and ringworm, 197–98; and salmonellosis, 188; tularemia, 183–84; and viral zoonoses, 188–93; zoonoses of, 181–99
Smallpox, 192; eradication of, 228; and monkeypox, 192
Smuggling, animals and animal products, 116

Sneezing, and pet allergies, 5
Sodium cromoglicate, for pet allergies, 9
Sodium cromolyn, for pet allergies, 9
Soduku (rat bite fever), 183
Somatic cell nuclear transfer (SCNT), 240, 242
Sooty mangabeys, 109
South Africa: and plague, 185; Rift Valley fever in, 89; tuberculosis in, 81
South America, yellow fever in, 82
Southeast Asia, and H1N1 influenza, 108
Spanish flu epidemic (1918), 108
Spirillum minus, 184, 187
Sporothrix schenckii, 176
Sporotrichinosis, 176
Spousal abuse, 66
Spring viremia, 112
Squirrels: as pets, 181; and plague, 170, 185
St. Louis encephalitis, 93, 213
Staphylococcus aureus, 83–84, 156; and resistant cows, 251
Staphylococcus intermedius, 34
Steroids, for pet allergies, 9–10
Stillbirths, 132
STLV. *See* Simian T-lymphotropic virus
Strawberries, clones of, 242
Streptobacillus moniliformes, 184, 187
Streptococcus, group B, and stillbirths, 132
Streptococcus pnemoniae, 187
Stress, in birds, 203
Sudan Expanded Programme on Immunization, 235
Sudden acute respiratory syndrome (SARS), 90; associated coronavirus, 107; 2003 outbreak economic impact, 113
Suffering, 66
Sugar gliders, 112; and bacterial zoonoses, 187; as pets, 181; and salmonella, 188
Swamp buffalo, clones of, 244

Swine: domestication of, 240; and *Lep-tospira*, 149; and Nipah virus, 88
"Swine flu," 79
Syphilis, 132

Taenia (multiple species), 195
Tahiti, and *Miconia*, 231
Tamarins, 46
Tannic acid, and pet allergies, 10
Tapeworm infections, 195
Tapeworms: *Dipylidium caninum*, 175; *Hymenolepis nana*, 194
Tarsiers, 44
T cells, 121; and HIV/AIDS, 126; in pregnant women, 127
Tenrecs, 115
Thailand: and H5N1 virus, 212; and wildlife exports to U.S., 114
Therapy animals: characteristics of, 21–24; dogs, 19–20
Ticks: Amblyomma, 213; and animal-assisted intervention animals, 23; and *Coxiella burnetti*, 172; *Ixodes*, 87; and Kyanasur forest disease, 102; and Lyme disease, 132; and tularemia, 176, 183–84
Tigers, 103
Togaviruses, 213–14
Tortoises, 115, 181; U.S. ban on, 113
Toxacara canis, 144–46, 148
Toxacariasis, 144–45
Toxoplasma gondii, 164–66; and pregnant women, 127–28
Toxoplasmosis, 126, 163–66
Transgenic animals, 250
Transplantation, 254
Trauma, and dog bite injuries, 35
Tree squirrels, ban on, 107
Trichophyton, 197
Trichophyton mentagrophytes, 167
Trixacara caviae, 195
Trixacarus mites, 195–96
Tuberculosis, 45–46, 81, 158–59; bovine, 101; in deer, 226–27. See also *Mycobacterium*
Tularemia, 187; and small mammals, 183–84

Turkeys: domestic, bred from wild, 247; and *Salmonella*, 123, 208; and salmonellosis, 111–12
Turtles: bans on, 115, 123; China consumption of, 111
Twins, 242
Type I diabetes, 256, 259
Type I hypersensitivity reactions, 2
Typhoid Mary, 133
Typhus, 186, 187, 195
Tyzzer's disease, 187

Ulceroglandular tularemia, 184
Ungulates, and Orf virus, 125
United Kingdom: bovine spongiform encephalopathy in, 90; and cryptosporidiosis outbreak (2008), 194; foot-and-mouth disease in, 113; and variant Creutzfeldt-Jakob disease, 90
United Nations Children's Fund, 223, 236
United States: animal bites in, 168; and cats and rabies, 174; and cryptosporidiosis, 155; dog bites in, 35; and dog rabies, 141; dogs and cats in, 34; exotic pet trade in, 104; H1N1 pandemic, 104–5; and hantavirus, 91, 193; households with dogs, 139; and invasive species, 232; and leptospirosis, 131; lymphocytic choriomeningitis epidemic (1973–1974), 191; methicillin-resistant *Staphylococcus aureus* infection, 156; monkeypox in, 88, 105, 107, 192; pet birds in, 201; pet owners and allergies, 1; pets in, 119; and plague, 79, 170, 171, 185; and rabies, 227; reptiles trade, 112; *Salmonella* infections in, 112; and salmonellosis, 154, 208; and tularemia, 184; and violence as public-health emergency, 52–53; West Nile virus in, 213; and WHO influenza surveillance, 229; wildlife and wildlife products importation, 104; wildlife import regulation, 114–16; and zebra mussel, 231

Ureaplasma urealyticum, and stillbirths, 132

Urine, pet, and allergies, 3, 4

U.S. Department of Agriculture (USDA): and rabies vaccines, 143; tortoise ban, 113; wildlife regulation, 114, 115

U.S. Fish and Wildlife Service (USFWS), 104; Office of Law Enforcement (OLE), 114; and wildlife imports, 114

U.S. Food and Drug Administration (FDA): ban on African rodents, 107; ban on turtles, 111, 123; on drivers of zoonotic emergence, 105; regulation of genetically engineered animals, 253

Utility workers, and dog bites, 34

Uveitis, 178

Vancouver Island, British Columbia, Canada, 85

Variant Creutzfeldt-Jakob Disease (vCJD), 90

Vector, 178

Vector-borne diseases, and wildlife trade, 113

Venezuelan equine encephalitis (VEE), 93, 213, 214

Veterinarians: and public health, 235, 236; and reporting animal abuse, 60–61

Veterinary forensic science, 62–63

Veterinary infrastructure, partnering with human health care, 235, 236

Vibrio cholerae, 76–77

Vietnam, H5N1 virus, 212

Violence, against animals and humans link, 52

Viral encephalomyelitides, 213

Viral hemorrhagic fevers (VHF), 91

Viral zoonoses: in birds, 211–14; and small mammals, 188–93

Virchow, Rudolph, 222–23

Virginia opossums, as pets, 181

Virus-Serum-Toxin Act, 48

Visceral larva migrans, 145–46, 175

Vision, and ocular larva migrans, 145

Walking dandruff mite. *See* Cheyletiella mites

Waterfowl: and avian influenza, 211; and H1N1 influenza, 108

Waterways, bacteria in, 233

Weil, Adolf, 148

West African rodents, bans on, 115

Western equine encephalitis (WEE), 93, 213, 214

West Nile virus (WNV), 92, 204, 206, 213, 214; in New York, 113; screening for in donated blood, 213

Wheaten terrier, soft-coated, 4

Wheezing, and pet allergies, 5, 6, 7

White blood cells, 120

Wild animals: as pets, 103; and plague, 185; and rabies, 227; and rabies vaccination baits, 228

Wild auroch, domestication of, 240

Wild Bird Conservation Act (1992), 115

Wild bird feeders, 204

Wild birds: illegal trade in and disease transmission, 108–9; U.S. import regulation, 115; and viral encephalomyelitides, 213

Wild boars, domestication of, 240

Wildcat, clones of, 244

Wild deer mice, and viral zoonoses, 189

Wildlife: conservation agreement (1973), 103; global trade in, 103; and human interface, 100–101; illegal trade in, 103; and medicines, 102–3; and pet trade regulations, 115–16; trade, demand, and health of, 99–117; translocation effects of, 104

Wildlife hunting and harvesting, 102

Wildlife reservoirs, *Yersinia pestis,* 170

Wildlife trade and extraction: global response to, 113–14; and infectious diseases, 104–13

Wild mice, and lymphocytic choriomeningitis virus, 190, 191

Wild rodents: and *Francisella,* 183; and hantavirus, 193; and hymenolepiasis, 194

Wisconsin, and monkeypox, 192
Wolf-dog hybrids, 47–48
Wolves, 139; and nomadic tribes, 239
Woodham, Luke 53
World Bank, and One Health, 223, 236
World Health Organization (WHO): on drivers of zoonotic emergence, 105; H1N1 pandemic, 104–5; and influenza vaccines, 212; and One Health, 223, 236
World Health Organization Global Influenza Surveillance Network, 229
World Organization for Animal Health: on drivers of zoonotic emergence, 105; and One Health, 223
Worms, and animal-assisted intervention animals, 23

XDR-TB, 96
Xenografts, 255
Xenotransplantation, 254–59; concerns about, 259; and genetically engineered animals, 257–59
Xoloitzcuintli, 4

Yellow fever, 81–82
Yemen, Rift Valley fever in, 89
Yersinia enerocolitica, 187
Yersinia pestis, 79, 169–70, 185, 187
Yersinia pseudotuberculosis, 187

Zebra mussel, 231
Zoo animals, 181
Zoonoses, 16, 222; and AIDS patients, 126–27; bacterial, and birds, 206–10; bacterial, and small mammals, 183–88; from cats, 161–77; from dogs, 139–59; fungal, in birds, 210–11; parasitic, in birds, 214–15; from pet birds, 201–16; potential in health-care settings, 29–30; of small mammals, 181–99; viral, in birds, 211–14; viral, and small mammals, 188–93; and wildlife, 104–13; and wildlife trade, 112–13
Zoonosis, 76
Zoonotic diseases, 41–43; emerging, 73–75, 76, 93, 221; prevention, 135; transmission, and nonhuman primates, 45. *See also* Tuberculosis
Zoonotic protozoa, and cats, 175
Zoophilia, 56, 66

About the Editor and Contributors

RADFORD G. DAVIS, DVM, MPH, DACVPM, is an Associate Professor of Public Health at Iowa State University, College of Veterinary Medicine. Dr. Davis has been a veterinarian for more than 20 years, practicing in small animal emergency medicine before taking the position at Iowa State University. Since 1998, he has taught and trained veterinary students, state and federal workers, and others in the fields of public health, zoonoses, bioterrorism, and One Health, with many publications in these same areas. Currently, he is active in improving animal and human health, alleviating hunger, and reducing poverty in developing countries around the world through the application of One Health concepts.

A. McKENZIE ANDRÉ, MD, MPH, is an internal medicine physician who graduated from Yale University and Howard University College of Medicine. He has dedicated his career to working in public health as an epidemiologist for the Centers for Disease Control and Prevention and the Food Safety Inspection Service of the Department of Agriculture, concentrating on foodborne illnesses and allergies. He has spent the last two years working in Bangladesh for Helen Keller International.

ZANDRA HOLLAWAY ANDRÉ, DVM, MPH, DACVPM, is a Senior Technical Adviser for the Office of Population, Health, Nutrition, and Education at the U.S. Agency for International Development in Dhaka, Bangladesh. Dr. André is a former small animal private practitioner and Centers for Disease Control and Prevention, Epidemic Intelligence Service, alumni who has conducted training, served as mentor, authored several publications, and given numerous presentations in the fields of zoonoses, environmental health, emerging infectious diseases, and international public health.

CARINA BLACKMORE, MS Vet. Med., PhD, DACVPM, is the State Public Health Veterinarian and State Environmental Epidemiologist with the Florida Department of Health. In her One Health public practice, she consults daily on diseases of infectious and environmental origin that affect animals and man. Dr. Blackmore is the author of a number of public health guidance documents and articles in peer-reviewed journals.

LOUISA J. CASTRODALE, DVM, MPH, DACVPM, is the Alaska State Public Health Veterinarian. She worked in a small animal practice in Maryland for two years before going to Alaska on a two-year federal field epidemiology training fellowship. For the past decade, Dr. Castrodale has worked in infectious disease epidemiology at the state level and has several publications in the identification and control of infectious disease outbreaks and the practice of public health.

KIRA A. CHRISTIAN, DVM, MPH, DACVPM, graduated from Michigan State University's College of Veterinary Medicine and University of Illinois at Chicago's School of Public Health, and is also a graduate of the Epidemic Intelligence Service with the Centers for Disease Control and Prevention. Dr. Christian practiced small animal medicine and surgery prior to her career in veterinary public health, and has published work related to zoonotic diseases and veterinary medical education.

EVGENIJ EVDOKIMOV, PhD, is a molecular biologist in the Animal Biotechnology Interdisciplinary Group at the Center for Veterinary Medicine (FDA), where he evaluates the products of animal biotechnology, including genetically engineered animals. Dr. Evdokimov received his doctorate degree from Georgetown University. Before joining FDA, Dr. Evdokimov investigated aspects of mouse embryogenesis at the National Cancer Institute.

JEFFERY JONES, DVM, PhD, is a Veterinary Medical Officer in the Animal Biotechnology Interdisciplinary Group at the U.S. Food and Drug Administration, Center for Veterinary Medicine. His primary activities focus on evaluation of the molecular biology and veterinary medical aspects of genetically engineered animals. Dr. Jones also sees small animal patients in private practice.

LILA MILLER, BS, DVM, has been working for the American Society for the Prevention of Cruelty to Animals (ASPCA) as a shelter veterinarian, director of one of their outpatient veterinary clinics, and as an adviser and instructor for more than 30 years since her graduation from Cornell University. She is adjunct faculty at the University of Pennsylvania and Cornell University and lectures at veterinary colleges and conferences about shelter medicine and animal cruelty topics. She received animal welfare awards from both the AVMA and AAHA and cofounded the Association of Shelter Veterinarians. She edited three textbooks and has written several articles on shelter medicine and continues to work to fight animal cruelty and improve the lives of shelter animals.

JEFFREY L. RHODY, DVM, is owner and chief veterinarian of the Lakeside Veterinary Center, LLC, in Laurel, Maryland. His caseload includes many small mammal patients including rabbits, ferrets, rodents, sugar gliders, and hedgehogs. He is an active member of the Association of Exotic Mammal Veterinarians.

LARISA RUDENKO, PhD, DABT, is the Senior Adviser for Biotechnology at the Center for Veterinary Medicine at the U.S. Food and Drug Administration, where she is also director of the Animal Biotechnology Interdisciplinary Program. She has developed science-based approaches for regulating the products of plant and animal biotechnology in both the private and public sectors for the past 25 years.

KRISTINE M. SMITH, DVM, DACZM, holds a doctor of veterinary medicine degree from Tufts University and is a Diplomate of the American College of Zoological Medicine. After completing her residency at the Bronx Zoo in New York, Dr. Smith worked as a field veterinarian conducting wild animal disease surveillance in Africa and Asia. She served as the Assistant Director for Field Programs with the Wildlife Conservation Society's Global Health Program (GHP), coordinating field surveillance activities around the globe. She currently is Associate Director for Health and Policy at EcoHealth Alliance, focusing on conservation and health impacts of the wildlife trade.

MIRANDA SPINDEL, DVM, MS, is Senior Director, Shelter Medicine Veterinary Outreach, American Society for the Prevention of Cruelty to Animals. Dr. Spindel believes that the world within an animal shelter is rich in opportunity for veterinary education and research integrated with improving the lives of animals. Dr. Spindel initiated and completed the first residency in shelter medicine offered though Colorado State University and has been teaching shelter medicine there for seven years. She is a two-term past president of the Association of Shelter Veterinarians, a member of the ASV Shelter Standards Task Force, and volunteers as a disaster responder. Dr. Spindel lives in Colorado and works with shelters across the country.

TEGWIN K. TAYLOR, DVM, MPH, DACVPM, received her Doctor of Veterinary Medicine degree from Iowa State University. She practiced small animal medicine before completing a residency in veterinary preventive medicine and public health with the University of Minnesota. Dr. Taylor returned to Iowa State as a veterinary specialist with the Center for Food Security and Public Health, authoring several online training modules for veterinarians in the areas of infectious disease, emergency response, and occupational health. She currently resides in West Virginia and continues to practice veterinary public health.

KEN THORLEY, BVSc, MVS, MACVSc, graduated from Sydney University in 1986, and spent the first five years of his career working in Australia and the United Kingdom, before landing in Hong Kong in 1992. That year he opened the first branch of Victoria Veterinary Clinics near the border with mainland China, and it has since grown to be one of Hong Kong's largest veterinary practices. He has a master's degree in small animal medicine and was awarded membership of the Australian College of Veterinary Scientists in the subject of medicine of cats. He is a feline medicine consultant for the Veterinary Information Network (VIN).

NIKLOS WEBER, DVM, DABVP (Avian, Canine, Feline), is the owner of a specialty veterinary hospital in northern California and has been a small animal and exotic pet veterinarian since 1995. Dr. Weber is the author of numerous articles in peer-reviewed veterinary journals and also researches homing pigeon exercise physiology.

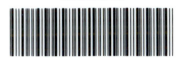